WHAT TO EXPECT®
EATING WELL
WHEN YOU'RE EXPECTING

2nd EDITION

by Heidi Murkoff

Workman Publishing • New York

To Erik, my everything and my always
To Emma and Wyatt for making me a mom
To Lennox and Sebastien for making me a grandmom
To Simon for making me a mom-in-law
To Arlene, forever
To all moms, dads, and babies everywhere—
and to all those who care for and about them.

———

Library of Congress Control Number: 2020937942

ISBN 978-1-5235-0139-7

Recipe consultants: Rena Coyle and Brierley E. Horton
Medical consultant: Erika F. Werner, MD, MS
Book design: Lisa Hollander
Main cover photograph © MattBeard.com
Additional photo credits appear on page 389.

Workman books are available at special discounts when purchased in bulk for premiums and sales promotions as well as for fund-raising or educational use. Special editions or book excerpts also can be created to specification. For details, contact the Special Sales Director at the address below, or send an email to specialmarkets@workman.com.

Workman Publishing Co., Inc.
225 Varick Street
New York, NY 10014-4381
workman.com

WORKMAN is a registered trademark of Workman Publishing Co., Inc.

Printed in the United States of America
First printing July 2020

10 9 8 7 6 5 4 3 2 1

Thanks Again!

....

I've often said that writing books is a little like making babies. You conceive. You do some seriously heavy lifting. Expend a lot of energy. Lose a lot of sleep. And finally . . . you deliver (hopefully, on time).

And you can't do either one on your own. Fortunately, I've never had to try. From day (and book) one, I've had support I could count on from more amazing people than I can count. But as always, I'll try. Thanks a million to:

Erik, literally What to Expect's baby daddy—the man who made me a mom to Emma and Wyatt, and with that, a mom to What to Expect, and a mom on a mission (a mission we've shared since the very beginning). You're my partner in life, love, work, advocacy, and everything What to Expect. Not to mention, the best partner in parenting (and grandparenting) a mom could ever have.

Maisie Tivnan, who has fearlessly stepped into some pretty big flats, picking up the mantle for my editor-forever, Suzanne Rafer, without missing a beat. Nobody said it was going to be easy to go with my frenetic flow of edits or take my pickiness (okay, nitpickiness) in stride, but you kind of make it look that way. And to Suzanne, whose contribution to What to Expect—and friendship—will always be treasured.

Everyone else at Workman who has helped birth this baby: To Vaughn Andrews and Lisa Hollander, for designing a book that's easy to read and good enough to eat, and for sifting through all those melons, muffins, shades of blue, and Emmas to create a cover that will make readers hungry for more. To Barbara Peragine, as always, for magically making text fit, and getting us out of some serious deadline tight spots. Beth Levy and Doug Wolf for your production values under endless pressure. My forever Workman family, Jenny Mandel and Emily Krasner. Peter Workman for creating the house my books have been born in, and Suzie Bolotin for growing and nurturing it.

Eating Well's first recipe consultant, Rena Coyle, for her dedication to all things delicious and nutritious. And to our latest one, Brierley Horton, for developing yummy recipes to fit a time-challenged mom's reality, and bringing a fresh perspective to cooking well (with a minimum of cooking). Who ever said that too many cooks spoiled the broth (or in this case, the carrot-ginger soup)?

Alan Nevins, of Renaissance Literary & Talent, for always going that extra mile (say, to Romania with us), for your friendship and support, and for always being so much fun to drink wine (or pretty much anything) with. To Marc Chamlin, for taking such good care of me, and more important, for caring so much about me—you're my friend and my lawyer, and that's an unlikely combination!

Our WhatToExpect.com dream team, led by Heidi Cho, Christine Mattheis, Michele Calhoun, and hopefully always, Kyle Humphries and Sara

Stefanik, for endless energy, enthusiasm, innovation, integrity, creativity, conviction, patience, passion, and shared purpose (and for believing in the power of purple). And for never forgetting the most important part of the QBR: Big hugs and big reds.

ACOG, for being tireless advocates for moms and babies everywhere, and to all the obs, midwives, nurses, doulas, and lactation consultants around the world helping to deliver a healthy beginning and a healthy future for our moms and babies. To the experts and advocates at the CDC—an organization devoted to the health and wellbeing of our global family, especially when it comes to our most vulnerable—for your shared mission and commitment to improving maternal and infant health.

Dr. Erika Werner for your thoughtful, thorough review of *Eating Well*—for making sure the facts about the impact of maternal nutrition on the health of moms and babies are stated, not overstated.

Howie Mandel, for always being the voice of reason and delivering compassionate care (and Lennox). Lauren Crosby, for being an invaluable source of information and common sense for so many parents (including Emma and Simon) and for the What to Expect family, as well your friendship.

The What to Expect Project, our incredibly passionate leader, Annie Toro, and our director of policy, strategy, research, and everything else, Wyatt Murkoff. Together, and in partnership with organizations who care just as much about maternal health (and nutrition) as WTEP does, we will make the world a healthier, happier, more nurtured place for moms and the babies they love to live in.

For inspiration and love, Wyatt, Emma (our beautiful cover mom), Simon, and of course Lennox, and Sebastien (who would happily eat this book if he could). Victor Shargai (I'll never stop missing you) and Craig Pascal (we'll never stop inviting you for Christmas).

Arlene Eisenberg, for everything you've given me, and continue to give to me every day. Your legacy lives on; you'll always be loved and never forgotten.

And most of all, to every mom and every baby, everywhere. You inspire me to do what I do and to never stop doing it, and I love you all (and only wish I could hug you all).

Thanks again, everybody and big hugs,

Heidi

Contents

....

════════════════════ **PART 1** ════════════════════
EATING WELL

========= PART 2 =========
COOKING WELL

The Dish
on Eating Well

E ver notice that when it comes to nutrition, the more things change, the more they stay the same? Sure, you can yo-yo with fad diets (low-carb? That's so last week . . . low-fat? Week before last . . . raw foods? . . . raw deal), but if you step off the diet treadmill and take stock, you'll notice that the basics of healthy eating haven't changed all that much over time. A balanced diet of lean protein, calcium-rich foods, whole grains, fruits and vegetables, and healthy fats is what nutritionists, doctors, and Mom herself have been quietly touting for years while the conflicting nutrition books duke it out on the bestseller lists, only to be forgotten the moment the newest diet craze makes headlines.

And what about for pregnant moms? Have the fundamentals of eating well when you're expecting changed much over the years? They haven't really—and mostly because eating well for two isn't all that much different from eating well for one. The proportions may shift a bit (to accommodate a growing baby's proportions), but the basics are still pretty basic.

So if eating well when you're expecting is really just a matter of sticking to a balanced diet, why would you need a book to show you how?

To answer that question, let me backtrack a few years. Make that 30 plus years. Six weeks into my first pregnancy (due to some cycle wrinkles, it was a little late in the game when I first got the news), I was determined to make up for lost time—and make the most of the rest of my seven-and-a-half months of baby growing. I was a healthy twenty-three-year-old who lived a healthy lifestyle and ate a healthy diet—and I was pretty sure I knew what it took to feed myself and my baby healthfully. So I stocked our fridge and prepared our meals with nature's best baby-building materials: fresh chicken breasts, fish, dairy, whole grains, and a plethora of produce.

And then I ran to the bathroom to throw up.

The chicken breasts, my usual protein of choice, were the first to go—victim of a sudden aversion to flesh foods (funny, I'd never thought of chicken as flesh before). The salmon didn't stand a chance, of course—the smell (that's before I even took the fillets out of the wrapper) sent me reeling (and back to the bathroom). Got milk? I did, but definitely couldn't bear the thought of drinking it. The whole grains were welcome to stay (in bread form, toasted within an inch of their life, thank you very much), as was the fruit (with the possible exception of the honeydew, which had somehow become a honey-don't). But the broccoli I used to gobble with a rabbit's abandon turned my stomach.

I knew that I was supposed to eat a certain number of green vegetables a day, but nobody (not even my OB) could tell me how to eat them without turning greener than they were. I knew protein was the building block of human cells (which meant that building a baby would take protein aplenty), but I had no idea that cottage cheese could stand in for those dreaded flesh foods until the first-trimester aversions had worn off. Or that microwaving the salmon zapped its offensive odor. Or that calcium did not have to come with a white mustache (and a side of bloat). Or that dried apricots quelled the queasies while simultaneously satisfying my baby's requirement for vitamin A (turns out babies don't need broccoli after all) or that I could drink my vitamin C in a smoothie instead of a glass of tummy-churning OJ. Or that I could take my baby out to eat almost anywhere (except maybe that Italian place, where just a whiff of the scampi could inflict third-degree heartburn).

So I spent the rest of my pregnancy eating the best I could—gagging down the milk, choking down the chicken, and, most of the time, worrying that my best wasn't nearly good enough. If only I knew then what I know now. That eating well when you're expecting doesn't have to be torture—and that it doesn't even have to be challenging. It can be fun, easy, and, most of all, delicious—no matter what pregnancy symptom has got you down (or is keeping food from staying down). You can coddle your cravings, pander to your aversions, mollify your morning sickness, indulge your indigestion—and still feed yourself and your growing baby exceptionally well.

Enter (way too late for me, but hopefully right on time for you) *Eating Well When You're Expecting*, everything you need to know to feed yourself and your baby well in the real world—the world where nausea dictates what's on the menu (even if that's two crackers and an extra-cold glass of ginger ale); where heartburn can burn a hole in your resolve to eat your vegetables; where temptations (glazed, iced, fried, chocolate-covered, creamed, or super-sized) lurk around every corner; where "lunch" meetings in the conference room are catered by Doughnuts-by-the-Dozen; where airline flights aren't catered at all. Everything you need to make eating for two half the effort and twice the pleasure—from savvy shopping to smart snacking, dining out strategies to pregnant party protocol, brown-bag lunches to breakfasts on the fly. Everything you need to put it all together, including 175 recipes that neatly package all your nutritional requirements into gourmet—yet quick and easy—dishes, while taking into account the special needs of your often tender tummy. In short, everything you need to eat well when you're expecting.

Wishing you a delicious and nutritious nine months of eating well!

heidi

PART 1

Eating Well

CHAPTER 1

Why Eat Well?

Congratulations! The pregnancy test (and the 3 you took afterward, just to be sure) is positive—and the big (but still very little) news has started to sink in. You're pregnant. As you sit back and take it all in, you're probably equal parts overjoyed and overwhelmed by the enormity of what has just happened . . . and what is about to happen. That and, more than likely, a little queasy.

Ready or not, you're about to grow a baby—from a shapeless blob of cells not yet visible to the human eye to a dimpled, suitable-for-snuggling newborn.

Much of that work will take place without you lifting a finger—or a fork. In many ways, your pregnant body (especially if it's a healthy one) will rely on biological-business-as-usual to transform the rapidly dividing bundle of cells that's just burrowed into your uterus into a warm bundle of baby you'll hold in your arms in about 8 months' time, give or take. Nature is good at what it does, no matter what a mom does or doesn't do—which means your baby already has an excellent chance of arriving in those welcoming arms of yours fully developed and completely healthy.

Still, there's no reason to take a backseat to your body's pregnancy auto-pilot. In fact, there are many convincing reasons to jump up front (while you can still jump), take the wheel, and help guide your baby to a healthy start in life and a healthy future.

How? Chances are, you probably know many of the basics of healthy baby making—and if you were planning this pregnancy, you may have implemented many (or all) of them before sperm even met egg: See an ob or midwife for regular prenatal care, adjust your lifestyle as needed (cut back on caffeine, cut out alcohol, smoking, marijuana, and any other recreational drug use), finesse your fitness routine, and take a close look at the supplements and medications you take, adjusting as recommended by your prenatal practitioner. And, of course, eat well.

Seeing as you've picked up this book, you're probably already committed to eating well when you're expecting—or at least, you're curious why you should think about committing. Maybe you don't need any facts or figures to convince you that feeding yourself and

My Baby, the Parasite?

Myth: A baby takes all the nutrients needed for growth and development from mom, no matter what she eats or doesn't eat.

Fact: It's true that most babies develop and grow well even when their moms don't eat particularly well. But they aren't parasites. When there aren't enough nutrients to go around—because mom's stores are low and she's not eating well enough to replenish them—mom gets first dibs. To ensure the survival of the species, Mother Nature swings in favor of the mother (who can live to reproduce again if she's well nourished and healthy)—not in favor of her baby. In fact, babies can be born with vitamin deficiencies to moms who show no signs of deficiency. The exception: When it comes to calcium, a developing baby's needs will be met first when mom doesn't sock away enough—even if it means draining her bones of this vital mineral to build her baby's bones.

your baby right during pregnancy is a priority.

But the connection between pregnancy eating and pregnancy health may be even more compelling and far-reaching than you'd imagine. And it's growing, too. Almost daily, scientists make a stronger case, discovering just how many aspects of a baby's development and future wellbeing can be influenced by a mom-to-be's diet. What's more, what's good for a baby is also good for mom. Research continues to show that healthy eating can make pregnancy safer, less likely to become complicated, and (important from where you're sitting, queasy, tired, gassy, constipated, and bloated) more comfortable. Talk about win-win . . . and more win!

Eating Well: What's in It for Baby

No news flash here: Your body will be changing plenty during the 40 weeks of pregnancy. And growing, too—in places you'd expect (your breasts, your belly), and places you probably wouldn't (like your feet). But consider how much your baby will be changing and growing over those same 40 weeks (really, 38 weeks counting from conception). Cells dividing at an unbelievable rate, organs (that heart, that brain, those lungs, that stomach) and systems (circulatory, urinary, digestive) rapidly developing, the senses (hearing, sight, taste, and smell) taking shape, along with those perfect 10 little fingers, 10 little toes, and those little girl and boy parts. Bones, muscle, skin, and eventually fat forming, hair sprouting. All in life's first and most fantastic journey, taking fertilized egg to blastocyst to embryo to fetus and finally, to ready-to-deliver baby.

CHEW ON THIS. If there's one thing that every culture and every generation shares—from the East to the West, from the ancient to the contemporary—it's the tradition of telling pregnant women what they should and shouldn't eat. Pregnancy is fertile ground for superstitions, folklore, and tales from old wives from around the world and through the ages . . . not to mention sketchy internet rumors, social media shaming, and public pregnancy policing ("you're going to eat *that*?").

The truth is, you can pass up most of that passed-along pregnancy advice, as well meaning or time honored (by old-timers) as it might be. Among the pregnancy food myths you can definitely discount:

- Eat salty or sour foods and your baby will be born with a sour personality.

- Spicy foods will make your baby hot tempered.

- Chow down on chilies and other spicy foods and your baby will be born bald.

- A teaspoon each of honey and vinegar, taken every morning during pregnancy, will help your baby grow more hair.

- Dark-colored foods will make a baby's skin darker, while light-colored foods (some say milk) will turn a baby's skin lighter.

- Eat fish and your baby could end up stupid as a salmon. (Ironically, of course, eating salmon and many other types of fish is linked to optimal baby brain development.)

- Eat rabbit and your baby might sleep with his or her eyes open.

Hungry for more pregnancy food fiction? You'll find "Chew on This" boxes throughout this book.

What fuels that journey? Actually, the fuel source is you. Your baby—and the complex, ingeniously designed baby-making factory your body runs—is fueled primarily by what you eat and what you drink. Vitamins, minerals, calories, protein, fluids, and other nutrients necessary for healthy baby production—and a healthy pregnancy—come mostly from your diet. Though your body can use backup reserves of some resources, like calcium from your bones and calories from stored fat, it'll spoon up (or suck up) most from what you're eating and drinking—and the more nutrients you take in, the more you'll dish out to your baby. Though most babies grow and develop normally even when their moms don't eat all that well, study after study shows that, on average, healthier eaters have healthier pregnancies and healthier babies.

Think of healthy eating as one of the first and best gifts you can give your baby-to-be. And it's a gift that keeps on giving. Your diet can impact many components of your little one's health in many ways—in both the short and the long term—including:

Your baby's organ development. With all those body parts developing from tiny cells (the heart, liver, lungs, kidneys, and nervous system, just to name a few), and only 9 months in which to accomplish this phenomenal growth, your baby-making factory is working full steam, day and night. Most of the raw materials needed to turn a fertilized egg into a fully equipped bouncing baby are supplied through your diet.

Fortunately, those raw materials aren't hard to come by. The average American diet provides enough of most nutrients to ensure a healthy, bouncing baby—but, not surprisingly, extra-good nutrition can offer extra insurance that all will develop according to plan. At the other extreme, a diet that's severely deficient in certain types of nutrients (uncommon in the United States) increases the risk that a baby may not develop normally. For instance, a deficiency in folic acid can result in neural tube defects (defects in the brain or spinal cord), such as spina bifida. Happily, the number of babies born with these defects has decreased since folic acid supplementation has become routinely recommended for women of childbearing age—a great case for taking a prenatal vitamin before and during pregnancy.

Your baby's brain development. While the development of most organs is relatively complete midway through pregnancy, your baby's brain will have its greatest growth spurt during the last trimester and beyond (brain development continues at a mind-boggling pace for the first 3 years of a baby's life). Since protein, calories, and omega-3 fatty acids are particularly crucial to optimal brain development, taking in enough of these nutrients—especially during those final 3 months of baby growing—may boost your baby's brainpower. So it's smart to reach for that bowl of walnuts or that dish of fish.

Your baby's birthweight. How much and how well you eat can impact how your baby measures up—and weighs in—at delivery. While genetics definitely plays a role in baby's birthweight and beyond, a mom's diet during pregnancy does, too. Eating too little can keep a baby from growing to potential in utero, sometimes resulting in a low birthweight (also known as small for gestational age or SGA). Eating too

much can lead to a baby growing too much too fast, and being born too large for gestational age. Very small babies have an increased risk of complications and health problems at birth and sometimes later on. Extra-large babies are more likely to arrive early and/or via c-section (because they're too big to fit through mom's pelvis) and are more likely to have complications and health problems, including low scores on the Apgar test (which measures a baby's wellbeing at birth), an increased risk of breathing problems and hypoglycemia, and a greater chance of needing a stay in the neonatal intensive care unit, or NICU. Very large babies are also predisposed to obesity and Type 2 diabetes later in life. Not surprisingly, following a just-right formula—eating a healthy number of calories and gaining about the right amount of weight—can help fuel just the right amount of growth for your baby. See Chapter 6 for more on weight gain.

But it's not only the quantity of food (or calories) you eat that matters to your baby's bottom line. The quality matters, too. Too little iron can slow a baby's growth. So can too little zinc. Falling short on folate (folic acid) or being generally malnourished can lead to restricted fetal growth (aka Intrauterine Growth Restriction or IUGR) and a baby being born small or even with signs of malnutrition. Eating the right amounts of the right foods will help give your baby what he or she needs to grow on—and contribute to a bouncing baby birthweight.

Your baby's arrival time. There are many reasons why a mom might deliver prematurely that have nothing to do with diet. Still, on average, moms who lack enough key nutrients like iron, zinc, vitamin C, vitamin D, and magnesium may be more likely to have a preterm birth than well-nourished moms. Ditto for moms who don't get enough folate in their diets. On the other hand, moms who eat well and gain the right amount of weight can boost their chances of carrying to term. Not surprisingly, full-term babies are more likely to be healthy babies.

Your baby's sleep habits. There's some evidence that newborns whose moms get their fill of omega-3 fatty acids during the last trimester are better overall sleepers than other babies. Does feasting on fish late in pregnancy guarantee you a full night's sleep in your baby's first months? No—and in fact, spoiler alert: Newborns aren't supposed to sleep through the night. But it may promote healthier sleep patterns. So may having a daily serving of dark chocolate during your last trimester, which some research links to babies who sleep better and cry less (and, obviously, to happier moms).

Your baby's eating habits. Fast-forward to future family dinners, and you can definitely see how your tastes might affect your baby's. After all, little monkeys tend to mimic their moms and dads in many ways, including whether they savor salad or favor fries. But did you know that how you eat during pregnancy can also help shape your baby's future eating habits? Because your baby's taste buds develop at about 16 weeks of pregnancy, he or she can become accustomed to flavors that make their way from your meals into the amniotic fluid he or she swallows. Which means that baby's food favorites can form before he or she even takes a first bite of solids. This concept, sometimes referred to as flavor learning, has been boosted not only by word of mom ("I ate nothing but watermelon, and my baby loves watermelon!" or "I craved hot sauce and so does my kid!"), but also by studies. For instance, one study found that babies of moms who drank a lot of carrot juice during pregnancy were more likely to lap up cereal mixed with carrot juice than those whose moms didn't touch the orange stuff. Other studies have shown that babies of moms who went gangbusters on garlic and other strong flavors while they were expecting were more likely to scarf down scampi or curry, and those of moms who brought on the broccoli and other "bitter" vegetables were more likely to be sweet on those bitter tastes. The moral of these studies: If you'd like your baby to eat his or her leafy greens later, consider going green now. And keep going green later, too, since flavor learning continues as baby becomes acclimated to the changing taste of breast milk, which is also flavored by a mom's diet.

Your baby's long-term health. So you know your baby has a lot of growing and developing to do during those 9 months in your womb. And you know that your little one is a miraculous work in progress—and that you can help that progress along by eating well and eating enough. But did you know that this early progress—and your efforts to fuel it—may go a long way beyond birth, laying the foundation not only for a healthy start in life, but also a healthy lifetime?

Researchers have provided plenty of food for thought on how a mom's diet during pregnancy (and even, to a certain extent, before conception) can affect her baby's long-term health. A person's predisposition to certain diseases (cancer, for instance, or schizophrenia) or to chronic conditions such as diabetes, hypertension, and heart disease may be related to his or her mom's nutritional intake during pregnancy.

A striking example: Studies show that babies who are undernourished in the first trimester or who are overfed in the third trimester may be at greater risk for obesity later in life. Other research suggests a link between a mom's low intake of calcium and other bone-building nutrients and her child's risk for osteoporosis later in life. Nutrition during pregnancy, say researchers, may influence a baby's health not only at birth, but years later, even into adulthood.

Eating Well: What's in It for You

Baby's not the only one benefiting every time you brake for breakfast, crunch on carrots, or choose the grilled chicken salad over the finger-licking nuggets and fries. There's plenty in eating well for you, too. Among the many possible perks of healthy pregnancy eating for moms-to-be:

More comfort. Let's face it: The average pregnant woman doesn't really walk around for 9 months with a rosy glow. In fact, in the first few months, she's more likely to walk around with a greenish tint. And morning sickness is just one of the many miseries pregnancy can serve up. Other uncomfortable symptoms your body may have in store for you: fatigue, constipation, hemorrhoids, heartburn, headaches, backaches, varicose veins, pregnancy pimples (even the dreaded bacne), bleeding gums, swollen ankles—and that's just naming a few. Will you have every symptom in the book or just a handful? Will they be majorly miserable or just moderately? Your individual pregnancy comfort (or discomfort) quotient will largely be decided by factors you can't control, like your genes (thanks, Mom!), the work you do (say, standing all day on the job), or the weather you're weathering (like sweltering heat and humidity). But at least some of it will be up to you—and influenced, to some extent, by how you eat. Grazing on the energy-boosting combo of protein and complex carbs can ease fatigue, minimize headaches and mood swings, even keep some of the queasies at bay. Filling up on fiber and fluids can clear up constipation, and curbing sugar while focusing on healthy fats may help clear up your complexion. Cutting the grease can cut back on heartburn. For more on eating well to feel well during pregnancy, see Chapter 7.

Fewer complications. It's as simple as this: Pregnancy complications are less common among moms who eat well. For instance, good dietary habits—eating plenty of fruits and vegetables, lean protein, beans, and whole grains, and limiting sugar and refined grains may lower the risk of gestational diabetes. Top-notch nutrition—including enough magnesium—may reduce the chances of developing preeclampsia. Staying well hydrated can help prevent excessive swelling and preterm contractions. Getting enough iron can help reduce the risk of anemia and postpartum complications. And because eating well is likely to lead to healthy weight gain, the risks of all kinds of pregnancy complications, from developing gestational diabetes to having a c-section, are lowered. Bottom line: A healthy pregnancy diet gives you the right balance of vitamins, minerals, and other vital nutrients, paving the way for a healthier pregnancy.

Birthing benefits. Can eating well help you order up an easier labor and delivery? Not exactly (though wouldn't that be a nice app to have?). But an overall healthy diet—one that provides a balance of baby-friendly nutrients and about the right number of calories (leading to the right amount of weight gain)—may help prevent a too-early birth. Especially beneficial when it comes to keeping a baby bun baking until term: iron, zinc, vitamin C, vitamin D, and magnesium. Deficiencies in those nutrients have been linked to premature labor. And though there are definitely no sure things when it comes to labor and delivery, here's another possible birthing room benefit: In general, moms who are well nourished handle whatever childbirth happens to hand them better than those who are low on nutrient stores—just as a well-nourished athlete is able to perform better and endure better than one who's nutrient-deprived. (And when it comes to athletic events, there's none more challenging than childbirth. Just ask any Iron Woman who's also a mom.)

A faster route to recovery. A baby's not the only thing you can expect after delivery, though it's definitely the best thing. No, you'll also take home a host of postpartum symptoms as your body attempts to recover from 9 long months of pregnancy, the grueling marathon of labor, and the pounding it might have taken while delivering 7, 8, or even more pounds of baby (or having major surgery, if you end up with a c-section). Add to your body's challenges overall exhaustion and the cumulative toll of new-parent sleep deprivation—plus the energy needed to care for and feed your baby (particularly if you're breastfeeding)—and you'll understand why it'll need all the help it can get. Eating well during pregnancy allows your body to store resources that will help you meet the physical and emotional challenges of new mom life, speed your postpartum recovery, and provide the get-up-and-go you'll need to keep on getting-up-and-going. That, and help supply your little one's fast-growing demand for breast milk. (See Chapter 10 for more on eating well postpartum.)

Better bone health. All ready to put your baby's needs ahead of your own? The truth is that your pregnant body has other plans when it comes to divvying up the nutrients from incoming food—giving you first dibs on most of them, then serving leftovers to your baby. One nutrient this mom-first policy doesn't cover: that essential bone-builder, calcium. If you don't take in enough calcium when you're pregnant, your body will drain this vital mineral from your own bones to help build baby's. This potential shortfall could set you up for bone loss later in life, and even for osteoporosis.

Better overall health. It's probably not a shocker, but healthy eating habits can improve overall health. Embracing healthy eating habits for baby's sake now can—if you stick with them later—gift you with a lowered risk of all kinds of diseases, from chronic hypertension to heart disease, Type 2 diabetes to cancer. Share those healthy eating habits at home, and you'll be sharing those possible long-term health benefits with your whole family—including your baby-to-be.

Ready to Get Started?

So now you know the "why" of eating well—it's best for you, your baby, and your pregnancy. But what about the "how"—and the know-how—you'll need to make it happen? It's all here in the pages that follow: The nutrition facts, and the facts about nutrition. The tips, advice, and recipes you'll need to eat your way through a healthy and comfortable pregnancy. How to prepare (or order up) meals and snacks that satisfy your cravings, tempt your taste buds, and fill your pregnant body's requirements while nurturing your baby's growth and development. Plus, how to keep your weight gain on the track that's right for you and your pregnancy.

Ready to get started? Sit back, sip a fruit smoothie, and read on to learn how to eat well when you're expecting.

CHAPTER 2

The Nutrients That Make a Baby

....

Y ou can't see them. You can't smell them. You can't even taste them. But they're in just about every bite you take. They're nutrients, substances your body needs to survive and thrive—the vitamins, minerals, protein, carbohydrates, and fats in the salmon and strawberries and broccoli and cereal (and yes, even in the ice cream, chips, and chocolate bars) you eat. Whether these nutrients find their way into foods naturally (like the vitamin C and lycopene in that juicy vine-ripe tomato) or thanks to fortification (for instance, the vitamin D in that glass of milk, the B vitamins added to that slice of bread), whether they're found in the healthiest sources (that kale salad) or the least healthy ones (those gummy bears), they all play an important role in the making of your little baby bun. Wondering how? Read on to learn what's behind all the nutrients in the foods you eat every day and what makes them so vital to the growth and development of a fetus. Don't want to get in the weeds with your nutrients, and just want to get busy eating well? Skip ahead to Chapter 3, "The Pregnancy Diet."

From A to Zinc: An Encyclopedia of Vitamins and Minerals

Few people digging into their morning oatmeal or tucking into their lunchtime sandwich give a first—never mind a second—thought to the vitamins and minerals they're about to consume and absorb. But every food you eat

What's an RDA, Anyway?

The Food and Nutrition Board of the Institute of Medicine, National Academy of Sciences may be a mouthful, but it's the organization that establishes principles and guidelines for approximately how much of each nutrient an average person requires—and approximately how many mouthfuls of a certain food you'll need to eat to meet that requirement. These guidelines are called the DRIs, or Dietary Reference Intakes. For the most part, they're also TMI (too much information). That's because they're just a little too specific for most consumers, even especially health-conscious ones, and definitely too specific for those who'd rather just consume food, not analyze the nutrients in it.

Still, there are 2 DRIs that apply in this chapter, at least, if you choose to apply them (you can also just look for foods that are high in a certain essential nutrient, and leave the analysis to the pros):

Recommended Dietary Allowance (RDA). The RDA is the amount of a nutrient needed per day to meet the nutrient requirements of nearly all healthy people (divided by sex) in a particular life stage (infant or child, for instance, or during pregnancy or lactation).

Adequate Intake (AI). The AI is the amount of a nutrient recommended per day when there is insufficient scientific evidence to develop an RDA. The AI is set at a level assumed to ensure nutritional adequacy, so it's not as reliable as an RDA, which is based on solid evidence, but it still gives good guidance.

For the latest information about the DRIs, go to health.gov/dietary guidelines.

---

contains at least some of these essential nutrients, each of them vital to your health (clearly, some foods deliver more nutrients and come in more nutritious packages than others). During pregnancy, the mission of the nutrients you consume becomes even more important, since they must fuel the needs of two bodies, including a rapidly growing one. Which means you'll need to take in more vitamins and minerals than ever before. You'll get a good supply from your prenatal vitamin-mineral supplement, but you'll benefit even more from getting nutrients from their natural sources. Knowing how each vitamin and mineral contributes to making a healthy baby—and where you can find them—can help inform (and, hey, inspire!) the food choices you make. Here's a guide to the most important nutrients your body needs.

Vitamins

Vitamins play leading roles when it comes to metabolism, cell production, tissue repair, and a variety of other vital processes. And while vitamins themselves are not sources of energy, they also help convert the carbs, fats, and proteins that you eat into energy. Quite simply, you can't live without them, and neither can your baby.

Not surprisingly, moms-to-be—who are nourishing not only themselves but also a rapidly growing baby—require more vitamins than the average adult

Can Your Body Store Vitamins?

Here's a fast fact about vitamins: They can be either fat-soluble or water-soluble.

Fat-soluble vitamins—vitamins A, D, E, and K, for instance—can be stored in the body, which means that you don't necessarily need a daily dose of them, assuming your body has backup to draw from. That's the good news. The bad news is that because the body can store these vitamins, taking too much of them (for instance, taking mega-doses of A or D supplements) can lead to toxic levels in your system, which can be particularly danger-ous if you're pregnant or planning to become pregnant. But (back to the good news), you can't overdose on these vitamins by eating foods that are naturally rich in them, even if you're also taking a prenatal.

Water-soluble vitamins—such as vitamins B and C—dissolve in water and therefore can't be stored in the body. Your body uses what it needs for the day and then you pee out the rest. Which means that you'll have to make sure you restock those water-soluble vitamins daily by eating a healthy vitamin-rich diet and taking that vital prenatal supplement.

female. Popping a prenatal vitamin sup-plement is always a good place to start, but eating well will also help you get your pregnancy share of vitamins.

Vitamin A. Vitamin A is a nutritional powerhouse—essential to many aspects of baby making, including the growth and development of cells, bones, skin, eyes (especially important for night vision), teeth, and immunity. Too little vitamin A in a mom-to-be's diet (plus the absence of a prenatal vitamin) has been linked to premature delivery and to slow growth in her baby, as well as to skin disorders and eye damage. But as with other fat-soluble vitamins, when taken in supplement form in very high doses for long periods of time, vita-min A can be toxic. Pregnant women who take very high doses of vitamin A (beyond what is included in a prenatal supplement) may increase the risk of birth defects in their unborn babies. But don't let that stand between you and the salad bar. You can't get too much vitamin A from your diet—not even if you pile your plate high with broccoli, carrots, and other vitamin A–rich foods.

The recommended dietary allow-ance (RDA) for vitamin A during preg-nancy is 770 mcg, but there's no need to calculate. It's easy to get what you need from a well-balanced diet, though your prenatal supplement will offer insurance in case you fall short. You'll find the best sources in the produce department (or in the frozen fruit and vegetable cases), and hue will clue you in: Look for vitamin A in yellow and orange vegetables and fruits (carrots, winter squash, sweet potatoes, pump-kin, cantaloupe, papaya, apricots) and dark green vegetables (spinach, kale, broccoli, collard greens). You'll also score smaller amounts of A in oatmeal and other whole grains, as well as in some animal sources, including eggs.

Vitamin B$_1$ (thiamin or thiamine). Nothing B-list about this B vitamin, which helps convert carbohydrates into energy, regulate the supply of carbohy-drates to your baby, aid in the produc-tion of red blood cells (which you and your baby need plenty of), and assist in the functioning of the nervous sys-tem. Thiamin also promotes a healthy appetite—something that can definitely

Ugh ... What's an Ug?

Maybe you're wondering how many bananas you'll need to eat to reach your goal of 1.9 mg of vitamin B_6 or how many carrots equal 770 mcg of vitamin A. And wait—why do you sometimes see vitamin measurements in "ug"s? What the heck is an "ug"?

Reading food labels (see the box on page 58) can help ensure you're filling your mg, mcg, and ug recommendations—if you're willing to struggle through the fine print. Better still, the Daily Dozen (page 32) lets you dispense with all the ug, mg, and mcg measurements and makes meeting your nutritional needs much easier.

But if you're still curious, this chart should help you make sense of what all these measurements mean:

g	gram	A unit of weight equal to about 0.03 of an ounce
mg	milligram	One-thousandth of a gram
mcg	microgram	One-millionth of a gram
ug	same as mcg	One-millionth of a gram

Now for some perspective: A paper clip weighs 1 gram. A single grain of salt is equal to approximately 120 mcg or 120 ug. (770 mcg isn't looking so daunting after all, is it?) In terms you can appreciate, and eat: A bowl of cereal and a banana has your B_6 bases covered for the day. Ugs . . . without the ugh.

come in handy when you're nourishing for two. Deficiencies (something that won't happen if you're taking your prenatal vitamin) can cause fatigue and weakness in a mom and slowed growth and heart irregularities in her baby.

The RDA for thiamin during pregnancy is 1.4 mg, and though your prenatal will offer you cover, you can easily score more by eating whole grains, brown rice, oatmeal, pork, fish, beans, peas, peanuts, raisins, cauliflower, corn, acorn squash, nuts, and sunflower seeds, among other healthy foods in your diet.

Vitamin B_2 (riboflavin). Riboflavin helps release energy (something every mom-to-be can always use more of) from fats, proteins, and carbohydrates. It also helps in cell division (remember, baby's cells are dividing at a remarkable rate), and in the growth and repair of tissues (those tiny baby tissues!).

Finally, riboflavin stabilizes appetite, promotes healthy skin and eyes for you and the development of healthy skin and eyes for baby, and boosts baby's brain growth (making a steady supply of this vital vitamin especially important in the third trimester). Deficiencies of riboflavin (something that won't happen if you're taking a prenatal vitamin) can cause problems with the formation of fetal bones, poor digestive function in the fetus, and a suppressed fetal immune system. For mom, a deficiency can lead to poor appetite and mouth sores. There's also some evidence that a deficiency may increase the risk of preeclampsia, but again, if you're taking a prenatal vitamin and eating healthy foods, you don't have to worry about a riboflavin deficiency.

The RDA for riboflavin during pregnancy is 1.4 mg. You'll find it in eggs (it's in both the yolk and the white), milk,

A Baby in the Making

In approximately 266 days, your baby is transformed from a single cell to a complete human being. During that time, miraculous changes are occurring, sometimes on an hourly basis—from the formation of crucial organs (heart, lungs, stomach) to the formation of vital systems (digestive system, urinary system, circulatory system), from the development of arms and legs (including those tiny fingers and toes!) to the development of the central nervous system and brain. Here are some highlights of that transformation:

The First Trimester. Soon after sperm meets egg, the fertilized ovum begins dividing rapidly as it moves down your fallopian tube. Approximately 5 days postconception, the bundle of cells (already more than 100 cells) implants in your uterus. The outer cells will form the placenta, while the inner cells (made up of 3 layers) will form your baby.

The cells of that newly implanted embryo are already starting to specialize, getting organized into distinct tissues and organs. The outer layer of cells (the ectoderm) will develop into the brain, nervous system, hair, eyes, and skin. The middle layer of cells (the mesoderm) will develop into the muscle, bones, and cardiovascular and excretory systems. The inner layer of cells (endoderm) will develop into the digestive tract, lungs, and glands. As your pregnancy progresses, your baby will develop a rudimentary brain and the beginnings of a spinal column. The heart starts to beat somewhere around the middle of week 5. Arm buds and leg buds begin to form. As the embryo grows to the size of a grain of rice, the liver, kidneys, and thyroid gland become visible. The eyelids begin to appear, as do the nose, ears, lips, gums, and jaws. Toward the middle of the first trimester, the kidneys begin to function, blood forms in the liver, and the stomach begins to produce some digestive juices. By the time the fetus has reached the size of a coffee bean, your baby

yogurt, meat, chicken, mushrooms, peas, beans, asparagus, broccoli, spinach, and quinoa.

Vitamin B₃ (niacin). Not only is niacin involved in releasing much-needed energy from the foods you eat, but it also boosts blood flow—and so, the circulation of nutrients to your baby—by widening blood vessels. The right amount of niacin helps build a healthy nervous system and digestive tract for your baby while promoting healthier skin for you. But watch out for overdoses—which, once again, you can't get from eating healthy foods, only from taking too much in supplement form. Too much niacin can trigger itchy skin (something

pregnant women definitely don't need more of) and tummy troubles (something else pregnant women don't need more of).

The RDA for niacin during pregnancy is 18 mg. Good sources include meat, chicken, fish, milk, eggs (there's more in the whites than the yolks), legumes, and mushrooms.

Vitamin B₆ (pyridoxine). Vitamin B₆ helps the body use protein to build tissue—a very good thing when there's so much tissue to build. Because it plays a major role in baby's brain and nervous system, adequate intake of B₆ reduces the risk of neural tube defects. It also helps form red and white blood

bean's skeleton has already formed, and fingers and toes have begun to form. Fingerprints appear, and internal organs continue to mature. By the end of the first trimester, your baby, looking more like a human being now, can make facial expressions. Vocal cords are developing, bones are beginning to calcify, nails are forming, and tiny tooth buds are present. Sex organs are also developing.

The Second Trimester. Bones continue to develop and harden, causing the fetus to straighten from its curled position. Hair is beginning to grow, and muscles are more developed. (You'll probably begin feeling those first kicks sometime around weeks 16 to 20.) Your baby can hear by the sixth month, and will react to loud noises with a startle. Lanugo (a downy coat of hair) appears on the skin, as does vernix caseosa, a waxy covering that protects the baby's skin during its long soak in an amniotic bath. By the end of the second trimester, your still very little one has regular periods of wakefulness and sleep and is making more coordinated movements. Baby's eyes open and close, reacting to light. A baby boy's testicles begin their descent from the abdominal cavity into the scrotum.

The Third Trimester. Your baby will gain an average of one-half to three-quarters of a pound each week during this trimester (almost as much as you're gaining). As the ounces accumulate, baby fat develops under the skin, filling out that cute little form and ironing out that wrinkled look. Hair on that sweet head is starting to fill in (more in some babies than in others), eyebrows and eyelashes are present, and nails are already set for a manicure, having grown beyond the tips of the fingers and toes. The lungs and the digestive tract are reaching the final stages of maturity, but the most remarkable growth is in the brain, which is working overtime on its development. Your baby's immune system is also getting stronger. And 38 weeks or so after the amazing transformation began, it's showtime: Baby is ready to be born.

cells and is involved in immune function. And an added bonus: B_6 has been shown to reduce morning sickness symptoms, as well as help clear up skin unsettled by pregnancy hormones.

The RDA for pyridoxine during pregnancy is 1.9 mg. Feasting on many of your favorites will ensure that intake: bananas, avocados, tomatoes, spinach, watermelon, potatoes, brown rice, bulgur, soybeans, chickpeas, oatmeal, chicken, meat, and fish.

Vitamin B₇ (biotin). Biotin is involved in the production of amino acids and helps digest fats, carbohydrates, and proteins. Even more important when growing a baby: The rapidly dividing cells of the developing fetus require biotin for DNA replication. Deficiencies (if you're not taking a prenatal or eating well) can exacerbate several pregnancy symptoms, including fatigue, nausea, skin problems, and muscle pain. It can also trigger something that isn't common during pregnancy: hair loss.

The RDA for biotin during pregnancy is 30 mcg. You'll find biotin aplenty in many favorites, including egg yolks, fish, soybeans, seeds, nuts, sweet potatoes, spinach, and broccoli.

Vitamin B₁₂. Vitamin B_{12} is fundamental in the formation of red blood cells, for building genetic material, and for the proper development and functioning

The Placenta at Work

The placenta is what makes the making-of-a-baby possible—sort of the mission control of the baby factory. A complex network of blood vessels and tissues attached to the uterine lining and to the baby via his or her umbilical cord, the placenta contains two blood supplies: yours and baby's. These blood supplies communicate but never touch.

The placenta takes on many important roles, including producing several of the hormones that regulate growth and development. But its most significant function is as a vital pipeline, shipping nutrients from you to your baby and waste products from your baby back to you for disposal. Here's how that pipeline works.

When you eat something, your body digests it, taking available nutrients and transferring them into your bloodstream. Once your body takes what it needs (mom gets first dibs on most nutrients), it sends the rest to the placenta, where the fetus's blood vessels distribute them, along with fluids, oxygen, and other important substances. After baby's been fed, the placenta deposits waste products that are eventually shipped back for excretion via your kidneys (so, you really are peeing for two).

As baby grows, the placenta grows—but not without your help. The growth of your baby's placenta is directly related to the quality and quantity of what you eat. A better-nourished mom, on average, produces a bigger, more productive placenta (and when it comes to placentas, size does matter).

---

of the nervous system—in other words, for the making of a healthy baby. It also partners with folate (keep reading)—another essential baby building block. Deficiencies can cause neural tube defects (such as spina bifida), digestive tract disorders, or neurological disorders in the fetus, as well as severe fatigue and anemia in the mother.

The pregnancy RDA for vitamin B_{12} is 2.6 mcg. The only natural dietary sources are animal products, such as meat, chicken, dairy products, and fish. If you're a vegan, you'll need to get your vitamin B_{12} from a supplement taken in addition to your prenatal supplement (ask your practitioner for guidelines) and/or from nutritional yeast or B_{12}-fortified soy milk.

Choline. It starts with a C, but choline is a valued (if not well-known) member of the vitamin B family, essential for a baby's neural tube and brain development. It will also help give your brain a boost (you'll say "thanks for the memory" when pregnancy forgetfulness kicks in). Low levels of choline during pregnancy increase the risk of birth defects in the newborn, which is why most prenatal vitamins contain this essential nutrient in their portfolio.

The pregnancy adequate intake (AI) for choline is 450 mg. Sources include egg yolks, meat, poultry, fish, dairy, nuts, seeds, legumes, whole grains, quinoa, mushrooms, potatoes, beans, cauliflower, and brussels sprouts.

Folate (folic acid). Another member of the B team (and probably one of the most valuable players on Team Baby), folate is crucial in the proper development of the neural tube (the embryonic

Folate versus Folic Acid

Wondering why folate and folic acid are often used interchangeably? Confused about the difference between the two? So are many people, especially after a Google search. Here's the short explanation of how these two terms for the same nutrient (actually B₉) differ:

Folate. Folate is the name of the naturally occurring vitamin. It comes from the Latin word "folium," which means "leaf"—something that makes a lot of sense, since some of the best dietary sources of folate are leafy vegetables.

Folic acid. Folic acid is the synthetic form of vitamin B₉ and is what's used in supplements and added to processed- and fortified-food products, such as bread or cereals.

Glad that's cleared up? Great. Now comes the potential for more confusion. Many experts now believe that lumping folate and folic acid together is a false equivalency, at least for part of the population. And it all comes down to genes. Moms-to-be with a mutation in their MTHFR gene (and no, that's not shorthand for an expletive, it's just the name of a gene) have a difficult time properly metabolizing folic acid into usable folate. People with a mutation are better served getting most of their folate/folic acid from foods (in the form of folate) than relying only on a prenatal supplement to provide folic acid. And that's why (whether you have the gene mutation or not, or if you're not sure whether you have the mutation or not) it's so important not only to take a prenatal supplement that contains folic acid, but also to eat a diet rich in folate foods. There are also some prenatal supplements that provide folate in the form of "folinic acid" (you may also see it listed as "folate" on the label). This form (the "active" form of folic acid) may provide better absorption of this vital vitamin.

---

structure that develops into the brain and spinal cord). In fact, studies show that low levels of folate in the first months of pregnancy are responsible for about 70 percent of all neural tube defects—which is why it's so important that you get the right amount of folic acid before and during pregnancy. But folate does more than prevent birth defects, and its starring role doesn't end in the first trimester, either. Folate also aids in cell division and in the formation of red blood cells (yours and baby's), which is why getting too little can lead to anemia. Getting plenty of folate later in pregnancy is associated with a lower risk of slow fetal growth and an increased birthweight for baby, and has been linked in some situations to lower rates of premature birth, congenital heart defects, and possibly preeclampsia. Some research has suggested that adequate folate intake might help prevent Down syndrome. Other research suggests that too little folate during pregnancy may be linked to attention deficit hyperactivity disorder or future obesity in a child.

Aim to get 600 mcg of folic acid daily both before (if possible) and during pregnancy. Good sources are most leafy green vegetables, romaine lettuce, brussels sprouts, asparagus, avocados, bananas, oranges and grapefruits (a glass of OJ or grapefruit juice will score even more), tomatoes (and tomato

Don't Do the Math

Just skimming through this chapter, you can clearly see how vitamins, minerals, and other nutrients help build a healthier baby. But remember that good nutrition is not just about numbers—it's about food. So instead of whipping out your calculator to see if your RDAs for this mineral or that vitamin add up, just follow the Pregnancy Diet in Chapter 3. It does all the calculating for you. Follow the guidelines there (no need to do the math), and you and your baby will get your share of every nutrient, from A to zinc. Try the recipes in Part 2, and you'll get more delight in every nutritious bite.

juice), black-eyed peas, green peas, beans, and peanuts. Most grain products are also fortified with folic acid.

Vitamin C. Probably the best known of all vitamins, vitamin C has a remarkable resume. For one thing, it's essential to the production of collagen. This protein is what gives structure and strength to a developing baby's cartilage, muscles, blood vessels, and bones, and it's also found in skin and eyes. For another, it's needed (by both you and baby) for tissue repair, wound healing, and various other metabolic processes. And there's more to C: It helps in the absorption of iron and may help you resist infection. Getting enough vitamin C during pregnancy has been linked to a healthy birthweight and a decreased risk of preterm premature rupture of the membranes (when a mom's water breaks too early, leading to preterm birth). Deficiencies of vitamin C (not usually an issue if you're popping a prenatal daily) can cause periodontal disease, aka gum

disease (which pregnant women are more susceptible to anyway).

The RDA for vitamin C during pregnancy is 85 mg—and you'll need a fresh supply daily. Besides the obvious orange, sources include other citrus fruits, broccoli, brussels sprouts, raw cabbage, cauliflower, kale, red and green peppers, sweet potatoes, tomatoes, cantaloupe, cranberries, honeydew, kiwis, mangoes, papayas, peaches, strawberries, and watermelon.

Vitamin D. Essential for maintaining healthy teeth and bone structure, vitamin D helps in the absorption of calcium and is especially important during pregnancy. A severe vitamin D deficiency (something that is rare these days) can lead to rickets (a softening of bones), muscle disease, and seizures in a newborn. Some research suggests a link between a deficiency of D and an increased risk for preeclampsia and a cesarean delivery. Women who get enough D may be less likely to go into preterm labor, deliver prematurely, or develop infections—though the evidence for these isn't so strong and more research is ongoing.

The pregnancy RDA for vitamin D is 600 IU (15 mcg). While the body produces vitamin D when exposed to sunlight, making enough can be challenging —especially for those with darker skin and those who live in less-sunny climates, don't get outdoors enough, wear sunscreen, or cover their skin.

Can you eat (or drink) your D? Not easily, since it isn't found in large amounts in any food. Fortified milk and juices contain some, as do salmon, sardines, and egg yolks, but not nearly enough to prevent a D deficit. Your best bet is to fill in any D gaps with your prenatal vitamin, plus possibly an additional D supplement prescribed by your practitioner.

Vitamin E. Vitamin E helps ward off cell-membrane damage. There is also some preliminary evidence that an adequate intake of vitamin E for a mom during pregnancy may help prevent allergies in her child later on. Too much of this fat-soluble vitamin can be toxic, so be sure to get your E from food sources and from your prenatal supplement only—don't take any extra supplements.

The RDA for vitamin E during pregnancy is 15 mg. Get your fill from canola and olive oils, nuts, seeds, green leafies (like kale, arugula, spinach, lettuce), broccoli, kiwis, mangoes, and tomatoes.

Vitamin K. Vitamin K is essential for blood clotting and prevents excess blood loss after injuries (and after childbirth). It also maintains healthy bones and helps heal bone fractures. Not getting enough vitamin K (something that's unlikely if you're taking a prenatal) can cause easy bleeding and bruising in both you and the baby. Too much vitamin K (which you could get only from oversupplementation, not from foods you eat) can be toxic. Because little vitamin K gets transferred from mom to fetus during pregnancy, newborn babies receive a vitamin K injection soon after birth.

The AI for vitamin K during pregnancy is 90 mcg. Good sources are canola oil, olive oil, beef, broccoli, kale, spinach, turnip and collard greens, arugula, lettuce, edamame, green beans, asparagus, avocados, kiwis, blueberries, pomegranates, and bananas.

Pantothenic acid. Pantothenic acid, yet another member of the vitamin B family (B$_5$, if you're keeping score), is important for the metabolism of fats, carbohydrates, and proteins and the production of steroid hormones. It also regulates the body's adrenal activity, helps make antibodies, and stimulates wound healing.

The pregnancy AI for pantothenic acid is 6 mg. Sources include beef, chicken, dairy products, eggs, whole grains, potatoes, broccoli, and mushrooms.

Minerals

Vitamins may get all the buzz, but you wouldn't get very far without minerals—elements that are necessary for the health and proper functioning of many systems in your body. Though they tend to get lumped together with vitamins (did your parents ever tell you to "take your minerals"?), minerals are different, and they're important in different ways. The body (including your baby's body) contains about 25 essential minerals. Not surprisingly, the need for certain minerals increases when you're pregnant.

Calcium. Calcium is well known for its contribution to strong bones and teeth (including tiny baby bones and teeth)—but this vital mineral is also necessary for muscle contraction, blood clotting, and normal heart rhythm, as well as nerve development and enzyme activity. While mom gets first dibs on most vitamins and minerals (if there's not enough to go around, mom's needs will be met before baby's), that's not so with calcium. If your calcium intake is low, your body will drain your bones in order to supply calcium to your growing baby—and that can set you up for bone loss later on in life. Still, deficiencies can cause bone problems for both mother and baby. Another reason to bone up on calcium during pregnancy: Optimal intake has been associated with a decreased risk of preeclampsia.

The RDA for calcium during pregnancy is 1,000 mg. Milk may be the

> **CHEW ON THIS.** Here's a tart tall tale from the old wives' club: Drinking lime water frequently while you're pregnant builds strong teeth in the unborn baby. There's only one problem with that one. Even if it did strengthen baby's teeth (and it does not), it might weaken yours—that is, if you're sucking on limes often or drinking lime water 24/7. That's because the acid from the limes can wear away enamel over time—unless, of course, you brush after drinking lime water or sucking on limes.

obvious source (cow's or goat's milk, or fortified soy, almond, and other nut milks all contain approximately the same amount, glass for glass), but you can also claim calcium from yogurt, cheese, and other dairy products, sardines, canned salmon with bones, sesame seeds, tofu, almonds, dark green leafies, bok choy, broccoli, fortified fruit juice, and dried figs.

Chromium. Chromium works with other substances to control insulin and maintain the normal regulation of blood sugar—a process that's particularly important during pregnancy, when baby needs a steady supply of fuel for growth and development. This versatile mineral also stimulates the synthesis of protein in tissues and is necessary for baby's muscle strength, brain function, and immunity. Deficiencies (which are rare) can lead to weight loss and poor blood glucose control in the mom (which can then lead to gestational diabetes and its associated risks) and glucose intolerance in the baby.

The AI for chromium during pregnancy is 30 mcg. Most prenatal supplements don't contain chromium, but you can get your share from food sources such as cheese, whole grains, meat, poultry, spinach, mushrooms, peas, broccoli, and beans.

Copper. Copper allies with iron to form red blood cells (though iron usually gets all the credit). It also aids tissue growth, glucose metabolism, and growth of healthy hair and is essential for the development of the fetus's heart, arteries, blood vessels, skeletal system, brain, and nervous system. Deficiencies, which are rare, can cause seizures and neurological abnormalities in the baby and anemia in the mom. Excess amounts of copper can be toxic.

The RDA for copper during pregnancy is 1,000 mcg. You can cash in on copper with your prenatal supplement (but check to make sure yours contains it, since not all do) and by eating lobster, crab, cooked oysters, potatoes, dark leafy greens, mushrooms, prunes, barley, beans, whole grains, brown rice, nuts, and seeds.

Fluoride. Everyone knows that fluoride is a tooth's best friend, helping to strengthen enamel and prevent cavities. But bones depend on fluoride, too, since it acts as a bonding agent for calcium and phosphorus. With baby building up a storm in the tooth and bone departments, getting enough fluoride in your diet helps get those important jobs done. It'll also help protect your bones and teeth (keep in mind that pregnant teeth are more susceptible to decay). Too much fluoride can cause fluorosis (mottling of teeth), especially in young children.

The AI for fluoride during pregnancy is 3 mg. And you won't find it just in your toothpaste, which you won't be swallowing anyway. It also shows up in kale, spinach, milk, seafood, and canned fish with bones, as well as in green and black tea. The easiest way to access fluoride: Drink fluoridated tap water.

Iodine. A component of the thyroid hormone thyroxine, iodine is needed for the proper functioning of the thyroid gland (responsible for regulating metabolism), as well as for a baby's nervous system development. Deficiencies (an intake of less than 10 to 20 mcg of iodine a day) can cause thyroxine levels to drop, resulting in a condition called goiter in a mom and possibly in her baby, as well. Low iodine intake is associated with restricted growth and neurodevelopmental problems in utero, as well as with a lowered IQ or learning problems later on for a child. Severe iodine deficiency (rare in the U.S.) is also linked with miscarriage and stillbirth.

The RDA for iodine during pregnancy is 220 mcg. Many people get what they need from iodized salt, but the mineral is also available in seafood, seaweed, and dairy products. Keep in mind that many varieties of salt are not iodized, and that not all prenatals contain iodine, either (see the box on this page).

Iron. Getting enough iron, the must-have mineral used to produce red blood cells and distribute oxygen throughout the body, is the greatest nutritional challenge a woman faces during her reproductive life, period—and not only because of those monthly periods. In fact, the challenges multiply when you're pregnant and not getting those periods. That's because of the dramatic increase in blood production during pregnancy, which requires more iron than ever. Low iron levels can result in iron-deficiency anemia, with symptoms that include feeling extremely weak, fatigued, and/or breathless (beyond what's normal in pregnancy).

Since it's very hard to fill the pregnancy requirement for this must-have

Give Iodine a Fair Shake

Time was, all it took to get enough iodine was a few shakes of iodized salt, once the salt standard in kitchens and on tables in the U.S. Today, however, the iodine content of an average American diet has dropped—even as sodium consumption has risen sharply. That's because the addition of iodine to salt isn't mandatory in the U.S. and the salt that's used in the high-sodium foods Americans like to eat—those baked goods, chips, and other processed foods—isn't iodized. Neither is sea salt, kosher salt, Himalayan salt, and other specialty salt. Which could mean that your iodine intake is lower than you think.

Because iodine is crucial during pregnancy, and because the iodine RDA increases during pregnancy, experts recommend that moms-to-be opt for iodized salt (check what you're shaking—many brands of table salt are still iodized) and take a daily prenatal supplement that contains 150 mcg of iodine (not all prenatals do, so be sure to check labels).

mineral through diet alone, or even from the iron that's added to a standard prenatal supplement, it's recommended that moms-to-be take a daily iron supplement beginning at week 20 (when blood volume begins to expand significantly), and continuing through the rest of pregnancy. Taking a slow-release supplement can be easier on your stomach.

The RDA for iron during pregnancy is 27 mg. You can get additional iron (beyond what's in your prenatal and/or the supplement prescribed by your practitioner) by eating beef, seafood, beans, lentils, chickpeas, tofu, peas, spinach, potatoes, dried apricots, prunes, dark chocolate, and oatmeal.

Magnesium. Another mineral that gives calcium an assist in the bone-building department, magnesium is also needed for nerve and muscle function, as well as for helping the body process carbohydrates. What's more, it's essential in the regulation of insulin and blood-sugar levels (so important during pregnancy) and needed for the removal of toxins from the body (ditto). Because magnesium relaxes muscles (as opposed to calcium, which stimulates muscles to contract), adequate levels of magnesium during pregnancy may help prevent premature contractions of the uterus (aka premature labor). Getting enough magnesium may help ward off leg cramps, constipation, and even morning sickness. Severe deficiencies are rare but can increase the risk of preeclampsia in a mom and stunted growth, muscle spasms, and congenital malformations in her baby.

The pregnancy RDA for magnesium is 350 mg (360 mg for moms-to-be over age 30). Most prenatals contain magnesium only in small amounts, so be sure

Another Strike Against Soda

Need one more reason to limit the pop, mom (besides all that sugar or all those artificial sweeteners)? Most sodas are loaded with phosphorus (listed as phosphoric acid), which lowers the level of calcium in the blood—with some sodas offering up to 500 mg of phosphorus per serving. So not only can a serious soda habit keep you from drinking your calcium-loaded milk, but it prevents the absorption of whatever calcium you do get from other sources.

to fill your requirement the natural way as well. Tasty sources include legumes, beans, nuts, seeds, tofu, yogurt, milk, whole grains, dried apricots, prunes, bananas, and dark green leafy vegetables.

Manganese. Not on many people's mineral radar (and often confused with magnesium) manganese is vital for the development of baby's bones, cartilage, and hearing. It's also necessary for good reproductive function. Deficiencies (very rare) can cause growth restriction in the fetus. Not all prenatal supplements contain manganese, so check the label to see if yours does.

The AI for manganese is 2 mg. Sources include strawberries, bananas, raisins, spinach, carrots, broccoli, whole grains, brown rice, legumes, nuts, and seeds.

Molybdenum. You probably haven't heard of this mineral before (and you almost certainly can't pronounce it), but humble molybdenum is thought to help in a monumentally important task: the transfer of oxygen from one molecule to another. It is also required for protein and fat metabolism, and it helps the baby use iron.

The RDA for molybdenum during pregnancy is 50 mcg. You can find it in legumes, beans, whole grains, and nuts. It's found in many, but not all, prenatal supplements.

Phosphorus. Another comrade of calcium, phosphorus is a component of healthy teeth and bones. It's also needed to maintain the right balance of body fluids and is essential for muscle contractions, normal heart rhythm, and blood clotting. Deficiencies, which are uncommon, can cause a loss of appetite (no good when you're pregnant), weakness (you're tired enough), and a loss of calcium from bones (your bones). Too

The Food Fortification Frenzy

Food enrichment (adding vitamins and minerals lost in processing back into a product) and fortification (adding extra vitamins and minerals that weren't naturally occurring in the first place) were introduced in the U.S. during the first half of the 20th century to prevent the thousands of deaths that resulted each year from severe vitamin and mineral deficiencies. It worked, big-time—such deficiencies have been virtually eradicated.

Fast-forward to the 21st century, and while enrichment is still humming away (replacing vital nutrients in white rice, white bread, and other refined baked goods), fortification is really on a roll. With manufacturers eager to cash in on the fortification frenzy, you'll find fortified foods and beverages in just about every aisle of your supermarket: calcium, vitamins A through E, zinc, even plant sterols (for a "heart healthy" bonus) in your OJ, added omega-3s in your peanut butter, phytochemicals in those gummies, amino acids in that chocolate,

and electrolytes plus protein (yes, protein) in that bottle of water.

Do the benefits of added nutrients add up? Sometimes—as when adding iodine to salt prevents goiter, adding vitamin D to milk prevents rickets, adding folic acid to grains prevents neural tube defects in developing babies. But often, those added nutrients add only to the product's cost—not its health benefits. They won't make an already nutritious food (that peanut butter) significantly more nutritious. And they definitely won't make an otherwise unwholesome food (those gummies) a health food.

The bottom line: Eating a diet of naturally healthy foods is the best way to fill your nutritional requirements and, now that you're expecting, your baby's. There's no harm in chowing down on enriched and fortified foods (and in some cases, there are significant protective perks, especially for the pregnant). But there's no reason to go out of your way—or out of your budget—to load up on them, either.

---

much phosphorus (which you might get from drinking too much soda; see the box on the facing page) can interfere with your body's ability to properly use both calcium and iron.

The RDA for phosphorus during pregnancy is 700 mg. Look for it in yogurt and cheese (where you'll also find your calcium), fish, meat, poultry, eggs, oatmeal, and lima beans.

Potassium. Potassium works with sodium to maintain fluid balance in cells (so vital during pregnancy, when fluid levels must increase significantly) and regulate blood pressure. It also maintains muscle tone, key in minimizing

pregnancy aches and pains, aiding in delivery, and speeding postpartum recovery.

The AI for pregnant women is 4,700 mg of potassium a day. There are many delicious sources of potassium, including avocados, bananas, dried apricots, oranges, peaches, pears, raisins, prunes, tomatoes, carrots, peas, pumpkin, spinach, squash, potatoes, lentils, kidney beans, peanuts, meat, fish, poultry, and dairy products.

Selenium. Selenium is important for your body's defense against disease—preventing cell damage, working with vitamin E as an antioxidant, and binding with toxins in the body, rendering them harmless (and protecting baby from them).

The pregnancy RDA for selenium is 60 mcg. Sources include Brazil nuts (half a nut supplies all the selenium you need for the day), fish, meat, poultry, eggs, dairy products, and whole grains.

Sodium. Sodium generally gets a bad rap—and not without good reason. But while too much sodium is a diet-don't for any body, so is too little sodium, especially when it comes to pregnant bodies. The right amount of sodium is needed to maintain the right amount of water in the body (essential when blood and fluid volumes are expanding rapidly), as well as the perfect balance of acids and bases in body fluids. It also helps nutrients cross cell membranes, a very valuable skill when there's a baby to be nourished.

Though your need for sodium increases slightly during pregnancy, it's unlikely you'll need to shake up your salt intake (though many moms-to-be find themselves craving salty foods, like pickles). After all, the average American diet includes more than enough (way more than enough) sodium to keep you covered. That said, unless your practitioner has suggested otherwise, there's no need to restrict your sodium intake.

The AI for sodium during pregnancy is 1,500 mg per day. You'll find sodium in almost every food in some amount (even unlikely sources, like celery), and in generous amounts in processed foods, pickles, sauces, and, of course, in your salt shaker. Just add iodine (see the box on page 21).

Zinc. Zinc is one of a developing baby's best mineral buddies, essential for cell division and tissue growth, as well as for hair, skin, and proper bone growth. It also helps in the perception of taste and works with insulin to regulate blood sugar. Touted for its reproductive benefits (boosting fertility in both women and men), some research has suggested pregnancy benefits, too. Deficiencies in this vital mineral can increase the risk of miscarriage, preterm delivery, low birthweight, and possibly birth defects such as spina bifida, cleft lip or palate (or both), and visual impairment. Luckily, a daily prenatal supplement will have you covered in the zinc department.

The RDA for zinc during pregnancy is 11 mg. Good sources include turkey, beef, cooked oysters and other shellfish, eggs (mostly in the yolk), yogurt, corn, wheat germ, oatmeal, and cashews.

> **CHEW ON THIS.** Old wives in Indonesia have spooned this theory up: A superstition there advises expectant mothers to avoid putting a spoon in the salt container. According to the tale, failure to keep their salt shaken, not stirred, may cause them to have problems in labor. Clearly, another one to be taken with a grain (or a shake, or a spoonful) of salt.

Beyond Vitamins and Minerals

Now that you know everything you could possibly ever know about vitamins and minerals and how they nourish bodies big (yours) and tiny (baby's), is your nutrition education complete? Not quite yet. There are many other nutrients that benefit your body and your baby's, including:

Fiber. Fiber is a nutrient that your body doesn't actually digest—but it's key to digestion. The most famous part of fiber's job description, and one a constipation-prone pregnant mom can really appreciate: It helps move waste through the intestines. But fiber has other talents, too, including the ability to help regulate blood sugar, possibly reducing the risk of gestational diabetes and preeclampsia. Sources of fiber include fruit, vegetables, beans, legumes, and whole grains.

Omega-3 fatty acids. These good fats are essential in the production of cell membranes, hormones, and prostaglandins. But they've received the most kudos for their important work in baby brain and eye development. Enough DHA (a type of omega-3) during pregnancy may reduce the chances of baby being born too early or being born at a low birthweight. Research also shows that eating foods rich in omega-3 may help boost your mood. How can you reach the recommended intake of around 1.4 mg of omega-3s a day during pregnancy? Chow down on fish, nuts and nut oil, and omega-3 eggs. Your prenatal supplement may also contain some. Read more on page 51.

Phytonutrients. They've been around since the first little sprout—but they're big news, for good reason. Phytonutrients is a broad name for compounds (beyond vitamins and minerals) that are found in plants—fruits, vegetables, grains. Each type of phytonutrient—and there are thousands—is believed to have different benefits for the body. You may have heard of phytonutrients by some of their names: antioxidants, phytochemicals, flavonoids, isoflavones, and carotenoids, for instance. Research has shown that phytonutrients help reduce disease risk and stimulate immunities. Every day, researchers are uncovering more and more benefits of these and other natural components of plants, which you can't find in supplements. Fruits and vegetables are super sources of phytochemicals.

Probiotics. It's all in the name: Probiotics are beneficial (or "pro") bacteria that bulk up the numbers of helpful bacteria and crowd out illness-causing bacteria. Beyond helping to counterbalance the negative effects of antibiotics (like diarrhea), probiotics may stimulate the intestinal bacteria to break down food better, aiding the digestive tract in its efforts to keep things moving. They also help strengthen the intestinal lining so that bad bugs can't cross into the bloodstream, and even change the intestinal environment, making it more acidic and therefore less hospitable to bad bacteria. Research suggests that probiotics may possibly combat sinus, respiratory, and urinary infections (all more common in pregnant women), as well as boost the immune system in general. Studies have also shown that probiotics during pregnancy (and breastfeeding) may reduce the risk of food allergies and eczema in early childhood. You'll find plenty of probiotics in yogurt and yogurt drinks that contain active cultures. You can also ask your practitioner to recommend a good probiotic supplement—in capsules, chewables, or a powder form.

CHAPTER 3

The Pregnancy Diet

W hat does it take to make a healthy baby? Nutrients, and lots of them. From the vitamin A that'll help those little eyes see you for the first time . . . to the manganese that'll help those little ears hear you. From the calcium that will build strong bones and teeth (and make those tiny finger- and toenails grow!) . . . to the omega-3 fatty acids that will boost the development of a brain that has so many things to learn in a lifetime.

But just how do you take all the nutrients you and your baby need during the next 9 months and put them together in an eating plan that's easy to follow, practical to live and work with, as nutritious as can be—and as delicious as possible, so you can have fun feeding yourself and your baby well? Welcome to the Pregnancy Diet.

Nine Ways to Eat Well When You're Expecting—and Beyond

E ating well may not be rocket science—but there are times when it can seem just as complicated. Pregnancy is one of those times—what with all those recommendations that need following (Skip the sushi! Drink your milk! Limit your caffeine!), those requirements that need filling, and those symptoms getting in the way of eating altogether. But eating well doesn't have to be so complicated, even when you're trying to eat well for two. In fact, it can be easily broken down into 9 basic principles. Follow these steps even loosely, and you can't help but feed your pregnant body and your growing baby well during the 9 months ahead. Stick with them after delivery, and you and your family will continue to collect benefits that can last a lifetime.

Choose calories you can count on. While it's true that a calorie is a calorie, it's also true that not all calories are created equal. Some calories are packed with nutrients (the calories in an avocado, for instance), but others are essentially empty of nutrients (the calories in a glazed donut). With pregnancy awarding you only about 300 extra calories a day (over your regular daily intake), and with requirements for protein, calcium, vitamins, and minerals increased, it's smart to spend most of your calories on foods with nutritional cachet. To snack on a 100-calorie bag of almonds instead of a 100-calorie bag of jellybeans. To invest 300 calories in a grilled cheese on whole-wheat instead of a hot dog on white. And to choose the 35 calories in a tablespoon of hummus and a handful of baby carrots over the same number of calories you'll get from munching on ¼ cup of potato chips (who can stop at ¼ cup anyway?).

Be an efficient eater. Packing all those recommended nutrients into a day's worth of eating can seem overwhelming—a stretch for even the hungriest (let alone the queasiest) and definitely a stretch for your time, your tummy, your budget, and possibly, your weight-gain goals.

How to meet this challenge? By becoming an efficient eater: Focus on foods that overachieve in overall nutrients and multitask in nutritional categories (filling 2 or more food groups in the same serving), and don't waste too many calories or too much space in your stomach.

For instance, looking for a calorie-efficient way to score a serving of protein? Choose a cup of low-fat cottage cheese (weighing in at 180 calories) over a cup of the full-fat variety (240

calories). Seeking a zesty topping for your chili that adds calcium to your bottom line? Reach for low-fat yogurt instead of sour cream—you'll get about twice the calcium for a quarter of the calories.

Another way to eat efficiently: Choose foods that do double (or even triple) nutritional duty, filling 2 or more buckets in a single serving. Like a serving of mango or cantaloupe, which serves up both vitamin C and vitamin A. Broccoli or kale, which do the same (with a calcium bonus), or dried apricots, which deliver iron, too. Greek yogurt, which checks off calcium and protein. Salmon, which satisfies protein and omega-3s (plus calcium, if you eat the canned variety mashed with the bones). High-protein whole-grain pasta, which provides protein plus complex carbs. Chickpea or lentil pasta, which adds even more protein.

If you're having trouble gaining weight, being an efficiency expert will come in handy as well, with a switch in strategy: Choose foods that are dense both nutritionally and in calories (see page 99).

Feed yourself, feed your baby. Maybe you've been a meal skipper since middle school. Or maybe it's a habit you've picked up on the job. Or maybe you're too nauseous or too tired these pregnant days to even think about preparing or eating those 3 squares a day. Still, while you may not miss the breakfasts (or lunches, or dinners) you're skipping, your baby will—especially as those growth-intensive second and third trimesters roll around. Once growing really gets going, your little one counts on you for a steady supply of energy and nutrients around the clock—he or she can't order in when you skip out on lunch. In fact, "more often" may actually be "more" when it comes to eating regularly.

Putting the Natural in Sugar Substitutes

Trying to put less sugar and fewer calories into your diet naturally? There are plenty of low-cal natural sugar substitutes to choose from now, derived from fruits and vegetables instead of from chemicals. Options that are probably safe for pregnancy use (check with your practitioner before reaching for these and others) include monk-fruit sweetener (derived from, you guessed it, monk fruit), BochaSweet (derived from kabocha, a type of pumpkin native to Japan), and allulose (a rare sugar found in fruits like raisins and figs). Calories aren't your concern? Then you'll have even more natural, pregnancy-safe sugar substitutes to choose from, including honey (ask your practitioner before using raw, unpasteurized honey), agave, fruit juice concentrate, coconut sugar, molasses, barley malt syrup, maple syrup, or rice syrup. Run these options by your doctor or dietitian if you have gestational diabetes, since all can impact blood-glucose levels, some more than others. For information about the safety of artificial sweeteners, see page 74.

Research suggests that eating frequently as pregnancy progresses (3 meals plus snacks or 6 small meals a day) may boost the odds of a mom-to-be carrying to term. Plus, eating early and often every day will help keep your blood sugar level (minimizing headaches, fatigue, mood slumps, and more), and ease queasiness and other digestive troubles.

Know the benefits of eating regularly, but have a hard time fitting frequent meals into your schedule and your tummy? Or can't stomach the idea of eating at all, never mind eating often? See Chapter 7 for strategies to help you get around obstacles to regular eating.

Be complex with carbs. Complex carbohydrates (such as whole-grain breads and cereals, brown rice, fruits and vegetables, beans and other legumes) contain energy-yielding and energy-sustaining nutrients that every pregnant body needs—especially those B (for baby-building!) vitamins. Complex carbs also pack a natural punch of fiber, which can not only kick constipation in the butt but may reduce the risk of gestational diabetes. On the other, less healthy hand, simple carbs (like white rice, white bread and other baked goods made with refined flour, and sugary foods) have lost their natural nutritional edge in processing or (in the case of sugar) never had any. So when going for carbs (as you should every day; see the box on page 30), go complex whenever you can.

Spare the sugar. Easily sweet-talked by sugary treats? Listen to this: Calories that come from refined sugar actually come without benefits. Yes, they're often found in foods that provide pleasure (in some cases, lots and lots of pleasure), but too often, those foods don't contain much in the way of nutritional value. Which means too much sugar can add up quickly in calories without adding to your nutritional bottom line, or your baby's. Fine as a treat, not so fine as a staple of a healthy diet, especially a healthy pregnancy diet. Plus, another minus: Research shows that moms-to-be who consume too many sugary foods and drinks during pregnancy increase the risk of their babies developing allergies and asthma.

Does this mean you have to cut your sweet tooth off entirely? Absolutely not. Cutting back on sugar is certainly a smart move to make, but cutting it out entirely isn't necessary unless you want to (or you know you're the kind of sweets addict who can't stop crushing the candy once you start). Plus, sweet foods don't always come in empty packages, or even in sugary ones, especially if they've come by their sweetness naturally (think a juicy summer peach, a slice of ripe melon, a perfect banana—hey, spread with peanut butter and dipped in dark chocolate if that helps make the case). Or if their package is whole grain (like the Triple Blueberry Muffins on page 205 or a batch of the oatmeal cookies on page 352). So that you can have your cake . . . and nutrients, too.

Feature fruits and vegetables. Everyone knows that fruits and vegetables are the mainstay of a healthy diet—and that everyone can benefit from eating more of them, especially a mom-to-be who needs all the vitamins (vitamins A, B, and C, folate . . .), minerals (including the ever-important potassium), fiber, and phytochemicals those yummy fruits and vegetables provide. Need another reason to up your veggie intake? Researchers have found that children born to women who eat plenty of vegetables during pregnancy have a lower risk of developing Type 1 diabetes. An added bonus: Most vegetables and many fruits are naturally low in fat and calories. Another bonus: They fight constipation.

The best way to make sure you're getting the most out of your diet is to follow the rainbow—at least, the one in your produce aisle. If your food palate is mostly brown and beige (as in burgers and fries, not as in whole-wheat bread or walnuts), it's time to add some color to your life—and to your dinner plate—by loading up on fruits and vegetables. The more vibrantly colored the fruits and vegetables are on the inside, the better—those are the ones packed with the nutrients most valued in baby making.

Produce-Phobic?

Is a fear of pesticide residue keeping you and produce apart? Don't let it. As long as you follow the basic principles of fruit and vegetable safety (always wash fruits and vegetables, choose organic when you can, vary the produce you eat, and, when in doubt, peel), you won't have to pay the price in pesticides. In fact, many types of fruits and vegetables actually contain natural substances that protect you and your baby against the effects of chemical contamination (not only from the produce you eat, but also from other sources in your environment). So fear not your produce. For more information on chemical residue and pesticides on produce, contact the Environmental Protection Agency National Pesticide Information Center at npic.orst.edu. For more on choosing organic produce, see page 66.

Start early in the day by blending a fruit (or veggie) smoothie. Toss some spinach and peppers into your eggs. Top your yogurt or oatmeal with a bounty of berries. Explore recipes that include more vegetables—say, soups, salads, and stir-fries. Think green (or red, yellow, orange, purple) by prepping some of your produce ahead (or buying it prepped) and storing cut-up fruits and veggies in sealed containers in the fridge, alongside a container of dip for extra incentive. Freeze bananas so they're smoothie ready, and grapes for easy popping.

Choose foods that remember their roots. What separates the peach you're about to eat from the day it was picked? A week at the farmers market, ripening

The Lowdown on Low-Carb, Raw, and Paleo

Are you paleo-friendly? Keto curious? Raring to go raw? There's a reason why low is not the way to go when it comes to carbs, why you should aim for better balance in your diet (not higher protein), and why you shouldn't revisit the raw roots of your prehistoric ancestors now that you're expecting.

Low-carb. A diet short on carbs (especially the complex kind) may be short on vital baby-making ingredients, such as the folate and other vitamins and minerals found in grains, fruits, and vegetables. It can also pack far more protein than your body needs, even when you're pregnant. Other downsides to downsizing your carbs: You'll be skimping on constipation-fighting fiber and on the B vitamins believed to battle morning sickness and pregnancy-unsettled skin. A balanced diet may not be buzz-worthy, but it's definitely baby-worthy.

Keto. Taking low-carb to a new low is the keto diet, which eliminates nearly all carbs, including fruits, whole grains, and some vegetables. The thinking behind the keto craze? Carbs are the body's preferred energy source, and when the body runs out of carbs to burn, it burns fat instead, a state called ketosis. This can lead to rapid weight loss—something that's never recommended during pregnancy. Another downside to ketosis: Ketones (the by-products of that fat breakdown) can cross the placenta, and it's unclear how a buildup of ketones can affect a developing baby. Adding to the case against keto for you: While the general science about this eating plan is very limited, the research is even scarcer when it comes to pregnancy. There haven't been any controlled studies done in pregnant humans, but babies of pregnant mice fed a ketogenic diet had complications, including slower growth and behavioral changes after birth. Need more convincing? It's a given that the lack of fiber in a keto diet will compound pregnancy constipation. By all means, choose your carbs carefully when you're making a baby, but for healthiest results, don't choose to cut out all carbs.

Paleo. What's old (really, really old) is new again, thanks to the much-hyped

in the sun? Or months in transport from Chile, cold storage in a warehouse, then more travel to the supermarket? Was it cut and flash-frozen or freeze-dried fresh days after picking, or cut, cooked with water, corn syrup, and sugars, and canned? No shocker here: Nature's finest doesn't fall far from the tree—and is at its finest when served up with its just-harvested goodness still intact (even if it was frozen or freeze-dried or minimally processed and canned just after harvest and served much later). Picking up that produce at a farm stand? Chances are the vegetable or fruit you're choosing remembers its roots. Shopping at a supermarket produce section? Gauge the freshness factor by checking not only a product's source (did it come from in-state . . . cross-country . . . or around the world?), but also its color, texture, and condition. Is the broccoli soft, pale, and anemic from its journey, or vibrant green and firm (almost certainly packing more nutrients, stalk for stalk)? Are the carrots soft, split, and faded, or brilliantly hued and begging to be crunched? Tomatoes or strawberries washed out from premature picking and subsequent storage and transport—or blushing a

paleo diet, which takes eaters back (way, way back) to the days when meat ruled and foraging was limited to whatever grew on bushes and trees. While some of the principles of the paleo diet, like cutting out refined sugar and processed foods, are good diet values in general (and in pregnancy), going all hunter-gatherer when you're growing a baby may not be so smart. Studies show that eating high amounts of red meat while going low on carbs during pregnancy can lead to low birthweight. Other risks for women who eat paleo while pregnant: low blood sugar and constipation (because of the lack of grains and the excess of protein). A modified paleo diet—lower on the proteins and higher on the carbs, particularly whole grains, beans, and other legumes—can fit the bill during pregnancy (and will look similar to the Pregnancy Diet). Another positive takeaway from the paleo diet you can feel free to take with you into pregnancy: Eat more nuts and seeds.

Raw. Another blast from our primitive past, eating a completely raw diet was a pregnant woman's only choice BC (before cooking). Today, of course, with dozens of cooking techniques at your fingertips (along with apps to deliver your food fully cooked), you've got options. Which is a good thing, because eating a raw-only diet may be a raw deal for you and your baby. First reason: Because some vitamins and minerals are absorbed only when they're cooked, it's hard to get all the nutrients you need during pregnancy when you're eating only raw. Second reason—and perhaps most important: There's always the possibility that raw foods may be contaminated with bacteria that cooking or pasteurizing (both taboo among raw eaters) would otherwise kill. That holds true not only for the obvious suspects—the ones you're not supposed to eat anyway during pregnancy (raw dairy products, raw juice, raw meat and fish)—but also for "raw" prepared foods sold in health food markets that aren't prepared or stored safely. So dig into those raw veggies (also have cooked vegetables to optimize absorption), savor those salads, and by all means eat that apple (and fresh peach, and fresh mango) a day—but also remember that some foods were made to be cooked (or heat-pasteurized), at least when you're baking a baby bun.

deep, vine-ripened red? When you can't find produce that's as fresh as nature intended, don't change your menu, just head to the frozen-food aisle. Quick-freezing is done almost immediately after harvesting, when produce is at the height of its nutritive value, so most frozen fruits and vegetables have as much to offer as their "fresh" counterparts—or even more. Just read labels to be sure nothing has been added to your frozen produce picks, such as sauces, sugar, salt, or other unwanted ingredients. Canned fruits and vegetables (without added salt or sugar) can be nutrition-packed and handy in a pinch, too. Also explore the growing assortment of crunchy freeze-dried fruits and vegetables, which offer the same nutritional benefits as fresh, with a far longer shelf life—not to mention, a long life in your car, your handbag, the deepest recesses of your office drawer, and ultimately, your diaper bag.

Carry the freshness principle over to the other aisles of the market, too. When possible, select rolled oats over packets of instant, fresh potatoes for mashing over flakes, natural cheese over those cellophane-wrapped slices.

Cave to the crave. Maybe you've always thought about food in 2 categories: food you want to eat (I shouldn't . . . but yum), and food you're supposed to eat (I should . . . but yuck). And now, with the responsibility of growing a healthy baby weighing heavily on your growing belly, maybe you're assuming your focus needs to be only on the foods you're supposed to eat. Not so. Always denying yourself the foods you want to eat will just leave you feeling grumpy— and hungry. So don't deprive yourself. Find ways to substitute like for like (see page 114 for some suggestions). Or, if you're craving ice cream, have a scoop or two (and choose your ice cream with an eye on calcium content—some varieties contain more than others, often for fewer calories). Longing for a chocolate bar? Munch on a mini instead of a king-size (or try switching to dark chocolate, which comes with health benefits). Just keep the amount of healthy foods higher than the less healthy ones, and add nutrition where you can (choose the brownie with walnuts instead of the one with chocolate chips, switch from fudge topping to fresh berries on your ice cream). Of course, if you find you can't stop once the lid's off the ice cream—or you can't stop at one brownie once there's a tray in front of you—it's probably smart to curb your enthusiasm . . . and your cravings.

Eat well family-style. How well you and your baby eat isn't directly impacted by how well the rest of your family is eating—but there's definitely a connection that goes both ways. First, it's always easier to eat well when those around you (at least those who live with you) eat well, too—chowing down on a bag of crunchy kale chips instead of a bag of sour-cream-and-onion, or savoring the salmon and brown rice bowl instead of the bowl of hot wings and fries. Second, it's win-win-win if eating well during pregnancy becomes a lasting family tradition: A win for baby (nurtured on a healthy pregnancy diet, then weaned on healthy foods and raised in a home where healthy eating habits are second nature). A win for you (no surprise, you'll be left with a healthier postpartum body if you eat well during pregnancy, and if those habits you develop now stick, you'll have a healthier body for life). And a win for your partner (who will be healthier, too—now and in the future). If your new and improved eating style becomes the new and improved family norm, everyone stands to gain long-term health benefits— including not gaining too many pounds over the years to come. Encouraging healthy eating habits can also lower your family's future risk of diet-influenced (and weight-influenced) diseases, such as diabetes and high blood pressure.

The Pregnancy Daily Dozen

No need to keep track of your K, add up your A, chart your chromium, monitor your magnesium, or follow your fiber. The Pregnancy Daily Dozen serves up all the vitamins, minerals, and nutrients you and baby need in 12 easy food groups. Just eat about the number of recommended servings from each of the 12 categories (keeping in mind that many foods overlap in 2 or more categories, cutting down on the number of portions you'll have to eat from each), and you're done for the day.

Calories: Approximately 300 extra daily. Never thought of calories as your friend? It's time to rethink that relationship. Calories represent the amount of energy supplied by the carbohydrates, protein, and fats in foods. They're essential to life, but especially essential in the life of a pregnant woman, who needs energy for so many things—from just staying on her feet (no easy feat when pregnancy has you beat) to fueling that baby-making factory.

Does your need for extra energy require you to eat extra calories? Yes—just maybe not as many as you might expect (or as the phrase "eating for two" suggests). Believe it or not, the making of a baby requires only about 300 extra calories a day (added to the number of daily calories required to maintain prepregnancy weight; see the box on page 34), and fewer than that during early pregnancy. A bonus, true, but not exactly the all-access ice-cream pass you might have been hoping for.

Now that you know how many calories you'll need every day for the rest of your pregnancy, forget it. Instead of keeping track of calories, just keep track of your weight gain. If you're gaining about the right amount of weight, you're eating about the right number of

The Pregnancy Daily Dozen in a Nutshell

Here are the 12 food groups that make up the Pregnancy Diet—the Pregnancy Daily Dozen:

Calories: Approximately 300 extra daily

Protein: 3 servings daily

Calcium: 4 servings daily

Vitamin C: 3 servings daily

Vitamin A: 3 to 4 servings daily

Other fruits and vegetables: 1 to 2 servings daily

Whole grains and legumes: 6 or more servings daily

Iron-rich foods: Some daily

Fat and high-fat foods: Some daily

Omega-3 fatty acids: Some daily

Fluids: At least 10 8-ounce glasses daily

Prenatal vitamin supplement: A pregnancy formula taken daily

calories. If you're not gaining enough weight, you're eating too few calories. If you're gaining too much weight (or gaining it too quickly), you're getting too many. Adjust as needed—and you're done and done.

Moms carrying more than one baby need more calories. See page 156 for details.

Protein: 3 servings daily. There's no material more essential to the making of a baby than protein's amino acids, the

Pregnancy Calorie Count

Over the course of 40 weeks, it takes an estimated 75,000 calories to make a baby. Just don't try to eat them all in one sitting.

The Truth About Eating for Two

Myth: You're eating for two during pregnancy. So that means you should take everything you usually eat and then double it.

Fact: While it's true you're eating for two people—you and your baby—remember that one of those two is very, very small. Feeding your baby and fueling your baby-making factory will require only about 100 extra calories a day during the first trimester, when your little one is extra little. As baby grows and your body works harder, that number will triple to about 300 calories—more, but definitely not double your usual.

building blocks of human tissue (your little human's tissues included). But does that mean you'll have to pack in extra protein when you're building a baby?

That depends on how much protein you're already getting. The pregnancy requirement for protein is about 75 grams, or 3 servings, a day—but many Americans eat at least that much protein without even trying, and those on high-protein diets consume much more. Chances are you, too, fit that protein-plentiful profile (unless you're a vegetarian, especially if you're a vegan; see the box on page 42).

Here's how easy it is to get your fill of protein. Have just 1 serving at each meal (for example, a cheese omelet for breakfast, a salad topped with grilled chicken for lunch, and a fish fillet for dinner), and you're done. Prefer to graze your day away? Six half servings of protein will fill the bill. Can't contemplate so much protein first thing in the morning? Fill in the protein gaps later on in the day—say, with 8 ounces of chicken for lunch or dinner. And if 8 ounces sounds like a lot, consider that it's just an average serving in most restaurants.

Not in a meat-eating mood? Look for protein in the dairy case—you'll find ⅓ of a serving in every glass of milk and every ounce of cheese, plus ⅔ of a serving in every cup of Greek yogurt. Score additional protein from whole-grain bread, cereal, and pasta (especially high-protein pastas, like those made from beans).

If You're Counting

You know you're supposed to add 300 calories to your daily intake now that you're pregnant, but what number are you supposed to add them to? Start with your prepregnancy weight (if you know it) and multiply it by 12 if you're sedentary, 15 if you're moderately active, and up to 22 if you're extremely active. That's approximately the number of calories it took to maintain your weight prepregnancy, and that's the number you'll be adding your 300 extra calories to. Because the rate at which calories are burned varies from person to person even during pregnancy, calorie requirements vary, too, so the figure you arrive at is just an estimate. In other words, don't count on it. Remember, the very best indicator of whether you're getting the right number of calories, or too many, or too few: your weight gain. See Chapter 6 for more.

Every day, try to have about 3 servings of the following foods (or any combination equal to 3 servings). If you're using dairy sources for protein, don't forget to give yourself credit for calcium, too (credit works both ways, so count up the protein in your calcium foods).

24 ounces (3 8-ounce cups) of cow's or goat's milk or buttermilk

3 ounces hard cheese (check out the freeze-dried varieties, too)

1 cup cottage cheese

1 cup Greek or Icelandic yogurt

3 cups regular yogurt

4 eggs

4 ounces cooked fresh fish (see page 72 for information on safe fish eating during pregnancy)

4 ounces cooked shellfish

3½ ounces canned tuna or sardines

4 ounces skinless chicken, turkey, duck, or other poultry

4 ounces lean beef, lamb, veal, pork, or buffalo (bison)

Have queasiness and aversions pushed meat and other animal products off the menu? Or are you vegan? There are plenty of protein sources beyond the animal kingdom. Many of the following also net a serving of complex carbs, and some add significant amounts of calcium or omega-3s:

Beans and Legumes
(half protein servings)

¾ cup cooked beans, lentils, split peas, or chickpeas (garbanzos)

½ cup cooked soybeans (or edamame)

2 ounces legume pasta

Visual Reality

Do your eyes deceive you when you're judging the serving of food on your plate? Chances are, they do. Most Americans, weaned on supersize fast-food portions, extra-large beverage containers, and all-you-can-eat buffets, are actually eating 2 to 3 times the recommended serving amount per food item. A plateful of spaghetti at a typical restaurant, for instance, is closer to 3 servings of grains than it is to 1. The hefty half pounder weighs in at 2 protein servings, even before you add the cheese and bacon. Having an entree-size salad for lunch? You'll be helping yourself to several servings of vegetables. So before you dig into your Daily Dozen, here's a visual reality check:

- A serving of meat, poultry, or fish (4 ounces) is equivalent to the size of a deck of cards.

- A serving of fruit or vegetables (around half a cup) is about the size of a light bulb.

- A serving of pasta (1 ounce) would fill an ice-cream scoop.

- A serving of butter or oil (1 tablespoon) would just cover the tip of your thumb.

In other words, you may find that your requirements aren't quite as filling as you thought—or that you're filling them far faster than you might expect. Not sure how much is in a serving of a particular food you're eating? Check the food label on the package—you'll find all your serving-size questions answered right there.

Pass the Peanuts

A peanut butter and jelly sandwich is as American as apple pie—probably more so. And the good news for those who crave this lunch-box staple: Researchers have found that eating peanuts while pregnant not only doesn't trigger peanut and other allergies in babies-to-be, but may actually prevent them. So as long as you're not personally allergic to peanuts, there's no need to pass on the peanut butter—and maybe more reason than ever to reach for it. Same goes for nuts and nut butters of all kinds. If you're not allergic, you're good to go nuts when you're expecting.

If you have a history of allergies, ask your practitioner whether you should restrict your pregnancy diet in any way. The recommendations may be slightly different for you.

2 ounces soy pasta

¾ cup green garden peas

1½ ounces peanuts or peanut butter

¼ cup miso

4 ounces tofu

3 ounces tempeh

1½ cups soy milk

¾ cup vegetarian "ground beef"

1–2 vegetarian "hot dogs" or "burgers"

Grains
(*half protein servings*)

3 ounces (before cooking) whole-wheat pasta or high-protein pasta

The Scoop on Protein Supplements

H oping to scoop up your protein requirement in a supplement? Supplement makers may have crowded the field, but nature—the first producer of protein—is still the best provider of this baby-building nutrient, and there are a few reasons why. First, supplements often contain a whopping amount of protein in a concentrated form, easily giving you too much of a good thing. Second, supplements usually come packaged with more than just protein. They may also contain ingredients (such as sugar substitutes, herbs, and enzymes) that may not be pregnancy-appropriate, or be fortified with megadoses of vitamins and minerals that can push your intake beyond what's considered pregnancy-safe. That can apply to all types of protein supplements (whey, pea, chickpea, and so on) and all forms (bars, powders, and shake mixes). Another point to consider when thinking about turning specifically to whey protein bars, powders, and shake mixes: Whey protein is made from cow's milk, which means it's not the way to go if you're lactose intolerant (who needs more gas?) or have a milk allergy.

It's probably best to get most of your protein the way nature intended: in foods that come by their protein naturally, instead of through fortification. Want to shake up your protein intake? Skip the mix and blend a shake with protein-rich Greek yogurt.

Not Feeling the Milk?

If milk leaves a sour taste in your mouth, no need to drink it straight up—or even at all. You can cash in on calcium by eating cheese or yogurt or sipping calcium-fortified juice or other nondairy beverages. Or by blending milk into soups, sauces, or smoothies. Or subbing milk for the water in your morning oatmeal (you'll never know it's there, but your bones will). It's not your mouth that milk leaves sour, but your tummy? You, too, have options. If you're lactose intolerant or think you might be, simply sub lactose-free dairy (and see page 148). Not the lactose that's doing your tummy in, but the protein in cow's milk? Reach for A2 milk, which comes from cows that naturally produce only the A2 protein and not the A1 that causes sensitivity in some people (see page 149 for more).

¾ cup oat bran

1 cup (uncooked) oats or oatmeal

Approximately 2 cups whole-grain ready-to-eat cereal

½ cup (uncooked) whole-wheat couscous, bulgur, buckwheat, farro, amaranth, freekeh, quinoa

4 slices whole-grain bread

Approximately 2–3 whole-grain pitas

Approximately 2 whole-grain English muffins

Nuts and seeds
(*half protein servings*)

3 ounces nuts, such as walnuts, pecans, and almonds

About 3–5 tablespoons nut butter

2 ounces sunflower, sesame, or pumpkin seeds

Calcium: 4 servings daily. Make no bones about it—calcium intake is crucial during pregnancy, not only for your baby's bones (approximately 200 mg of calcium per day is deposited into your baby's skeleton during the last trimester of pregnancy), but also for yours. Women begin to lose bone mass in their 30s, and they'll lose it faster if calcium is drained from their own bones to help build baby's. Getting the right amount of calcium daily (especially during pregnancy) will keep your bones healthy and help prevent osteoporosis later in life. Getting enough calcium is also believed to lower the risk of developing preeclampsia. So it's clear that calcium does a mom-to-be's body (and her baby's) good.

Milk is the most well-known source of calcium, and a very efficient one, too. So if you "got milk," and you love drinking it, great—you'll have no problem meeting your calcium requirement. If

CHEW ON THIS. In ancient Rome, pregnant women were advised that if they wanted their baby to be born with dark eyes, they should eat mice often. While a mouse might be an interesting protein choice (if you're a pregnant snake, that is), this is clearly a case where you wouldn't want to do as the Romans did—even if you did happen to be in Rome.

Milking the Nondairy Alternatives

Cruising the dairy case, but you'd prefer to sport an alternative-milk mustache? Whether your reason for staying away from traditional sources of milk (cows, goats) are philosophical (you're vegan, or concerned about dairy farming's impact on the planet) or physical (you're allergic to dairy or are lactose intolerant), you're in luck. The number of nondairy "milks" on store shelves (and at coffee bars) is booming—which means there's no need to have your cereal dry or your coffee black . . . or to chase your cookies down with orange juice. But how do these milk alternatives stack up against the real thing? Results vary depending on variety, but also on brand. None mimic milk in flavor (some would argue that's a plus), or in naturally occurring nutrition (especially when it comes to protein and calcium), or even in texture (most aren't as creamy), but some perform better than others. Here's a quick introduction to some of the options:

Soy milk. Of all the milk alternatives, soy milk is considered the most similar to cow's milk. Its taste is subtle and beanlike, its texture is creamy, and it contains comparable amounts of protein and calcium (though it comes by its calcium through fortification). It is also fortified, as cow's milk is, with vitamin D and vitamin A. Though the evidence is limited, some experts recommend restricting the amount of unfermented soy products (such as soy milk) during pregnancy because they contain isoflavones—chemicals that mimic the hormone estrogen in the body.

Almond milk. With a slightly sweet and subtle nutty taste, almond milk gets top ratings because of its versatility. It's also often fortified with calcium, vitamin A, vitamin D, and vitamin E (check the label for specifics), raising its nutritional profile, but it is far lower in protein than cow's milk or soy milk. Choose those that are fortified with calcium and vitamin D.

Coconut milk. Also labeled as "coconut milk beverage," this milk alternative (it's different from the coconut milk that comes in cans, which is high in fat and calories and is used to replace cream, not milk) has a sweet coconut flavor that's almost tropical. Some brands are fortified with calcium (though less than other milk alternatives), vitamin D, vitamin B_{12}, and other vitamins. Something you won't find in coconut milk beverage: protein.

Rice milk. Low in fat and protein but high in calories, rice milk has a texture similar to skim milk with a barely-there rice flavor. Rice milk is the safest option

your tummy can tolerate milk, but you can't stand its taste, also no problem—it's easily disguised. It can be downed in delicious milkshakes, smoothies, soups, skim milk decaf lattes, or low-fat chocolate milk. It can be eaten in hot or cold cereal, too. No tolerance for lactose? No problem. Milk and dairy products of all varieties (including cheese, cottage cheese, yogurt, sour cream, ice cream, and cream cheese) come in lactose-free form.

Just not that into milk? Calcium is supplied by many other dairy sources, from yogurt to cheese. For vegans (or others who prefer not to take their calcium in dairy form), there's no shortage of nondairy sources.

for those with allergies or intolerances to dairy, soy, or nuts. But because rice contains low levels of arsenic, it's best to limit the amount of rice milk you consume in general, and especially when you're expecting.

Cashew milk. Like almond milk, this nut-based milk alternative is sweet with a faint nutty flavor. Though cashew milk contains about one-third of the calories of cow's milk and half the fat, it's actually creamier than cow's milk, making it a great alternative in "cream" sauces. Look for ones that are fortified with calcium and vitamin D.

Pea milk. Derived from yellow pea protein, creamy-textured pea milk has a similar amount of protein and twice as much calcium as cow's milk. And because many brands boost their pea milk with sunflower oil or algal oil, it also contains omega-3 fatty acids. Another fortification bonus in some brands: vitamin B_{12}. Pea milk is allergy-friendly, too, since it's not made from nuts or soy.

Hemp milk. High in omega-3 and omega-6 fatty acids, hemp milk is thin with a hint of grassy flavor. Most brands have thickeners in them and a funky taste. Hemp milk contains a similar amount of fat to cow's milk, but around half the calories and protein. See the box on page 76 for caveats about hemp when you're pregnant.

Flax milk. Like hemp milk, flax milk is a seed-based nondairy milk. It has a creamy texture and is a good source of omega-3 fatty acids. Unfortunately, flax milk may not be the best choice for a mom-to-be (see the box on page 75 for reasons why).

And if that's not enough alt-milk options for you, not to worry. Scan the store shelves these days and you'll find a host of others, from quinoa and oat milk to peanut milk, hazelnut milk, macadamia milk, and even banana milk. Not all provide the same amount of nutrients (like the all-important baby-building calcium and vitamin D), so be sure to check labels before you toss them into your shopping cart.

A few other potential pitfalls in the alt-milk department: First, while cow's milk comes by its sweetness naturally in the form of lactose, many milk alternatives can be loaded with added sugars, so consider opting for the unsweetened kinds. Second, some alt-milks contain thickeners (like carrageenan) and other additives (like gellan gum), so scan labels before choosing brands that add those unneeded extras. You'll also want to choose milk alternatives that are as close as possible nutritionally to calcium-rich cow's milk, looking for those that contain important mom-to-be nutrients. Be sure to shake before using, because the added nutrients sink to the bottom.

Too much caffeine, salt, or soda (or more accurately, the phosphorus soda contains) can interfere with calcium absorption, a good reason to order your latte half-caf. Alcohol, diuretic pills, and laxatives can do the same, but those aren't recommended during pregnancy anyway. Since a lot of dietary fiber can take calcium down the chute before

it can be absorbed, try not to take the bulk of your fiber with the bulk of your calcium. (For instance, if you're counting on that calcium in your milk, you might not want to dunk bran muffins in it.)

Choose 4 servings daily from the following list of calcium-rich foods. And don't forget that many of the dairy

Divide, Combine, and Conquer

Can't drain the whole glass of milk? Had your fill halfway through your cup of yogurt? Just because they don't add up to a full serving doesn't mean they can't be added to your daily total. When a full serving is just too much, combine ½ (or ⅓, or ¼) servings together instead. For instance, that 1 egg (¼ protein serving), plus 1 slice of whole-grain toast (¼ protein serving), plus ½ cup of soy milk (½ protein serving) equals a full protein serving—and you don't even have to eat them all in the same sitting (just in the same day). Divide, combine, and conquer—and you'll have to do a lot less eating to finish up your Daily Dozen.

sources (and the seafood ones) also provide protein and that some of the non-dairy provide vitamin C and vitamin A:

1 cup cow's or goat's milk or buttermilk

1 cup yogurt

1 cup Greek or Icelandic yogurt

⅔ cup kefir

1 ounce hard cheese (check out the freeze-dried varieties, too)

1 cup calcium-fortified beverages (juice, soy, nut, and other plant-based milk; check labels for varieties that have 30 percent or more of the DV for calcium)

1½ cups cottage cheese

3 ounces canned sardines with bones

4 ounces canned salmon with bones

½ cup ricotta cheese

Tofu (check the label, some tofu is higher in calcium)

Other calcium sources

Sesame seeds

Greens, such as kale or collard

Bok choy

Spinach

Edamame

Beans

Almonds or almond butter

Dried figs

Broccoli

Vitamin C: 3 servings daily. Because the body doesn't store vitamin C, you and baby will need a fresh supply every day. Easy enough, since vitamin C comes naturally in a wide variety of tasty packages. Effective ones, as well, since many vitamin C–listers play on the vitamin A team, too.

Shake It Up, Baby

Much of the calcium in calcium-fortified beverages (juice, soy milk, almond milk, and calcium-added milk) tends to settle at the bottom of a container—good if you're getting the last sip, not so good if you're getting the first. To make sure the calcium is evenly distributed from first sip to last, shake these beverages thoroughly before each use.

Can't stop at 3 servings of C? Help yourself to extra servings. Choose from the following (listed in order from highest to lowest vitamin C content):

Guava

Red, yellow, green, or orange bell pepper

Kiwi

Orange

Papaya

Broccoli

Kohlrabi

Parsley

Pineapple

Grapefruit

Brussels sprouts

Broccoli slaw

Daikon (Chinese radish)

Mango

Snap peas

Green garden peas

Strawberries

Cantaloupe

Tangerine

Coleslaw mix

Green or red cabbage

Cauliflower

Bok choy

Greens, such as kale, collard, mustard, or turnip greens

Rutabaga

Honeydew

Blackberries or raspberries

Plantain

Count 'Em Once, Count 'Em Twice

Sometimes, you'll even be able to count them thrice. Many of your favorite foods may fill more than 1 Daily Dozen requirement in each serving. Case in delicious point: A slice of cantaloupe fills a Vitamin A plus a C. Same goes for a tangerine. Broccoli covers A and C with a calcium bonus. Greek yogurt delivers calcium and protein. So don't forget to give yourself credit where credit is due. Count them once, count them twice.

Tomato

Sweet potato, baked in skin

Okra

Vitamin A: 3 to 4 servings daily. These A-plus powerhouses are the superstars of the produce section—serving up whopping quantities of vitamin A. It comes in the form of phytochemicals called carotenoids, including alpha-carotene, beta-carotene, lutein, zeaxanthin, and

CHEW ON THIS. Here are a couple of old wives' tales that may well have been generated by old vegetarians: Chinese folklore maintains that a woman should avoid eating both rabbit and chicken during her pregnancy—or else her baby will be born with a hoarse voice. Eating squid and crab are also discouraged, according to Chinese tradition. Squid, so the tale goes, is believed to cause the uterus to "stick" during delivery, and eating crab will result in a mischievous child.

If You're a Vegetarian or a Vegan

Got a beef with beef (or chicken, fish, eggs, or dairy)? No worries. Vegetarians of just about all varieties, including vegans, can have pregnancies and babies that are at least as healthy as those of carnivores . . . or even healthier. So no need to swap out your all-veggie burger for an all-beef patty, or even to add cheese to it. But because diets without animal products tend to be low in fat and high in fiber, you may find it hard to pile on enough pounds. If so, up the weight shortfall by adding more fat servings to your diet, eating smaller amounts more often, and choosing foods that are particularly dense in both calories and nutrition (think avocados, nuts and nut butters, seeds, beans, peas, and dried fruit).

Vegetarian moms easily score more of some nutrients (most B vitamins, folate, vitamins A and C, and more) from their grain and veggie-rich diet than pregnant meat eaters typically do. But without a little extra effort, it's also possible to fall short on a few important baby-building blocks, including:

- Protein. Vegetarians who include eggs and milk products in their diet usually have little trouble getting enough protein, but vegans may find it a stretch. If you're a vegan, net your protein share by eating protein-rich grains, beans, peas, and lentils (and pastas made from them), and tofu and other soy products.

- Vitamin B_{12}. Since vitamin B_{12} is found only in foods that come from animals, vegans will have to look elsewhere for their B_{12}. A supplement can pick up the slack (ask your practitioner if you need more than what's provided in your prenatal vitamin), but you can also get an extra shot of this vital vitamin from fortified soy and other plant milks, fortified cereals, nutritional yeast, and fortified meat substitutes.

beta-cryptoxanthin—all important in the making of a baby. To get the best mix of these phytochemicals, add a good mix of yellow and green vegetables into your diet each day.

And there are more good reasons to make green and deep yellow your Team Baby colors. The greens and deep yellows are also excellent suppliers of vitamin E, riboflavin, B_6, folate, magnesium, and a host of other essential minerals—plus a bonus of fiber.

Maybe you've never been the type to volunteer for vegetables or choose a side salad over fries. Or maybe green describes how you've been feeling these days, not so much what you feel like eating. No need for kale coercion or to cozy up to collards (that is, unless you're up for the challenge). Instead, turn to soothing shades of yellow and orange: carrots, sweet potatoes, butternut squash, pumpkin. Or get sneaky with yourself, cleverly concealing finely minced veggies in your spaghetti sauce, meat loaf, lasagna, casseroles, and soups. Or skip the vegetables altogether for now, and get fruity. Cantaloupe and mango can be sweet revenge if you're feeling bitter about broccoli, filling requirements for vitamin A and vitamin C as well as any green can. Or sip a vegetable or veggie-fruit juice or smoothie.

Try to have at least 3 to 4 servings from the following fruits and veggies every day, ideally including at least 1

- Iron. It's not easy for anyone (except big red-meat eaters) to get enough iron from their diets, especially during pregnancy, when iron's in high demand. For those who stick to plant foods, it's next to impossible. If you're a vegetarian—and especially if you're a vegan—you'll need to be extra diligent about taking your practitioner-recommended iron supplement. If you haven't been prescribed one, ask.

- Calcium. For vegetarians who eat dairy products, cashing in on calcium is easy (just say cheese! Milk! Yogurt!). For vegans, getting enough calcium may be a taller order, but it's definitely not out of reach. Though dairy products are the most well-known sources of calcium, they're not the only ones. Calcium-fortified almond, other nut, and plant milks and calcium-fortified juices, for instance, offer as much calcium as milk, ounce for ounce—making any a perfect, perfectly vegan source of this essential mineral. Other non-dairy sources of calcium include dark green leafy vegetables, sesame seeds, almonds, and calcium-fortified soy products. Still, adding a calcium supplement is probably good insurance for pregnant vegans. Ask your practitioner for a recommendation, preferably one that adds vitamin D (see below) and magnesium to the mix.

- Vitamin D. Since the best dietary source of vitamin D is milk, non-milk drinkers will have to depend on their supplements (or fortified milk alternatives, cheese, or juice) to provide them with all they need of this very valuable vitamin. Also look for breads and cereals that are fortified with it. Your best bet: Ask your practitioner about testing your vitamin D levels and prescribing a supplement if needed.

green and 1 yellow. Mix up your prep, too, if you can—eating some raw, some cooked. Keep in mind that in the case of many, you'll also be filling your vitamin C in the same serving:

Carrot

Sweet potato or yam

Pumpkin

Green leafy lettuce, such as romaine, arugula, red or green leaf, or field greens

Cantaloupe

Spinach

Parsley

Red bell pepper

Greens, such as Swiss chard, kale, or collards

Apricot

Pink or ruby red grapefruit

CHEW ON THIS. Here's an ancient custom that has modern applications, particularly for pregnant women: It was customary for the Romans to precede their banquets with refreshing salads, which they believed enhanced the appetite. Here's one that may not: In Elizabethan times, dried lettuce juice was used to aid sleep.

An Apple
(and Two Carrots and a Cup of Broccoli) a Day

For salad bar buffs and fruit fanatics, filling the various produce requirements of pregnancy may be a job they can't wait to sink their teeth into. But for those who've struggled to manage even an apple a day, packing in all that produce may seem daunting. It can also be a challenge for the easily bored (with steamed broccoli, tossed salad, that piece of fresh fruit). Here are some tips for fitting more fruits and vegetables into anyone's day:

- Top pancakes or waffles with sliced berries instead of syrup.

- Add mashed banana or blueberries to pancake batter.

- Whip up some fruit smoothies and drinks (see the recipes starting on page 342).

- Add peaches, bananas, strawberries, or blueberries to your cereal. Or pop freeze-dried fruit right out of the bag and into your mouth.

- Add mushrooms, peppers, broccoli, or tomato to your omelet (see page 193).

- Make friends with cauliflower rice—sautéed, it makes a super side or a delicious bed for just about any entree. Baked, it works well as pizza crust.

- Stuff a baked sweet potato with broccoli or mushrooms and cheese.

- Grab a bag of sweet potato, zucchini, or butternut squash "noodles" or make your own with a spiralizer—then sauté and sauce as you'd prepare pasta.

- Toss kale leaves with olive oil, salt, and pepper, and then roast until crispy. Bingo—it's kale chips! Or, just open a bag of kale chips.

- Bake carrot muffins (see page 206).

- Add chopped dried apricots into anything you're baking.

- Grill vegetables on skewers. Fruit, too.

- Add carrots, tomatoes, peppers, mangoes, or strawberries to your salad.

- Make pesto out of parsley and toss with whole-wheat, brown rice, or another type of whole-grain pasta.

- Add lettuce and tomatoes to your sandwiches.

Bok choy	Prune
Persimmon	Tangerine
Mango	Red cabbage
Vegetable juice	Okra
Tomato	Green beans
Winter squash	Broccoli
Papaya	Plum

- Layer spinach, avocado, and portobello mushroom into your grilled cheese.

- Toss cauliflower, broccoli, squash, mushrooms, or really any vegetable into your lasagna. Want to go extra veggie? Use sliced eggplant instead of pasta sheets.

- Stir grated carrot into your meat loaf mix.

- Create a burrito bowl out of kale, avocado salsa verde, seasoned black beans, cherry tomatoes, and brown rice.

- Add fresh vegetables to low-sodium canned soups.

- Add pumpkin puree, diced red bell peppers, minced carrot, parsley, or kale to your tomato sauce—sauté first and you'll never notice them.

- Toss wedges of sweet potatoes with olive oil, salt, and pepper, and roast for sweet potato fries.

- Top chicken or seafood with a mango salsa (see page 296).

- Add peas, red peppers, asparagus, squash, or other colorful vegetables (roasted or raw) to quinoa, farro, or brown rice.

- Put nutrition—and dinner—on the fast track by stirring up a veggie-filled stir-fry.

- Add dried fruit to stuffing.

- Pop some brussels sprouts into an air fryer with a spritz of olive oil and some salt. Add to the top of your salad for crunch, or eat as a snack.

- Blend a bowl of gazpacho (see page 226) or carrot soup (see page 224).

- Sauté mirepoix (diced carrots, onions, and celery), add any kind of roasted vegetables (butternut squash, broccoli, mushrooms, cauliflower), cover with broth, and simmer until soft. Blend until smooth for a delicious soup.

- Dip baby carrots, broccoli, cauliflower, green beans, or peppers in salsa, hummus, or guacamole.

- Stuff walnuts, raisins, and cinnamon into an apple and bake or microwave for a sweet snack or dessert.

- Toss pomegranate seeds into a salad of kale, shaved brussels sprouts, and red cabbage.

- Have a virgin Bloody Mary (tomato or vegetable juice and spices, minus the vodka) as a predinner mocktail.

Nectarine

Yellow peach

Celery

Other fruits and vegetables: 1 to 2 servings daily. So they're not the A-list, or the C-list—but they dabble well in a variety of well-known nutrients, with some excelling in emerging categories, too.

From that apple a day (full of fiber) to blueberries (abundant in antioxidants) and bananas (packed with potassium), you'll get more than you'd expect from these other fruits and vegetables.

Aim for 1 to 2 servings of the following delicious choices every day:

Apple

Applesauce

The Truth About Grain

Yes, you know that whole grains are a healthier choice than refined grains. But do you know why? Understanding how white bread gets its color (or lack of it) may help you see why whole grains take the cake nutritionally. All grains start out whole (that's the way nature grows them). It's during their processing into refined bread, rolls, cereals, pasta, and white rice that the nutritious parts of the grains are removed (including the vitamin-and-mineral-packed germ and the fiber-packed bran). Just how much difference does a whole grain make? Compare whole-wheat flour to white flour: Whole-wheat flour contains 4 times more fiber, 2 times more copper, 6 times more magnesium, 3 times more potassium, 2 times more selenium, 4 times more zinc, and 20 times more vitamin E than white flour. That's a pretty convincing profile.

Though enrichment of refined grain (as required by law) tosses back in a handful of the vitamins and minerals found naturally in whole grains, it leaves out about 20 other nutrients (likely even more, including ones that haven't yet been discovered—that's how good nature is). Also missing: that naturally occurring fiber. In other words, nature's recipe for grainy goodness will probably never be duplicated.

Is white always wrong and brown always right? Not necessarily. Color doesn't always tell the whole story when it comes to whole grains. A brown bread can get its wholesome-looking hue from coloring, not just from whole-grain flour. Names may deceive you, too: The label "wheat" on a loaf of bread tells you only the type of grain it's baked with, not whether it's a whole grain. To make sure you're getting the whole wheat and nothing but the whole wheat, read the label and the ingredients carefully (see page 58 for more).

Apple juice

Banana

Blueberries

Cherries

Cranberries

CHEW ON THIS. Here's another old wives' tale to help you figure out if you're carrying a boy or a girl: Eat a clove of raw garlic. If the smell of garlic seeps out of your pores, it's a boy. If no garlic smell is detected at all, it's a girl. There's a 50 percent chance this method will work, of course, but probably a much higher chance that it will leave you with heartburn.

Figs

White peach

Pear

Pomegranate juice

Pomegranate seeds

Rhubarb

Dates

Grapes or raisins

Avocado

Water chestnuts

Beets

Sweet corn

Cucumber

Eggplant

Iceberg lettuce

Mushrooms

Onion

Parsnip

Turnip

Zucchini

Radishes

Radicchio

Whole grains and legumes: 6 or more servings daily. These days, it isn't easy being grains. Once valued as the staff of life—the most important link on the human food chain, a dietary staple around the world and throughout history, and yes, the breakfast of champions—bread, cereal, rice, and pasta have been shelved by a generation of carbo-phobes. Unfair to carbs, unnecessary for those who love them (and really, who doesn't?). The truth is, while refined grains don't stack up, whole grains of all kinds (and in all forms), as well as legumes, should be a healthy mainstay of just about every diet, especially every pregnancy diet. These complex carbohydrates contain a wealth of vitamins, particularly vitamin E and the B vitamins so essential for every part of your baby's developing body. They're rich in trace minerals, such as zinc, selenium, chromium, and magnesium. Full of constipation-fighting fiber. And for many queasy moms-to-be, their starchy, bland goodness is just the ticket to comfort. For some, maybe the only ticket.

Go for the whole-grain varieties of these whenever you can (see the box on the previous page for all the reasons why; see the box on page 48 for a list of great grains to choose from). Choose from the following (serving sizes vary, so check labels):

½ cup cooked brown, other whole-grain, or wild rice

½ cup cooked quinoa, farro, barley, bulgur, buckwheat groats (kasha), whole-grain couscous, spelt, wheatberries, or other cooked whole grains (see box, page 48)

½ cup cooked whole-grain or legume pasta

½ cup cooked oatmeal or other whole-grain hot cereal*

1 cup whole-grain, ready-to-eat cereal*

¼ cup granola*

1 slice whole-wheat or other whole-grain bread

Whole-grain corn or flour tortilla (1 small or ½ large)*

Whole-grain wrap*

Whole-grain pita (1 small or ½ large)*

½ whole-grain English muffin or bagel

Whole-grain crackers or crispbreads*

Whole-grain corn or bean chips

Brown-rice cakes or crackers^

2 cups popcorn

¼ cup oats

¼ cup whole-grain cornmeal, grits, or polenta (non-degerminated)

¼ whole-grain flour

2 tablespoons ground flaxseed or chia seed

½ cup cooked beans, lentils, or split peas

½ cup cooked edamame (soybeans)

Toasted chickpeas, soybeans, lentils, or other beans and legumes*

Great Grains

Looking for a change of whole-grain pace? Here are a few to look for, either on their own or in combos with other grains in baked goods or cereals or in ready-to-cook form. They're all loaded with vitamins and minerals:

Amaranth has a nutty flavor and sticky texture and is rich in protein, iron, calcium, B vitamins, and fiber. It's a nutritious gluten-free substitute.

Barley is a delicious stand-in for rice in salads and side dishes. Opt for hulled barley (it's whole grain) over pearled (refined)—just plan for extra cooking time. Whole-grain barley flour can also sub for all-purpose flour in most recipes.

Buckwheat isn't actually a grain—it's a seed that cooks and eats like a nutty grain. It also doesn't have any relation to wheat, so it's gluten-free. Use buckwheat groats (also called kasha) as a cooked cereal or side dish (see Three-in-One Pilaf, page 341). You can also use buckwheat flour in a variety of baked goods.

Bulgur is a whole grain made from dried, cracked wheat. It's best known for its starring role in Mediterranean dishes such as tabbouleh, but can also substitute for rice or couscous in pilafs, stews, casseroles, soups, and stuffings—or for oats as a whole grain cereal. Bonus: It cooks up quickly.

Corn is the only cereal grain native to the Americas. Unfortunately, most corn-based products sold in the U.S. today are stripped of their whole grain goodness (aka degerminated). Look for baked goods that contain non-degerminated or whole grain corn, or for whole-grain cornmeal when you're baking up cornbread, stirring up polenta or grits, or breading chicken or fish.

Farro has been a crowd-pleasing grain at Italian tables for centuries—now available at a market near you. Its chewy texture stands up to soups, stews, and salads, as a bed for just about any meat, fish, or poultry, in a starring role in a pilaf, or as a satisfying hot cereal.

Kamut is a high-protein Ancient grain that was once a Pharaoh fan favorite—one taste and you'll likely be a fan, too. Its toothsome chew and nutty, slightly sweet taste holds its own in salads, stuffing, and side dishes of all kinds (sub it for the bulgur in tabbouleh). Or cook it up for breakfast.

Millet is another whole-grain that's actually a seed. It's crunchy and mild-tasting, plus it's gluten-free. Look for

---

Iron-rich foods: some daily. Your body will be working overtime to generate enough red blood cells to keep up with the demands of baby making while trying to keep you from developing iron-deficiency anemia. Pumping up your blood supply will require pumping up your iron intake. Since it's hard to fill the pregnancy requirement for this must-have mineral through diet alone, your practitioner will likely recommend that you take a daily supplement of iron (in addition to what's in your regular prenatal) beginning at week 20 and continuing through the rest of pregnancy. To maximize iron absorption, take your supplement with a vitamin C food or drink to enhance iron absorption. On the flip side, chasing down your iron supplement with milk or

it in cereals and baked goods. While millet can be served like rice or quinoa in salads, pilaf, or as a stuffing (try it in Red Pepper Stuffed with Millet Pilaf), and side dishes, it's not the easiest grain to DIY—so check out the package directions before committing.

Oats are, of course, well-known for their breakfast potential (in hot and cold cereal), though perhaps best loved for their cookies. They're naturally high in fiber, and may help regulate both blood sugar and blood pressure, giving the humble bowl of oatmeal some impressive health credentials. Look for rolled or old-fashioned oats (pass by the instant when you can), or whole-grain oat flour. Have time on your hands? Cook up an extra batch of slow-cooked oats—Irish or Scottish are especially chewy and satisfying. Oats are considered gluten-free but with caveats for some with celiac disease (see page 150).

Quinoa (KEEN-wah), has a unique fluffy texture and a delicate taste, but it's a heavyweight when it comes to nutrients, especially protein. It's also a quick cook and can be used in pilaf, salads, soups, or in any recipe that calls for rice or another grain. It plays well with other grains, too (check out Three in One Pilaf, page 341).

Rice clearly needs no introduction, but its many whole-grain forms may.

Since white rice has been stripped of fiber and nutrients, explore rice varieties that haven't been milled—you'll be surprised at how many options you'll discover beyond the basic brown, including brown basmati, red rice, purple rice, black rice, and wild rice (this chewy grain isn't actually a rice at all, but a grass). Use whole grain rice of all varieties just as you would use white rice—just plan to add a little extra simmer time.

Spelt is an ancient grain that's undergone a culinary renaissance. Its nutty taste and chewy texture makes it an intriguing alternative to more common varieties of wheat—plus it's higher in protein. Use hulled spelt as a cooked grain, rolled spelt as a cereal, and spelt flour for pancakes, waffles, or just about anything you're baking.

Wheat berries have a crunchy chew and a nutty, slightly sweet taste, but they adapt deliciously to both sweet and savory recipes. High in protein and fiber, they can be added to hot cereal, pilafs, soups, stuffing, stews, breads, muffins, and other baked goods. They're yummy in salads, too. Fun fact about wheat berries: wheat flour comes from wheat berries that are milled and ground. Because wheat berries are hard, they take some time to cook, but soaking speeds that process.

---

other calcium-rich foods (or with antacids that contain calcium, like Tums) may block iron absorption. Ditto high-fiber foods.

While iron comes from both the animal and plant kingdoms, it's much more absorbable when it comes from an animal source (that steak) than when it comes from a plant source (those beans). Good news if you're a meat eater, not

such good news if you're a vegetarian or are meat-averse at the moment.

These foods are naturally high in iron:

Beef

Poultry

Cooked clams, oysters, mussels, and shrimp

Salt Sense

Classic cravings have you reaching for the pickle jar—and then emptying it, down to the last sip of zesty juice? Your body may actually be doing you a solid with those salty cravings: propelling you to drink more liquids. An adequate sodium intake is required to accommodate pregnancy's higher fluid volume, and overly restricting salt intake can disrupt that delicate fluid balance. What's more, contrary to popular belief, it's not the sodium that makes you puffy during pregnancy—it's the hormones. A certain amount of swelling is your body's way of ensuring it has enough fluids on board for baby making, and that's healthy and normal (if not so swell from a comfort perspective).

So go ahead and get busy with those pickles. Give yourself a fair shake from the saltshaker (doing it to taste, instead of routinely, will naturally moderate what you shake). Just remember that many of the fast and processed foods that give sodium a bad name actually earn their less-than-wholesome reputation for other reasons (they're full of fat, sugar, and questionable chemicals, they're low in nutrients and fiber). Those are definitely worth limiting or skipping. Also remember that, especially as you close in on the end of pregnancy, too much salt can lead to too much swelling—and a lot more discomfort than you'll probably care to experience. There's no need to hold the pickles or the pickle juice—just moderate where you can, and don't sweat the rest.

To meet the increased need for iodine in pregnancy (see the box on page 21), use iodized salt in cooking and at the table (unless your practitioner recommends otherwise in your case— for instance, because you're hyperthyroid). The label will tell you whether a salt you're selecting has iodine added— unfortunately, many popular salts (including most sea salts and kosher salt) don't. That's a concern, since about a third of moms-to-be are deficient in iodine, a nutrient needed for healthy baby brain development. Some prenatal vitamins also contain iodine.

Sardines

Cooked dried beans

Soybeans (edamame) and soy products

Barley, bulgur, quinoa

Pumpkin seeds

Jerusalem artichokes

Spinach, kale, and collard and turnip greens

Seaweed

Dried fruit

Fat and high-fat foods: about 4 servings daily (more if you're having trouble gaining weight, less if you're gaining too fast). Here's a fact about fat: Most people get more fat than they need without even trying—and many get more than they need even when they're trying (really, really hard) not to. After all, when stacked against other nutritional requirements, fat comes in relatively small packages (when it comes to oil or butter, for instance, just a tablespoon per serving).

But here's another fact about fat: Your body needs it, especially when you're pregnant. Essential fatty acids are—wait for it—essential for a baby's growth and development. Especially important in the last month of pregnancy and first few months of breastfeeding are omega-3 fatty acids, since this form of fat is needed for optimal brain development (see below).

The foods listed below are composed completely (or mostly) of fat. Though they won't be the only source of fat in your diet (you'll get extra fat from dairy products, nuts, avocado, meat, poultry, and more), they're the only ones you'll need to keep track of. Keeping track will be easier if you keep an eye out for the many places fat ends up (the mayo on your chicken salad sandwich, the oil in your salad dressing, the butter on your roll).

If you're gaining weight too quickly, you can cut back by 1 or 2 fat servings. You might also want to consider cutting way back on foods that are prepared with a lot of fat (anything fried or swimming in a pool of butter). If you're gaining weight too slowly, you may want to add a fat serving—as well as some extra high-fat foods (preferably nutritious ones, like nuts and avocados). One serving equals about a tablespoon of the following:

Oil, such as vegetable, olive, canola, avocado, walnut, and sesame

Butter

Mayonnaise

Regular salad dressing

Peanut, almond, or other nut butter

Omega-3 fatty acids: some daily. Here's a fat you can really feel good about eating, particularly while you're eating for two: omega-3 polyunsaturated fatty acids (such as DHA). Touted for a variety of general health benefits,

Fatten Up Your Salad

Fat-phobics, it's time to confront your fears. And to start drizzling fats on your salads and steamed vegetables. Turns out that a little fat actually brings out the best in broccoli (or romaine, or carrots). Though it's tempting to save yourself a few calories by pouring on the fat-free dressings or opting for a virtuous squeeze of lemon, research has shown that sparing the fat spoils the nutrients. Scientists have found that many of the vital dietary properties in vegetables (like alpha-carotene, beta-carotene, or lycopene) aren't well absorbed without a side of fat. So add some real dressing to your salad, dip for your carrots, oil to your stir-fry—or just a handful of nuts or a few slices of avocado to any veggie dish. Just remember as you drizzle and douse, sauté and stir-fry, that a little fat goes a long way—say, a tablespoon of dressing on your lettuce, not ¼ cup.

DHA is a major component of the brain and retina and is needed for proper brain growth and eye development in fetuses and young babies. Getting enough of this vital baby brain fuel in your diet is especially important during the last trimester (when your baby's brain grows at a phenomenal pace) and during breastfeeding (the DHA content of a baby's brain triples during the first 3 months of life).

Other potential perks? Getting enough DHA during pregnancy may reduce the chances of baby being born too early or being born at a low birthweight. And what's good for the expected is also good for the expecting.

Didn't Make the List?

Can't find your favorite fruit, grain, or protein source on these food lists? Just because a food isn't listed doesn't mean it isn't worth a place in your diet. For reasons of space (and so you don't have to spend 9 months flipping through pages to find the food you're looking for), only more common foods and beverages are listed in this chapter. If your inquiring mind wants to know more, you can check out the USDA's National Nutrient Database website at fdc.nal.usda.gov.

Luckily, DHA is found in plenty of foods you probably already eat—and like to eat:

Salmon and other higher-fat fish, such as sardines

Canned light tuna

Walnuts and walnut oil

Brazil nuts

Seeds (pumpkin, sunflower, chia, and flax)

Seaweed

DHA-rich eggs (often called omega-3 eggs)

Omega-3 fortified milk alternatives and juice

Grass-fed beef, buffalo, and lamb

Crab and shrimp

Pasture-raised or omega-3 chicken

You can also ask your practitioner about pregnancy-safe mercury-free DHA supplements (many prenatal supplements contain up to 200 to 300 mg of DHA already). Not a fan of the fishy aftertaste (and the fishy burps) some DHA supplements leave behind? There are vegetarian and vegan alternatives that are fish-free.

Fluids: at least 10 8-ounce glasses daily. Water—essential for almost every function in your body—is especially essential during pregnancy, when there's another little body on board. That little body will need water to build cells, for its developing circulatory system, for the delivery of nutrients, and for the excretion of wastes. Your body, too, will require more fluids during pregnancy, to help combat constipation, prevent dry skin, regulate body temperature, and reduce the risk of urinary tract infection. And because water also helps your body flush out waste products, drinking enough can actually keep you from retaining too much fluid (aka swelling). All good reasons to aim for at least 10 8-ounce glasses of fluid daily. You may need more during hot weather, if you're working out a lot, or if you've been vomiting a lot. How will you know you're getting enough liquid in? When enough is coming out, in the form of pale or clear urine. Pee that's dark or scant means you need to step up your fluid intake.

When tallying your fluid intake, remember to also count fluids that don't come from the tap (or your water bottle). Milk (which is two-thirds water), juice, soups, and broths also figure in. Fruits and vegetables count, too—5 typical servings equal about 2 servings of fluid, with some (such as watermelon, cucumber, and lettuce, which are all about 95 percent water) outperforming on fluids. Count sparkling water, as well as decaffeinated coffee or tea, but don't count caffeinated beverages, since they act as diuretics, causing calcium and other key pregnancy nutrients to be

Water, Water Everywhere

Never been a big drinker—of water? Here are some tips to help you get in the water habit:

- Carry a refillable water bottle with you wherever you go. Drink while you're in the car, on social media, waiting in line at the market, riding the commuter train.

- Fill a 24-ounce container with water and keep it with you all day, on the job or at home. You'll need to fill it only one more time to get just over half of your fluids requirement. Top it off with some servings of fruit, a salad, a bowl of soup, a glass of almond milk—and you've met your goal (plus covered a few other Daily Dozen bases).

- Aim to drink 1 glass of water every 2 hours during the day.

- Use larger glasses or mugs, so you'll drink more at each sitting.

- When eating out, down a glass of water before you leave for the restaurant. And down another one at the table while you're waiting for your food.

- Blend up a breakfast smoothie to start your day juiced on fluids— you'll score extra fluids from the ice and the juicy fruit you use.

- Remember to look for water, water everywhere in the produce department, too. You'll find plenty of fluids in watermelon (obviously), other melons, lettuce, cucumbers, celery, tomatoes, strawberries, grapefruit, and oranges.

washed out of your system before they can be thoroughly absorbed.

Are frequent trips to the bathroom tempting you to cut back on fluids? Don't let them. All that pee is serving a vital (if annoying) purpose: flushing waste products from your system and your baby's.

Prenatal vitamin supplements: a pregnancy formula taken daily. Sometimes, despite your best intentions and your best efforts (you did try to eat that bowl of cereal between trips to the bathroom to throw up), your diet may be lacking in a vitamin one day, a mineral or two another day.

That's where a prenatal vitamin-mineral supplement comes in. Not to stand in for a healthy diet (a supplement can't, since it doesn't provide many of the nutrients a healthy pregnancy needs and a healthy pregnancy diet contains, from calories and fiber to phytonutrients and certain vital minerals), but to fill in the nutritional blanks when what you eat comes up short. Not so you can intentionally let your diet slide, but for those days (and early months) when it inevitably does slide, maybe because you're too busy to eat well or you're too sick to eat well. To keep you covered on nutrients that are just plain hard to get enough of from diet alone, like iron (and for vegans, calcium, vitamin D, and vitamin B_{12}). Or on ones that are so vital to baby's development that extra insurance makes extra sense, especially folic acid. Studies show that women who take prenatal vitamins before and during pregnancy dramatically lower the risks of having babies with

Take Your Iron with a Side of C

Chances are you'll get another pill prescribed by your practitioner midway through your pregnancy—an iron supplement, to be taken in addition to your regular prenatal supplement. It's to refill those stores of red blood cells needed as your blood volume increases. Try to avoid eating or drinking something high in calcium when you take your iron supplement, since calcium interferes with iron absorption. Instead, accompany your iron with food or drink high in vitamin C, which will aid in iron absorption.

spina bifida and cleft palate (probably because of the folic acid content of the supplements).

The formula you take should be especially designed for pregnancy. Ask your practitioner to prescribe one or suggest an over-the-counter one, or select one yourself that contains the vitamins and minerals in approximately the same dosages as these:

- No more than 4,000 IU (800 mcg) of vitamin A

- At least 400 to 600 mcg of folic acid, folate, or folinic acid

CHEW ON THIS. Pregnancy superstitions run the gamut from possibly plausible to downright peculiar. Definitely falling into the latter category is this one: Pregnant women centuries ago were told that if they didn't drink enough water, their babies would be born dirty. (Care for some soap with that glass of water?) While there's clearly no truth to this tale, there is some obvious wisdom behind the advice: Getting enough water is important during pregnancy, even if you're not superstitious.

- 250 mcg of calcium. If you're not getting enough calcium in your diet, you will need additional supplementation to reach the 1,000 mg needed during pregnancy. Don't take an iron supplement at the same time as or within 2 hours of a supplement containing more than 250 mg of calcium, since it interferes with iron absorption.

- 30 mg of iron

- 50 to 80 mg of vitamin C

- 15 mg of zinc

- 2 mg of copper

- 2 mg of vitamin B_6

- At least 400 IU of vitamin D

- Approximately the RDA for vitamin E (15 mg), thiamin (1.4 mg), riboflavin (1.4 mg), niacin (18 mg), and vitamin B_{12} (2.6 mcg). Most prenatal supplements contain 2 to 3 times these amounts, and those higher doses aren't considered harmful.

- 150 mcg of iodine (not all prenatals contain iodine or this amount of it)

- Some formulas may also contain magnesium, selenium, fluoride, biotin, choline, phosphorous, pantothenic acid, extra B_6 and ginger (to combat queasiness), and/or DHA.

Bar None?

They fit neatly in a handbag, glove compartment, desk drawer, even your pocket. Many are loaded with protein, fiber, vitamins, and minerals, and are filling enough to keep you going when you're on the run. But do nutrition bars set a high enough bar when it comes to pregnancy nutrition? Do they really have what it takes to serve as a healthy snack, never mind a healthy meal replacement?

Well, that depends. Some bars definitely stack up better than others. When shopping the bar aisle, scout for ones that are made with real food, like oats and other grains, nuts and seeds, eggs, and fruit. Look for little or no added sugar (some bars rival candy bars in the sugar department), and bypass bars sweetened the artificial way ("sugar alcohols" on the nutrition label will clue you in). A little fortification is fine, a lot is unnecessary (especially if you're already taking a prenatal supplement, plus eating a healthy diet). If you're perusing a protein bar, check to see where the protein comes from: Eggs? Grains, nuts, and seeds? Or some lab-synthesized protein? Remember, too, that it's possible to pack too much protein, especially if you're eating protein bars and shakes on top of an already protein-rich diet. Avoid bars or jerky made from meat, poultry, or fish since there is the possibility of bacterial contamination.

Now that you know which nutrition bars to reach for, how often should you reach for them? While snacking on one occasionally (or even daily) is fine, especially when you're on the go, using them to regularly replace real food in your diet isn't. Use them for a quick and convenient lift, but not as a meal. And add on when you can: When you grab a bar, also grab a piece of fresh fruit. And look beyond the bar, too, for other nonperishable snacks that are easy to tote, like nuts and seeds, freeze-dried fruit and vegetables, and freeze-dried cheese.

If you're a queasy mom, the best time to take a prenatal is when you're best able to keep it down—and that's typically at night, with dinner or a bedtime snack (of course, your results may vary—so go with your gut). Check out the tips on page 112 for more on taking vitamins while combating morning sickness. Even if your stomach's not particularly sensitive, it makes sense to take the supplement with a meal or snack that contains some fat—some oil, some peanut butter, some nuts or avocado— to help you absorb those fat-soluble vitamins (A, D, E, and K). And make sure you chase it with plenty of fluids to help it dissolve well. Wondering if more vitamins, minerals, and other nutrients might be more beneficial to your body, your pregnancy, and your baby? Scarf down as many as you care to in food form (double up on veggies, fruit, salad), but don't take any extras in supplement form without your practitioner's approval. Some nutrients, such as vitamins A and D, are toxic in doses higher than those found in prenatal vitamins. And since some supplements may contain herbs that aren't known to be safe in pregnancy, be sure to scan the ingredients (or run them past your practitioner) before choosing a particular brand.

Good Enough Is Good Enough

Here's some straight talk about a pregnancy diet. There are plenty of reasons why eating well is good for you and good for your baby. But eating well enough, especially when that's the best you can do right now, is also good . . . really good. Eat a mostly balanced diet most of the time, with an eye to a nice mix of fruits, vegetables, whole grains, healthy fats, and protein, and don't stress about the rest of the time. Reach for the nutritional sky, by all means, but don't give up if you reach for the brownie you were craving instead. Look at each day as a new opportunity to aim higher, not as a reason to beat yourself up over yesterday's fast-food frenzy. Blend yourself a smoothie, build yourself a salad, or cut up some cantaloupe . . . and move on.

CHAPTER 4

Selecting Well to Eat Well

W hether you're browsing groceries online, braving the superstore, shopping the corner quickie mart, or foraging at the farmers market, chances are you have options—likely, a dizzying array of options, and a whole lot of competing packages, each promising to deliver on taste and nutrition. Happily, more and more of the products vying for your attention are healthy ones—which means that filling your cart (and your belly) with the best foods for you and your baby is easier than ever. Another plus to all those options: Eating well doesn't have to be monotonous, Mom (at least once morning sickness has returned your appetite and released your taste buds from cracker captivity). Here's to choosing well to eat well.

Shopping for Two

H opefully you've got your comfy shoes on (or your comfy sweats on if you're shopping online), because it's time to fill your fridge, freezer, pantry, snack containers, handbag, gym bag, glove compartment, and office drawer or locker with all the food you'll need to eat well. But even if you're just doing the supermarket sprint on the way home from a long day on the job, it'll help to keep these shopping do's and don'ts in mind as you fill your cart.

- Do make a list. How long a list depends on how often you'll be doing your food shopping—and how many meals and snacks you're planning to create from the list. If you're extra-organized and motivated, writing down your menus for the week and generating the list from there (or letting an app generate it from recipes you choose) is ideal—it'll keep you focused, on track, and on point nutritionally. Plus, it'll help avoid those otherwise inevitable

Reading Food Labels

How does a product stand out in a sea of similar products? With a label, of course. A label will tell you just about everything you need to know about a product before you decide to drop it into your cart—that is, if you know where on the label to look. Front and center? Not so much. That's where you'll find the pretty pictures and the enticing descriptions—but not where you'll find a lot of real food facts. That's because manufacturers, for the most part, design their labels (no surprise) to sell products, not inform consumers—at least, beyond what regulations require. To do this, they highlight in big print the hype they'd like you to notice ("great taste!" "wholesome!" "made with natural ingredients!" "no cholesterol!") and bury the details they'd rather you overlook on the side or back of the package in small print. Here are some clues to keep in mind when you're playing label detective:

Ingredients list. You'll find out a lot about a product just by skimming this list—and you may often be surprised at what you find. All ingredients in a product must be listed on the package in order of predominance, with the first ingredient the most plentiful (by weight) and the last the least. So a fruit bar that lists "sugar" and "high-fructose corn syrup" before "mixed berry puree" clearly has a lot more sugar than it does fruit. A bread that boasts "made with whole-wheat" but lists "wheat flour" and "sugar" before "whole-wheat flour" on the ingredients list is more white bread than whole-wheat.

You should also scan the list for ingredients the manufacturer is not likely to brag about elsewhere on the label, such as starchy fillers and artificial preservatives, colorings, and flavorings.

Serving size. What's in a serving? The nutrition information provided on a food label is based on the serving size listed. But get that product home, and the size of the serving can vary a whole lot, depending on who's dishing it out and who's eating it. So if the label says that a serving is half a cup and it's likely you'll eat a cup and a half, remember that all the numbers will triple (including the calories). And if the serving size is for a cup and you'll be eating only half a cup, you'll have to halve the nutrient numbers promised on the label.

Nutrition information. If you're looking for nutrition facts, don't look for them on the front of the box, where manufacturers aren't compelled to share them. After all, have you ever seen a label that boasts "loaded with saturated fats" or "now with lots more sugar" or "made with zero whole grains"? Instead, turn to the back or the side for the evidence you're searching for. "Nutrition Facts" gives an excellent nutritional profile of the product you're thinking about buying. It tells you how many calories, grams (or milligrams) of fiber, sugar, sodium, fat, protein, vitamins, minerals, cholesterol,

food fails (like forgetting milk for your cereal, handy snacks to take to work, or anything to eat for dinner)—all more likely as you add forgetfulness to your list of pregnancy symptoms. But even if you shop one day at a time, a list in hand will prevent you from getting sucked into the shopper's twilight zone—wandering the aisles aimlessly looking for inspiration and finding it in a half gallon of mint chocolate chip. For best results, organize your lists by

and carbohydrates each serving of the food contains. It also tells you the percentage of the DV (daily value) of these nutrients provided in a serving.

Now, this may seem like a lot more than you need to know about a product—and probably a lot more than you know what to do with. But the point of reading nutrition labels isn't so that you can calculate grams or add up percentages. After all, the Pregnancy Diet already ensures that you're getting the amounts of nutrients you need, without doing the math—not to mention that the DV for pregnancy is often different from that listed on the label. It's to figure out whether the product you're picking up is worth dropping into your cart.

The big type. Is the big type on a label just hype? It depends on the words being highlighted. The FDA (Food and Drug Administration) regulates words that describe a food's nutrient content (such as "light," "low-fat," and "high-fiber") to make sure they're accurate. But other terms—including "natural," "wholesome," "humanely raised," and "smart"—are still unregulated, so they can mean anything or nothing at all. Even "healthy" may not be—making it fair game for fooling a consumer (that "healthy" cereal could be packed with sugar, refined grains, and artificial colors and flavors). And goodness knows, "made with goodness" doesn't tell you anything about what's inside the package you're picking up. Here are some other tricks of the label trade:

- "Fortified with 6 vitamins and iron" looks impressive, especially in that extra-large print. And for the most part, fortification with vitamins and minerals is a good thing. But fortification alone does not make a food healthy—especially if it's just tossing some vitamins and minerals into a food that's weak in nutrition to begin with. Just about all processed food, after all, is fortified.

- "Cheddar and other natural flavors" looks impressive on that box of macaroni and cheese. But it's anybody's guess what the "natural flavors" are (that's unregulated). Plus, having "natural flavors" doesn't mean a product is free of artificial flavors or colors (you'll discover those in the ingredients list). And just how far down the list is that cheddar, anyway?

- "No preservatives" or "no artificial flavors" tells you only what isn't in a product. To find out what is in it (for instance, artificial colors), you'll have to read on.

- "Bran muffins" have to be full of bran, right? Actually, they don't have to be. A pinch of bran is all it takes for a bran muffin to earn its designation. So you'll have to go back to the ingredients list to see if these bran muffins really are. Does bran come second, after whole-wheat flour? Or fourth, after enriched white flour, sugar, corn syrup? Now you know what you're buying into.

For more tips on how to make sense of food labels, check out greenerchoices .org/labels/.

department or aisle—that way you won't end up visiting the produce section 3 times in the same trip, or making a last-minute dash back to retrieve an item when you're already halfway through the checkout line.

- Do stick to the list. Supermarkets, even virtual ones, are full of temptations. And advertising and marketing ploys. And sales that entice you to buy what you don't need and maybe shouldn't have—or just more than you need or can use. Resist with your list. Also consider that coupons (or rebate apps) can clip your healthy eating plans if you don't clip with care and choose foods that come not just with savings but also with nutritional redemption.

■ Do think outside the box. Yes, you've come equipped with your list—but don't let that stop you from picking up a healthy food that's new to you. A baby vegetable you've never seen, an exotic tropical fruit, an intriguing grain to add to your pilaf, a seed to snack on.

■ Don't shop when you're about to drop. When you can avoid it, try not to schedule in big-time marketing when you're on your last legs (and possibly swollen ankles) of the day.

■ Don't go hungry. Have a snack before you go shopping. A growling stomach will lead you off list—and down the snack aisle—every time.

Selecting for Two

You're motivated to eat well, you're ready to get started on the Pregnancy Diet, and you're eager to select the best foods for your health and your baby's. Here's what to keep in mind as you do your choosing.

Meat and Poultry

Not sure which cuts of meat and poultry make the cut? Aim for the leanest cuts of beef, pork, and lamb—look for the words "lean" or "extra lean," choose cuts that are graded "choice" or "select" ("prime" will usually have more fat), and select cuts with the least amount of visible fat (marbling). That's not only because less fat means fewer calories, but because fat is where any chemicals an animal ingests accumulate (this isn't a concern when it comes to organically raised animals; keep reading). As a rule of thumb, anything labeled "loin," "sirloin," or "round" is lean, with the leanest cuts of beef being eye round, top round, round tip, top sirloin, bottom round, top loin, and tenderloin. When selecting lean or extra-lean ground beef, also check the percentage of fat and choose the lowest fat percentage when you can. You'll pay more for less fat, but the meat will cook down less, leaving you with more meat by weight. Chicken or turkey on the menu? Reach for breasts, preferably skinless (or remove the skin, which is 85 percent fat, before cooking—or, if that's not possible, before eating). Or ground chicken or turkey breast, instead of the ground dark meat.

When it's available and your budget permits, consider buying meat and poultry that has been raised organically. The label "organic" on animal products means that the animals were fed organic food and not given antibiotics, growth hormones, or other drugs—a definite plus, since the antibiotics, hormones, pesticides, and chemicals you consume through your diet are shared with your baby both in utero and through breast milk. It makes even more sense to reach for organic when you're buying a fattier cut of meat or poultry (a marbled steak, chicken thighs, pork shoulder). Though an organic beef short rib will still contain as many calories as a short rib from a conventionally raised cow, it won't contain all the chemicals that may be stored in a conventionally raised animal's fat.

Also consider buying meat that's grass-fed (keeping in mind that organic meat isn't exclusively grass-fed unless it specifies so on the label, and grass-fed isn't always organic). Grass-fed cows (organic or not) eat the old-fashioned way, by grazing on the range. Not only is their diet vegetarian, but they have to work for it, resulting in leaner, lower-calorie meat. What's more, grass-fed beef is higher in omega-3 fatty acids, vitamin E, and beta-carotene than grain-fed—all excellent reasons to reach for grass-fed instead of conventional. Is springing for grass-fed not in your budget? No need to stress: Even though there are more nutrients in grass-fed than in conventional meats, the difference is small. One serving (4 ounces) of grass-fed top sirloin contains about 65 to 100 milligrams of omega-3 fats, while regular beef has about 30 to 50 milligrams of omega-3s per serving. A difference, yes, but not a significant one—especially when you consider that a 4-ounce serving of salmon has over 1,000 milligrams of that baby-brain-boosting nutrient. So by all means, choose grass-fed when you can, but don't worry if you can't find it or can't afford it.

Something else to consider when selecting meat and poultry: There aren't government standards when it comes to the terms "free-range," "grass-fed," or "pasture-raised"—which means it's not always clear what you're getting. Free-range, a label specifically for chickens, is supposed to indicate that the animals have access to the outdoors and are less likely contaminated with chemicals. Grass-fed is supposed to mean that animals are fed a diet that consists mostly of grass, not grains. Pasture-raised is supposed to mean that animals spend some of their time outdoors, feeding on grass

in the pasture. But without standards for these designations, there's no way to know exactly how much time those pasture-raised cows actually spent in the pasture or what kind of conditions the grass-fed cows actually lived in (never mind how much grain they received in addition to the grass) or how much time the free-range chicken spent free on the range (it could have been mere minutes a day).

Want to keep closer tabs on what your dinner ate for dinner, or on how it was treated? Don't rely on the "grass-fed" or "pasture-raised" label. For a more meaningful description, look for meat and poultry (and even dairy and eggs; see page 186) labeling that shows that higher standards were met, and that the animals were raised exclusively on a pasture or range and never fed grain. These include "American Grassfed," "Animal Welfare Approved," "PCO Certified 100% GrassFed," "NOFA-NY 100% Grass Fed," or "Global Animal Partnership Step 4-5+." The Certified Humane Raised seal means that higher standards were met, but not as high as those of the other labels. Keep in mind that in some cases, grass-fed, pasture-raised, or free-range (even with these higher-standard labels) doesn't mean organic. The grass the animals grazed on, for instance, may have been treated with pesticides or other chemicals, or exposed to runoff.

Fish

Loaded with baby-brain-boosting omega-3 fats, vitamins D and B$_{12}$, and a host of healthy minerals, fish should ideally make the menu cut at least 2 to 3 times a week when you're expecting (assuming you're a fish fan and you're not feeling too green around the gills to eat it). But what should you look for when you're in the market for fish? That depends on what you're fishing for. When selecting fresh fish, use your senses—especially your pregnancy-sensitive nose, which will quickly warn you if something's fishy (it should smell like an ocean breeze, not like a bait box). Fresh fish should look fresh, and if it's whole, it should have moist gills, shiny skin, and clear, bright eyes. Fillets should also be shiny, not dull, and the flesh should spring back without leaving an indentation when pressed lightly with a finger. Hopefully the fish will be labeled as "fresh" or "previously frozen," but if it isn't, just ask. Fish that was quickly frozen after being caught and then thawed carefully may actually be "fresher" than fish that was caught, stored, and shipped fresh. If the fish was previously frozen, don't refreeze it once you get home (you can freeze fish that has never been frozen). Buying fish that's already frozen? Just make sure you keep it frozen until you're ready to use it (thaw in the fridge before preparing). For a list of pregnancy-safe fish to choose and fish to avoid, see page 72.

Should you go wild (that is, caught in its natural habitat, whether that's an ocean, river, or lake) or farm raised (raised in a large tank)? That's not an easy call. Wild fish (wild salmon, for instance) may be lower in calories and higher in minerals, though farmed fish usually has an edge on omega-3s (because of fortified feed). Wild fish may also contain fewer contaminants than farmed, but either can contain mercury (which is why you should stick to low-mercury fish). Where the fish is sourced from (which farm, which ocean) can also impact the level of contaminants, since some countries are more lax than others when it comes to regulation of both farms and natural bodies of water. It can also impact the nutrients it contains (fish are what they eat).

If debates about which fish to buy don't mean much to you, either because farmed is the only option at your market

or because you can't afford to go wild, just remember this: Any fish (as long as it's a safe fish) is better than no fish at all.

Wondering whether you should buy organic fish? You really can't. Though some fish may be labeled as organic, there's no official U.S. government standard for "organic" seafood certification, which means it's hard to know what that designation actually means. Some states don't even allow the "organic" label on fish.

Eggs

Like your eggs any style? There's plenty to like: They're inexpensive, versatile, and packed with protein, and they're a solid source of nutrients from vitamin A, B_{12}, and D to selenium and zinc. But did you know that some eggs also provide more baby-brain-nourishing DHA than others? That's right. DHA eggs, also called omega-3 eggs, come from chickens fed a diet containing sources of omega-3s, such as flaxseed or marine algae. You'll also find plenty to crow about when it comes to pasture-raised eggs (even ones not marked "omega-3 eggs"). Compared with conventional eggs, they're higher in DHA, have more vitamins A and D and double the vitamin E. So if you're looking to make a good egg better, look for "omega-3," "DHA," or "pasture-raised" on the carton. Words that don't mean much nutritionally:

- "Cage-free" means only that the hens weren't completely confined to cages—there's zero guarantee that they had any access to the outdoors.

- "Free-range" means the hens had access to the outdoors, but not that they actually ever went outdoors.

- "Natural" (all eggs are natural).

- "Farm fresh" means only that they came from a farm (all eggs do).

Dairy

When selecting dairy, you'll score as much protein and calcium for fewer calories when you opt for low-fat or nonfat varieties. If your budget allows—and it's readily available at your market—choose organic dairy products over conventional, for a couple of reasons. First, because organically raised cows (and goats and sheep) are never given antibiotics or hormones, the milk they produce won't contain them (though most conventional milk won't contain them either; keep reading). Second, organic dairy products contain more omega-3 fatty acids than conventional dairy. That's because all USDA Certified Organic milk comes from animals that are grass-fed to some extent, with the rest of their feed grown without chemical fertilizers, pesticides, or genetically modified products. Milk that comes from 100 percent grass-fed animals may be even richer in omega-3s.

Can't find—or can't afford—organic dairy? The good news is that the FDA requires all milk—even conventional—to be checked for antibiotic residue (any milk that contains it can't be sold). Which means that there won't be any antibiotics in conventional milk you buy, whether it says so on the label or not. Growth hormones (BGH) are rarely used these days, and most conventional milk will specify "hormone-free." What's more, most tests show that there are practically no detectable levels of pesticides in conventional milk, either.

Other labels to consider: lactose-free if you're sensitive to the lactose in milk (see the box on page 37 for more), A2 milk if you have an intolerance to a certain protein in cow's milk (see page 149), calcium fortified for an extra dose of this bone-building mineral in every glass, and DHA omega-3 milk, which gives a boost of DHA through the addition of refined fish oil or algal oil (ask your practitioner if it makes sense for you to drink DHA-enriched milk).

Pasteurized, Please

Pasteurization may be the best thing that ever happened to a glass of milk (or a wedge of cheese), but it shouldn't stop at dairy products. Eggs come pasteurized, too (eliminating the risk of salmonella)—a good choice if you're whipping up a homemade Caesar dressing or prefer your yolks runny or your scrambles soft. Juices you drink should also be pasteurized (to eliminate E. coli and other harmful bacteria). Most (but not all) commercially packaged juices are pasteurized, so always check the label before you buy. Not sure if a juice is pasteurized or pretty sure it isn't (say, because it's freshly squeezed at the juice bar)? Don't drink it. Ditto for smoothies made with juice, unless you're sure it's pasteurized. Fresh coconuts cut open right in front of you and served with a straw are fine to drink since the coconut water is sterile and well protected inside the hard coconut shell. Look for pasteurized apple cider vinegar, too. (Just keep in mind that if you're turning to apple cider vinegar because you've heard claims that it will heal what ails you—from morning sickness to gestational diabetes—those claims are not backed up by science.)

Wondering about the label "flash-pasteurized"? It's a faster yet just as effective pasteurization process that kills bacteria while preserving flavor. And how about juicing you do at home? That's all good (and yummy, and nutritious)—as long as you've thoroughly washed the produce before juicing.

A Fresh Approach to Dried

When it comes to picking the most nutritious foods, nothing compares with fresh, right? Maybe not. Freeze-dried fruits, vegetables, and even cheese pack a nutritional punch equal to the fresh varieties. The freeze-drying process removes nearly all the water content of a food (around 98 percent), leaving it crunchy, more intensely flavored, and—key when you're snacking on the run or at your desk—not perishable. No spoiling, no need for refrigeration, and no preparation or cooking necessary. Open the package, open your mouth, and start popping everything from strawberries to mango, broccoli to carrots, cheddar to mozzarella.

Wondering how much freeze-dried fruit differs from traditionally dried? A lot, actually. First, freeze-dried is crunchy, while dried (aka dehydrated) is chewy. Dried fruit is higher in calories than freeze-dried, and often lower in nutrients (the dehydration process requires the use of heat, which can strip foods of naturally occurring nutrients, especially heat-sensitive ones like vitamin C). There may be sugar added to some dried fruits (particularly tropical fruits like pineapple, plus cherries, cranberries and other berries), as well as preservatives and oil. Even dried fruit that doesn't contain added sugar may be more likely to contribute to tooth decay and gum troubles (that's because it's so sticky).

Craving something crispy and salty? Seeking a snack you can take anywhere, including to bed? Freeze-dried cheese (like Moon Cheese) provides protein, calcium, and a satisfying, nutritious alternative to that bag of chips. And, unlike fresh cheese, you can keep it in your gym bag or your car without worrying about refrigeration. Looking for a blood-sugar-sustaining or quease-easing combo of protein and complex carbs you can tote for emergency snacking? Pack a bag of freeze-dried cheese and a bag of freeze-dried fruit, and you're good to go . . . anywhere, anytime.

All dairy products you select should be pasteurized, for safety's sake (see the box on page 63 for reasons why).

Looking for nondairy milks? See the box on page 38 for a list of options.

Fruits and Vegetables

Green means go. And when it comes to fruits and vegetables, so does red, yellow, blue, orange, and purple. When selecting fresh fruits and vegetables, pick the most ripe, richly colored, and fragrant options. And try to think seasonally—although most fruits and vegetables are available year-round, produce will be more flavorful, more nutritious, and probably cost less in season.

Check out these rainbow hot hues in the produce aisle:

- Red. Red is the color of lycopene, one of nature's superstar phytonutrients. Tomatoes, both raw and cooked (though cooking pumps up their nutritional content), are a great source. So, too, are ruby red (or pink) grapefruit, watermelon, persimmon, and guava. Another reason to see (and eat) red is the high antioxidant content of red fruit favorites like strawberries, cranberries, cherries, and pomegranates.

- Orange and yellow. Fruits and vegetables that are orange or yellow are usually rich in baby-friendly vitamin A (or more precisely beta-carotene).

The Biotech Boom

Heard that you should avoid GMOs, but not sure why—or even, what GMOs are? Here are a few fast facts. GMOs, or genetically modified organisms, are plants that have had their DNA modified. It's not technically a new process—farmers have been finessing their crops for thousands of years, breeding them to be hardier, tastier, more adaptable, and more resistant to pests—but this far higher level of crop engineering has definitely become a far higher tech process, as well as a far bigger business. Not to mention, a major source of controversy among consumers and consumer groups concerned about the safety of GMOs.

What are the benefits of GMOs—or at least, the potential benefits? Crops that are designed to acquire more desirable traits, like the ability to grow faster and less expensively under harsher weather conditions, stay fresher longer, be more nutritious, or to resist pests or disease without (again, potentially) the use of as many pesticides. These days, anything from corn to plums, potatoes to rice, can be genetically modified in the United States (the practice is banned in Europe), with soybeans being by far the most commonly grown GMO crop.

So is this biotech boom a boon or a bane, or somewhere in between, especially from where you're sitting—pregnant and legitimately concerned about the food you eat and share with your baby? From the research so far—and there has been a lot of research done—it appears that GMOs are not harmful. The consensus of the vast majority of scientists (including, among others, those in the American Medical Association, the World Health Organization, and the National Academy of Sciences) is that such biotechnological advances are safe, and that their responsible development may ultimately result in a healthier population and planet. So there's a significant upside to the GMO boom long-term, they say, and no particular downside in the meantime. That is, as long as consumers choose healthy GMO products (those huge crops of soybeans often end up in less healthy foods). Still, many consumer groups remain critical of GMOs, insisting that there are too many unanswered questions about how these changes in our food supply will impact our health.

Just feel better about staying GMO free? The FDA requires that foods that are genetically modified or contain GMOs be labeled as such, so avoiding GMOs is as easy as avoiding foods with a GMO label. You can also look for foods labeled "free of GMOs" or ones certified by the Non-GMO Project. Or choose certified organic products, which the FDA says are required to be GMO free.

Color your world with winter squash (from butternut to kabocha to delicata), carrots, sweet potatoes, apricots, yellow peaches, cantaloupes, mangoes, papayas, pumpkins, and yellow and orange peppers. Other oranges and yellows, such as oranges, tangerines, lemons, and pineapples, are also high in vitamin C.

■ Green. Some dark green varieties of produce are excellent sources of carotenoids (lutein and zeaxanthin) that may help reduce the risk of slow fetal growth and premature delivery. These carotenoids also play a role in the healthy development of vision and the nervous system. Leafy greens help you score some baby-friendly

---

When Organic Makes a Difference

Can't always spring for organic produce, or can't always find it at your market? Knowing when organic makes a difference and when it doesn't can help prioritize your purchases:

- Certain produce carries higher levels of pesticide than others, even after washing. So it's best to buy organic strawberries, spinach, kale, nectarines, peaches, apples, pears, grapes, cherries, tomatoes, celery, and potatoes.

- Other fruits and vegetables generally don't contain pesticide residue, which means it's a safe bet to buy them conventionally grown. They include cantaloupe, honeydew, pineapples, kiwis, avocados, corn, peas, onions, papayas, eggplant, asparagus, cabbage, cauliflower, broccoli, and mushrooms.

---

folate (folic acid), too. Besides lettuces, stock up on spinach, kale, Swiss chard, broccoli, artichokes, green peas, green beans, brussels sprouts, green peppers, zucchini, okra, avocados, honeydew, green grapes, kiwis, and parsley.

- Blue. The antioxidant anthocyanin makes the blueberry blue and is a powerful cancer fighter. Clearly, you won't find it in those boxes of Froot Loops—that blue (and pink, and yellow, and green) comes by its color in an entirely different way.

- Purple. Purple (or red) grapes contain lutein and zeaxanthin; plums, prunes, blackberries, and purple cabbage are also rich in antioxidants. Beets are rich in the antioxidant betacyanin. And acai (pronounced ah-sa-EE) berries—nicknamed "purple gold" (think of them as somewhere between a grape and a blueberry)—get their purple color from good-for-you phytonutrients, including polysterols and anthocyanins. In fact, acai packs more antioxidants than cranberries, raspberries, blackberries, strawberries, or blueberries (but eat acai in moderation and don't take it in supplement form, since its safety in pregnancy hasn't been studied). Other purple produce to color your world with: purple asparagus, purple carrots, purple figs, purple cauliflower, purple brussels sprouts, purple peppers, purple potatoes, and purple sweet potatoes.

- White. They're not exactly colorful, but don't overlook paler fruits and vegetables. Garlic, onions, shallots, scallions, and leeks contain compounds that protect DNA. Cauliflower contains a hearty dose of vitamin C, manganese, and phytonutrients (including antioxidants). And endive, mushrooms (particularly wild varieties), celery, and pears are rich in flavonoids (another phytonutrient) that protect cell membranes. You can't go wrong with that, baby!

What about organic? Is the heftier price tag that comes with the organic designation worth it? Does organic produce have an edge nutritionally? The latest research indicates that organic crops do not have higher levels of most vitamins compared with conventionally grown produce, though they do have substantially higher concentrations of antioxidants and phytonutrients. But let's face it—most people don't buy organic fruits and vegetables for their nutritional content, especially when that content doesn't always offer significant differences. They shop for organic produce because of what it doesn't contain:

Spotting Organic

It's usually easy to spot an organic product—just look for the word "organic" or the USDA Organic seal. But what about fresh produce that doesn't come neatly packaged and labeled? Here's a little trick: Look for the small sticker with a printed code. If the code has 4 digits, the produce is conventional. If the code has 5 digits and starts with a 9, the produce is certified organic.

pesticides and chemicals . . . a definite plus, since the pesticides and chemicals you consume through your diet are shared with your baby both in utero and through breast milk. And while taste isn't usually directly impacted by how produce is grown, organic fruits and vegetables are usually fresher than conventional when they hit the market. That's because they're more perishable and must be rushed to the market within days (conventional produce can tough it out during long stays in warehouses).

With that in mind, if organic products are available locally and you can afford the premium price, make it your choice—just keep in mind as you load up your shopping cart that organic produce will have a much shorter shelf life than conventional. If price is an object, pick organic selectively (see the box on the previous page). And remember: While organic produce won't be contaminated with pesticides, it could—like any produce—be contaminated with bacteria. That's why thorough washing is a step you shouldn't skip just because you've sprung for organic. In other words, no nibbling on those farmers market blueberries before they've been brought home for a thorough rinse. And of course

washing or peeling conventional produce can eliminate or greatly decrease pesticide residue. Remember, too, that what you eat overall matters more than whether you're eating conventional or organic foods. The benefits of eating more (even conventional) fruits and vegetables will outweigh the possible risks from pesticide exposure.

For more information on the USDA's organic products regulations, check out ams.usda.gov/grades-standards/organic-standards. Wondering about genetically modified produce? See the box on page 65 for the lowdown.

Whole Grains

Finding whole wheat in the bakery department is as easy as scanning the shelf for bread and rolls labeled "wheat," right? Not exactly. Wheat (or oat, or corn) specifies only the type of grain, not whether it's whole. Instead, look for the "100% whole wheat" banner on the packaging, and also make sure that the first ingredient is "whole-wheat flour." Take a closer look when you see a product tagged "multigrain," "seven-grain," or "nutri-grain"—this lets you know only that it contains multiple grains, not necessarily whole grains. Check the ingredients list to see whether all (or any) of those featured grains are actually whole.

The same rules apply to cereals and other grain products as well. Read up on your favorite cereals to be sure that the "oat" cereal you're buying is made from "whole-grain oats," not just "oats."

The following glossary should help you in the screening process:

- "Wheat flour" isn't whole wheat. It means the flour is made by grinding wheat and typically does not contain the bran or germ.

- "Enriched flour (wheat)" is wheat flour (no bran or germ) that has been

White Whole Wheat

Not a wholehearted fan of whole wheat? There may be something on the supermarket aisles just for you. White whole-wheat breads are made with whole white wheat, a grain that has a milder, sweeter taste than the red wheat that regular whole wheat is made from. Is white whole wheat the best thing since sliced bread? It may well be if you're a white bread fan, since it offers the same nutritional benefits of regular whole wheat—including the bran—with that just-like-white taste and texture. Just be sure to read labels, since white wheat bread isn't whole grain unless it says so. You can also find white whole wheat in flour form—use it instead of regular whole-wheat flour for lighter, less dense baked goods, pancakes, and more.

enriched with nutrients that are lost during the refining process.

- "Enriched flour (flour)" can be any type of grain flour (rye, oats, barley, or soybeans, for instance) that has been enriched with nutrients—and unless it specifies that it's whole-grain, you can be sure it isn't.

- "Milled" (for instance, "milled corn") sounds promisingly wholesome, but is actually often a sign that the grain is refined.

- "Stone-ground wheat flour" describes merely how the wheat grain (without the bran or germ) was milled. Whether it was ground by stones or machines, it's still refined if it doesn't specify "whole."

- "Whole-wheat flour" is wheat flour that includes the bran and germ. Look, too, for whole oat, whole barley, and whole rye flour for a whole lot of naturally occurring nutrition.

Pasta That Packs in Protein

Back off, beef. Step aside, poultry and pork. There's a new protein source in town: legume pasta. Made from chickpeas, lentils, black beans, and more, and available in a variety of shapes—from spaghetti to penne— these pastas are super high in protein, fiber, and iron, lower in carbohydrates (making them the perfect pasta for diabetics or those at risk for gestational diabetes), and often gluten-free. The texture is a little different from grain-based pasta, but close enough to pass (just make sure you don't overcook it). Toss legume linguini with marinara sauce, penne with broccoli and cheese, or (if you're feeling the meat love after all) spaghetti with meatballs.

Looking for rice that's nice and high in protein, plus grain-free? Look to chickpea rice (you'll find it in the rice aisle).

Tabled for Two

....

Now you know what to eat when you're expecting. But what about all the foods and drinks you shouldn't be consuming . . . or should be limiting? The ones that are off-limits entirely? The ones that are considered safe when they're cooked but are red-lighted when raw? The ones that are questionable, and the ones you have questions about? Happily, most foods and drinks can find their place on a mom-to-be's menu. But it's always best to play it safe when you're playing for two, so you'll also need to know which foods and beverages should be tabled during your 9 months and which can safely appear on your table in moderation. This chapter will clue you in on what should be off the menu when you're expecting.

What to Limit When You're Expecting

Bracing for the bad news about your morning coffee? Or your tea for two? Or maybe concerns about chemicals in your pregnancy diet have you second-guessing your Splenda, passing up ingredients you can't pronounce, or fearing fish? There's really more good news than you might think: Many of the foods and drinks you love (but may be worrying about consuming now that you're expecting) are safe to consume, especially in moderation. Here's the lowdown on what to limit.

Coffee

Maybe you're the type who can't get through the day without joe by your side (in a bottomless mug). Maybe a cup or two will see you through, at least on most days. Maybe it's not the pick-me-up you need, but the creamy deliciousness of that caramel macchiato that you crave . . . at least twice a day. Or maybe you're somewhere in between. No matter where you land on the caffeine map—or if you're all over the map, depending on the day you're

Caffeine Counts

You'd be surprised at how quickly the caffeine adds up even when coffee's not on the menu. Caffeine hides not only in coffee, but also in caffeinated soft drinks (too many Mountain Dews are a pregnancy don't), coffee ice cream and yogurt, many varieties of tea, energy bars and drinks, and chocolate (the darker the chocolate, the more caffeine it packs). Here's the approximate amount of caffeine you can expect to find in some of your favorites:

- 1 cup brewed coffee (8 ounces) = 135 mg

- 1 cup instant coffee = 95 mg

- 1 cup decaf coffee = 5 to 30 mg

- 1 shot espresso (or any drink made with 1 shot) = 90 mg

- 1 cup tea = 40 to 60 mg (green tea has less caffeine than black tea)

- 1 cup matcha = 70 mg

- 1 can cola (12 ounces) = about 35 mg

- 1 can diet cola = 45 mg

- 1 can energy drink = 50 to 350 mg

- 1 ounce milk chocolate = 6 mg

- 1 ounce dark chocolate = 20 mg

- 1 cup chocolate milk = 5 mg

- ½ cup coffee ice cream = 20 to 40 mg

---

having or how much sleep you got the night before—you're probably wondering if you'll have to cut out coffee altogether now that you're expecting.

Well, java lovers (and cravers of caffeine in other forms), get ready to rejoice—in moderation. Most evidence suggests that drinking up to about 200 mg of caffeine a day is perfectly safe for your little bean. What does that break down to exactly? Possibly not as much as you'd hope—about 12 ounces of brewed coffee (2 small cups or 1 "tall") or about 2 shots of espresso. Drink more, however, and there's less cause for celebration. Heavy caffeine intake (more than 5 cups of coffee a day) has been linked to miscarriage.

Other reasons to stick to the recommended limit? For one, too much caffeine can irritate your bladder, which may step up the number of those already-too-frequent trips you make to the bathroom and possibly lead to urinary tract infections. It can also irritate your emotions—exacerbating normal pregnancy mood swings and preventing you from getting the rest you need (especially when you drink it after noon). As if all that's not enough, caffeine interferes with your body's ability to absorb iron that both you and your baby need. And here's a potential downside to high consumption of caffeine you probably wouldn't expect: Research has found that an intake of 300 mg or more per day may be linked to a baby growing too big and too fast during his or her first year, and to an increased risk of being overweight throughout the toddler years and beyond.

Bottom line: There's no need to cut joe out of your life entirely when you're expecting (unless you really want to)—as long as you stick to the recommended 200 mg per day. One to two cups of coffee doesn't satisfy? You can stretch the 2 into 3 or more by adding more milk to each cup (you'll get a calcium bonus) or by ordering half-caf twice as

Energy in a Can?

Looking for a pick-me-up now that pregnancy fatigue's got you down? Wondering whether a jolt from one of the many energy drinks lining supermarket shelves may be just the ticket? Well, think (and read the labels) before you drink. Though a jolt-in-a-can energy drink might pick you up briefly, that blood-sugar high will be followed by a free-falling crash, leaving you dragging more than ever. Plus, many canned energy drinks may contain dietary supplements that aren't safe for pregnancy use, as well as a whopping amount of caffeine. So pass on the cans, and seek your energy boost the natural way instead (see page 125).

Herbal Tea

Had an extra long day? Feel like curling up on the sofa with a good book and a steaming cup of herbal tea? Before you reach for those herbal tea leaves, it's wise to read them—or at least the packaging they come in. The effects of herbs in pregnancy have not been well researched, and until more is known, the FDA advises that pregnant (and breastfeeding) women use herbal teas with caution. Another reason why it's smart to proceed with caution when contemplating a cup of herbal tea? Because herbs aren't regulated by the FDA, some herbal blends may contain contaminants or ingredients that aren't listed on the label. Some brews that sound like they're fruit- or spice-based (with names like "Lemon Ginger" or "Orange Spice") may actually be blended with herbs (another case for being a careful label reader).

How can you tell if you're brewing up trouble with your tea? It's actually not that easy, even if you're a label reader. While some herbal teas are probably safe in moderate doses, there's no scientific consensus on which ones are, which ones aren't, and what "moderate" means. You can ask your

often. Need tips for cutting back on caffeine? See *What to Expect When You're Expecting*.

Prefer to get your caffeine kick from an endless stream of Mountain Dew or Diet Coke? See the box on the facing page for a caffeine breakdown of your favorite beverage.

Herbs You Don't Have to Curb

Think no-go when you think herbs during pregnancy? That depends on what kind of herbs you're thinking. Medicinal herbs (like all drugs) should not be taken (or in the case of herbal tea, drunk) without the advice of a medical practitioner who knows that you're pregnant. Parsley, sage, rosemary, and thyme? They—along with other culinary herbs, from that basil and dill to

that cilantro and mint—are entirely safe to eat. And they add not only flavor, but also nutrients. Basil, for instance, packs in vitamin A, vitamin K, lutein, and zeaxanthin, among other essential vitamins and minerals. So chop some fresh basil and parsley into your spaghetti sauce, toss your cucumbers with cilantro and mint, stuff your chicken breasts with sage, and go rosemary, baby.

practitioner for a list of which teas to enjoy and which to avoid, or you can play it extra safe by sticking to regular (black) tea that comes flavored, or adding any of the following to boiling water or regular tea: slices of fruit (lemon, orange, apple, pear); fruit juice; mint leaves; cinnamon, nutmeg, cloves, or ginger (an effective calmer of queasy tummies). And (of course), never brew up homemade tea from a plant growing in your backyard unless you're absolutely certain what it is and that it's safe for use during pregnancy.

Eager for an easier labor, or impatient for one that's overdue to begin? Then you may have heard that raspberry leaf or black or blue cohosh can fast-track your trip to the birthing room. See the box on page 141 to find out if there's truth to that tea tale.

Green Tea

It's long been touted for its health benefits. But the jury's still out on whether green tea gets the green light during pregnancy. That's because green tea can decrease the effectiveness of folic acid, that vital pregnancy vitamin. If you're a green-tea drinker, drink it in (you guessed it) moderation, and ask your practitioner for a specific recommendation.

Matcha—ground green tea leaves in a powder form—is known for its antioxidants and anti-inflammatory properties. It can be used to make tea, sprinkled into smoothies, or mixed into cookies and other baked goods. But again, because green tea in large amounts can decrease the effectiveness of folic acid, and because you're using the leaves themselves (instead of merely steeping green tea leaves in water and then discarding), causing you to consume a larger dose of the active ingredients of green tea, you'll want to drink matcha in moderation when you're pregnant. Another reason to moderate your matcha: One cup of matcha has about 70 mg of caffeine, a little over one-third of the daily limit for caffeine intake during pregnancy.

Fish

It's an excellent source of lean protein, baby-brain-boosting omega-3 fats, and vitamins D and B_{12}, plus a host of healthy minerals, from iron and iodine to selenium and zinc—all good reasons to keep fish (and other seafood) on your pregnancy menu, or even to consider adding it if you've never been a fish fan before. In fact, experts—including the pregnancy experts, ACOG (the American College of Obstetricians and Gynecologists)—agree that pregnant and breastfeeding women should aim to eat 8 to 12 ounces of fish and seafood a week, or about 2 to 3 servings (a serving is 4 to 6 ounces).

So go fish, by all means. But when you're casting your net at the seafood department, be sure to fish selectively, sticking to those varieties that are lower in mercury—a chemical that in large, accumulated doses may be harmful to a fetus's developing nervous system.

According to expert guidelines, during pregnancy and lactation, you should:

EAT UP (*2 to 3 servings per week*)

- Anchovy
- Atlantic croaker
- Atlantic mackerel
- Black sea bass
- Butterfish
- Catfish

> **CHEW ON THIS.** In Nigeria, lore has it that eating snails during pregnancy can make your baby sluggish. In other words, that escargot may end up being more like escar-not-go. Sounds fishy.

- Clams
- Cod
- Crab
- Crawfish
- Flounder
- Haddock
- Hake
- Herring
- Lobster (American and spiny)
- Mullet
- Oyster
- Pacific chub mackerel
- Perch (freshwater and ocean)
- Pickerel
- Plaice
- Pollack
- Salmon
- Sardines
- Scallops
- Shad
- Shrimp
- Skate
- Smelt
- Sole
- Squid

- Tilapia
- Trout (freshwater)
- Tuna, canned light (includes skipjack)
- Whitefish
- Whiting

EAT IN MODERATION
(no more than 1 serving a week)

- Bluefish
- Buffalofish
- Carp
- Chilean sea bass/Patagonian toothfish
- Grouper
- Halibut
- Mahi-mahi/Dolphinfish
- Monkfish
- Rockfish
- Sablefish
- Sheepshead
- Snapper
- Spanish mackerel
- Striped ocean bass
- Atlantic tilefish
- Tuna, albacore/white tuna, canned, and fresh or frozen
- Tuna, yellowfin
- Weakfish/sea trout
- White croaker/Pacific croaker
- Fish caught recreationally: Limit to 1 serving a week and don't eat other fish that week (unless you've checked with the local fishing advisories or the EPA about the safety of the fish caught in local waters).

AVOID ENTIRELY

- King mackerel

- Marlin

- Orange roughy

- Shark

- Swordfish

- Tilefish (from the Gulf of Mexico)

- Tuna steaks, bigeye

For the latest information on fish safety visit fda.gov (search for "fish").

Sugar Substitutes

Hoping to spare those empty sugar calories by choosing an artificial sweetener? Sugar substitutes are a mixed bag when you're expecting—not only when it comes to their composition (some are straight-up chemical compounds, others are derived from natural sources but processed in a lab), but also to their calorie content and the way they're metabolized. Though most are considered safe, others should probably be consumed with a side of caution. Here's what's known about the most popular sugar substitutes so far:

Sucralose (Splenda). Made from sugar, but chemically converted to a form that's not absorbable by the body, sucralose appears to be the best bet safety-wise for pregnant women seeking sweetness with no calories and little aftertaste (it has been approved by the FDA for pregnant women to consume). Sweeten your coffee, tea, yogurt, and smoothies with it if you want, or use foods and drinks presweetened with it. It's also stable for cooking and baking (unlike aspartame), making that sugar-free chocolate cake less pipe dream, more possibility. Still, moderation is probably smart, even with sucralose.

Aspartame (Equal, NutraSweet). The research jury's still out on this zero-calorie artificial sweetener. Many practitioners consider it harmless and will okay light or moderate use in pregnancy. While the FDA has approved aspartame for pregnant women, it does recommend that moms-to-be limit consumption. A packet or two of the blue stuff now and then, a can of Diet Coke every once in a while—no problem. Just avoid consuming aspartame in large amounts during pregnancy. Women with PKU—phenylketonuria—must limit their intake of phenylalanine and are generally advised not to use aspartame.

Saccharin (Sweet'N Low). The FDA has deemed saccharin safe, but some studies suggest that this zero-calorie artificial sweetener reaches the placenta and that when it does, it's slow to leave. For that reason, you might want to stay away from the pink packets—or pick them up only occasionally (say, when there's no yellow in sight). Don't worry, however, about saccharin you had before finding out that you're pregnant, since the risks, if any, are extremely slight.

Acesulfame-K (Sunett). This artificial sweetener, 200 times sweeter than sugar, is approved for use in baked goods, gelatin desserts, chewing gum, and soft drinks. The FDA says it's okay to use in moderation during pregnancy, but since few studies have been done to prove its safety, ask your practitioner for guidelines before gobbling the stuff up.

Sorbitol. This "sugar alcohol" is found naturally in many fruits and berries, but its life as a commercial sweetener usually begins as corn syrup that undergoes chemical conversion in the lab. With half the sweetness of sugar (but more calories than most sugar substitutes), it is used in a wide range of foods and beverages and is safe for use in pregnancy in moderate amounts. But it does present a problem in large doses: Too much can cause bloating, gas pains, and diarrhea—a digestive trio no pregnant woman needs.

Mannitol. Less sweet than sugar, mannitol is another form of sugar alcohol that is poorly absorbed by the body. Like sorbitol, it contains fewer calories than sugar but more than most sugar substitutes. Mannitol, too, is considered safe in modest amounts, but large quantities can cause diarrhea.

Xylitol. A sugar alcohol derived from plants, xylitol can be found in chewing gum, toothpaste, candies, and some foods. Considered safe during pregnancy in moderate amounts, it has 40 percent fewer calories than sugar (still, 10 calories per teaspoon) and has been shown to prevent tooth decay—a good reason to grab a stick of xylitol-sweetened gum after meals and snacks when you can't brush.

Erythritol (Swerve). This sweetener is a fermented sugar alcohol that's found in grapes and pears. It has nearly zero calories, is about 70 percent as sweet as table sugar, and can be used in cooking and baking. Studies have shown that this sweetener, like xylitol, also prevents tooth decay. Erythritol is probably safe when you're expecting, but check with your practitioner before you reach for it, since there is limited data on its use during pregnancy.

Stevia (SweetLeaf, Truvia). This zero-calorie sweetener is made from erythritol and the leaf of the stevia plant. Though it's far sweeter than sugar (so you'll have to adjust the amount you use in cooking and baking), it can have a bitter aftertaste. Stevia is believed to be safe during pregnancy, but check with

your practitioner before you dip deeply (again, there's little data on it).

There are plenty of natural sugar substitutes hitting the market (and your coffee) as well. Monk-fruit sweetener (sometimes found in blends with erythritol), BochaSweet, allulose, lactose, Whey Low, agave, and many others are probably safe for use during pregnancy (most are derived from fruits or vegetables), but it doesn't hurt to ask your practitioner for the green light . . . just in case. A check-in with your doctor or dietitian about these sweeteners (and others) is also wise if you have gestational diabetes. Some (like allulose) are calorie-free, while others (like agave) contain even more calories than sugar.

Some Health Foods

Are health foods extra healthy when you're expecting—and super-foods extra super? Most probably are—but as in so many other departments, it's smart to proceed with caution down the health food aisle, browsing this list before you browse those shelves:

Flaxseed. There seems to be a health benefit for everyone in flaxseed (and products made from it), with research linking consumption to a lower risk of diabetes, heart disease, and cancer. And its high level of baby-friendly omega-3 fatty acids makes flaxseed sound like a natural for expectant moms, too—and it probably is. But because it's also a source of phytoestrogens (an estrogen-like substance found naturally in some plants), some practitioners recommend limiting the amount of flax expectant moms consume in oil, seed, or supplement form. Other practitioners say moderate amounts (up to 4 to 6 tablespoons per day) of flax, blended in your smoothie or spooned into your cereal,

Safe Right from the Tap?

Some would say it's the best drink in the house (or the restaurant), especially because it's free. But is tap water safe to drink when you're expecting? Most often, it is. Still, water safety varies from community to community, home to home—and can even vary because of storms or other natural disasters (for instance, flooding can contaminate drinking water), a lapse in oversight, or lax regulations. To find out if you should be drinking the water that flows from your tap (or your community's taps, including those in your favorite restaurants), check with your local water supplier or health department, the Environmental Protection Agency (EPA; epa.gov), or a consumer advocacy group. If there is a possibility that your home's or your community's water supply is unsafe (because of pipe deterioration, a contaminated water source, or proximity to a waste disposal area, or

because of odd taste or color), arrange to have it tested. Your local EPA or health department can tell you how.

If testing reveals that your water contains unsafe contaminants—or if your community has been alerted to system-wide issues—invest in a filter (the kind you get depends on what's in your water) or use bottled water or purified water delivery for drinking and cooking (keep reading for more on bottled water safety). Some potential contaminants: bacteria, microorganisms, chemical or industrial runoff, and pesticides.

Of most concern when you're expecting—and when there are little ones drinking the water in your home and community—is lead, which can leach from lead pipes or be present in the water supply even if your pipes aren't made from lead. High levels of lead in your body can cause serious problems during pregnancy, like

---

are safe and healthy during pregnancy. Unsure whether to reach for the flax or in what amounts? Check with your practitioner.

Hemp. Hemp seed, hemp food products, and hemp seed oil in moderation (1 to 2 servings a day) are probably safe for expectant moms—and a good source of protein, fiber, and fatty acids. But since hemp's use during pregnancy has not been well studied, it makes sense to avoid it in large concentrations (as in a supplement). See the box on page 39 for info on hemp milk.

Chia. Chia seeds are an excellent source of fiber, omega-3 fatty acids, protein, calcium, and iron—but while a sprinkle on a salad, yogurt, or cereal, or in

a smoothie is likely a safe and nutritious bet, check in with your practitioner before you chow down on large amounts of chia. Its safety in pregnancy hasn't been studied.

Spirulina. The pregnancy safety of spirulina (a natural algae powder that's high in protein and calcium and a good source of antioxidants, B vitamins, and other nutrients) also hasn't been established, leading some practitioners to suggest that moms-to-be limit or even avoid using this nutrient-packed powder. It's also sometimes contaminated with toxins, including heavy metals, as well as harmful bacteria—another reason to avoid it during pregnancy. Ditto for a close relative of spirulina: chlorella.

premature birth, low birthweight, and miscarriage. Lead will also cross the placenta and can impact the healthy development of your baby's brain and nervous system. Lead exposure during pregnancy and childhood has also been associated with reduced cognitive function, lower IQ, and increased attention-related behavioral problems. If testing shows lead in your water, switch to bottled water or water that comes from a filtration system certified to reduce or eliminate lead for cooking, drinking, and brushing your teeth. If you use well water, contact the EPA's Safe Drinking Water Hotline at (800) 426-4791 or epa.gov/ground-water-and-drinking-water/safe-drinking-water-information for information on testing your water for lead.

While there's no harm from the small amount of chlorine that's in your tap water (it acts as a disinfectant), the right kind of filter will remove chlorine before it reaches your cup. If your water smells and/or tastes like chlorine, boiling it or letting it stand, uncovered, for 24 hours will allow much of the chemical to evaporate.

Are you always better off—and safer—opening a bottle of water than turning on the tap? The reality is that bottled waters vary a lot, too, with some brands containing more impurities than tap water, and some actually coming directly from a tap before being purified—so much for that "natural spring." Also keep in mind that most bottled water doesn't contain fluoride (it'll say so on the label if it does), a mineral that's vital for growing teeth (your baby's). To check the purity of a particular brand, search for it at NSF International (nsf.org) or check the bottle's label for NSF certification. Also look for bottles that don't contain BPA by checking for the recycling code "1" on the bottom. Avoid distilled water, since the distillation process removes all beneficial minerals.

Raw cacao powder. Made by cold-pressing unroasted cacao beans, raw cacao is high in antioxidants and minerals. Don't confuse it with cocoa powder, which is cacao that's been roasted at high temperatures, effectively killing all the natural enzymes found in the cacao bean. But is mixing it into your morning smoothie or nibbling on cacao nibs safe during pregnancy? While dark chocolate is safe—and even beneficial—during pregnancy, it's less clear whether raw cacao, which contains much higher levels of caffeine and theobromine (a stimulant), is also safe. The jury is still out, but most experts would suggest a path of moderation when it comes to nibbling on those nibs—especially because roasting cacao beans is what destroys harmful bacteria, leaving the raw version susceptible to bacteria and other types of contamination.

Wheat grass. Wheat grass doesn't get a pregnancy pass—not only because there's no proof that it's safe during pregnancy, but because it can be contaminated with bacteria.

Maca. Maca powder may be touted as a fertility enhancer, but without any studies to show its safety during pregnancy, experts say it's best to avoid when you're expecting.

Moringa. This purported super-food comes from a plant native to Africa and India. It's packed with nutrients, but because it acts as a natural form of birth control and may cause the uterus to contract (which could lead to miscarriage), moringa in all forms should be avoided completely during pregnancy.

Already tossed back a few wheatgrass shots or sucked down some spirulina shakes? Not to worry—the potential risks (besides of bacterial infection, but you'd know if you'd developed one of those) haven't been proved, and probably wouldn't apply to average intake anyway.

Some Chemicals

Do you usually run for cover (or at least for the nearest Whole Foods) at the mention of the word "chemical"? If so, you might want to sit back down and continue reading. Not every food that lists chemicals on its ingredients list is necessarily bad (or dangerous) for you, just as not every food that doesn't list any is automatically safe and healthy.

But first, a chemistry lesson. All foods, from garden-variety tomatoes to laboratory-variety tomato-flavored sauces, are made of chemicals. A just-picked, organically grown strawberry, for instance, is composed of (among other chemicals) pelargonidin 3-glucoside, citric acid, malic acid, ellagic acid, auxin, methyl butanoate, ethyl butanoate, butyl ethanoate, methyl hexanoate, ethyl hexanoate, (Z)-3-hexenol, hexanal, (E)-2-hexenal, and (Z)-3-hexenal. How's that for a chemical profile?

Chemical additives found in processed foods are synthesized in the lab from a wide variety of organic and inorganic materials, or extracted from completely natural sources (sodium caseinate from milk, lecithin from soybeans). Some are suspected of being harmful (those that are indisputably proved to be harmful are taken off the market). But the good news is that more are believed to be harmless—and some are even beneficial, such as the chemical ascorbic acid, otherwise known as vitamin C. From what is known right now, potential risk to a developing fetus from chemical additives in the average diet is extremely remote.

Still, many processed foods are far from nutritious—and typically, the greater the number of unpronounceable additives a product contains, the less wholesome it is. Keep that in mind when selecting processed foods. Whenever possible, cook from scratch with fresh ingredients, or use frozen or packaged organic ready-to-eat foods. You'll avoid many questionable additives found in processed foods, and your meals will be more nutritious, too. Whenever you have a choice (and clearly you won't always), choose foods that are free of artificial additives (colorings, flavorings, and preservatives). Read labels to screen for foods that are either additive-free or use natural additives (a cheddar cheese cracker that gets its orange hue from annatto instead of red dye no. 40, and its flavor from real cheese instead of artificial cheese flavoring). For a listing of questionable and safe additives, go to cspinet.org.

What to Skip When You're Expecting

It's only 9 months, but when you're kept apart from your favorite foods and drinks, it can seem like forever (and at least a day). Even when you know that your sacrifice is in the name of a safe pregnancy, played extra safe. Even when

Wine in Dinner?

Hungry for some coq au vin or beer-braised short ribs, but not sure whether the pregnancy alcohol ban carries over from the bar to the stove? Feast away, within reason. Although alcohol does not cook out completely when you add it to a stew or baked dish (the amount of alcohol that actually cooks off depends on how long the food has been cooked; keep reading), the alcohol that remains will not add up to much in the context of a single serving. So unless you're planning to sip 3 cups of sauced sauce, you've got nothing to worry about. To be extra safe, stick to recipes that require cooking times of at least half an hour, avoiding those that expose the alcohol to only passing heat (such as flambeed cherries), or choose alcohol substitutions in your recipes instead (see the box on page 80).

IF YOU BAKE OR SIMMER FOR	THE AMOUNT OF ALCOHOL REMAINING IS
15 minutes	40 percent
30 minutes	35 percent
1 hour	25 percent
1½ hours	20 percent
2 hours	10 percent
2½ hours	5 percent

you're all in (if not super happy) giving up what you shouldn't have. Hopefully, you won't find too many of your favorites on this list of foods and drinks that are tabled when you're expecting, but chances are (sorry!) you'll find a few.

Alcohol

Wine with dinner? Cocktail before? Beer at the barbecue? As you probably already know, total teetotaling during pregnancy is recommended not only by doctors, midwives, and all health organizations, but also by the U.S. surgeon general (in the form of labels plastered on all containers of wine, beer, and other alcoholic beverages). And for good reason. Alcohol crosses the placenta in concentrations almost identical to those in the mother's blood—which means she shares each drink with her baby, and due to baby's tiny size, a higher share proportionately. What's more, it takes a fetus twice as long to eliminate the alcohol from its system. Drinking heavily throughout pregnancy or binge drinking (having 4 or more drinks at a time, even occasionally) can result not only in serious complications of pregnancy, but in fetal alcohol syndrome. This condition produces babies who are born small for gestational age, with facial deformities and with brain damage (which later shows up as tremors, motor development problems, attention deficits, learning disabilities, lower IQ, and possibly other mental deficiencies). But even drinking moderately throughout pregnancy can increase the risk of miscarriage and stillbirth, as well as the risk of developmental and behavioral problems in a child.

Since no "safe" limit of alcohol consumption has been determined—and even occasional light drinking hasn't been completely cleared—you're definitely safest staying on the wagon during your 9 months.

Standing in for the Sauce

Is your kitchen an alcohol-free zone now that you're expecting? Here are some ways to stir comparable flavor into your favorite recipes, without the sauce:

INSTEAD OF	TRY
Amaretto (2 tablespoons)	Almond extract (½ teaspoon)
Beer	Ginger ale or chicken broth
Brandy	Apple cider, apricot juice
Calvados	Apple juice concentrate
Champagne	Ginger ale or sparkling white grape juice
Cognac	Peach, apricot, or pear juice
Dry red wine	Grape or cranberry juice (cut the sweetness with red wine vinegar), or beef broth
Framboise	Raspberry juice
Cassis	Cherry, blueberry, or pomegranate juice
Frangelico	Hazelnut or almond extract
Grand Marnier	Orange juice concentrate; orange marmalade
Kirsch	Raspberry or cherry juice; cider
Port wine (or sweet sherry)	Grape or pomegranate juice
Rum	White grape juice or pineapple juice
Sake	Seasoned rice vinegar
Sherry or bourbon	Vanilla extract; orange or pineapple juice
Vermouth (sweet)	Apple or grape juice
Vermouth (dry)	White grape juice mixed with white wine vinegar
White wine	Chicken broth, diluted cider vinegar, or white wine vinegar

Which doesn't mean that you should worry about the wine, beer, or cocktails you drank before you found out you were expecting. What it does mean is that you should give up alcohol the moment you know you're pregnant (in the best of all possible pregnancy scenarios, you'd give it up when you first start trying to conceive). If you decide to take a very occasional celebratory sip or two, do so with food, which slows the absorption of alcohol into the system. For tips on giving up alcohol, see *What to Expect When You're Expecting.*

Raw Fish and Seafood

You probably knew this was coming—and if you're a raw seafood fan, you've probably already sighed deeply (maybe even cried a little) over the loss of your sushi and oyster bar privileges. Off the menu during pregnancy according to the FDA, EPA, ACOG, and other leading medical authorities: all raw or rare fish and seafood. That includes sashimi and sushi rolls that contain raw fish, fish tartare, carpaccio, or crudo, raw oysters, clams, and other seafood, as well as any fish or seafood that's served "seared" or "rare" but not cooked through (as salmon, tuna, and scallops often are). Why this rule? It's to protect pregnant women from bacteria, viruses, parasites, and other microscopic organisms that can cause infections, from food poisoning to hepatitis, if they're not killed by thorough cooking (and yes, anyone can get sick from eating raw fish or seafood, but pregnant women are at extra risk when they do). Marinating fish and seafood (say, in ceviche or poke) or dipping it in even the hottest of hot sauce doesn't kill those organisms, so those preps don't offer protection. Even pregnancy-safe varieties of fish (see page 72) should be cooked until they easily flake with a fork and reach the appropriate temperature (145°F). Seafood should be cooked through and firm.

Smoked and Cured Fish

Refrigerated smoked seafood—such as salmon, trout, whitefish, cod, tuna, or mackerel—most often labeled as "kippered," "smoked," "nova-style," "lox," or "jerky"—are also off the menu when you're expecting, because they can harbor the pregnancy-dangerous bacteria Listeria. Ditto, salt-cured fish (aka gravlax), pickled fish, or cured fish that

---

Champagne Dreams and Caviar Wishes

Champagne is definitely off the menu when you're expecting, but what about caviar? As with raw fish, there's a risk that caviar may be contaminated with Listeria. You can avoid that risk by picking pasteurized caviar.

---

isn't cooked or heated to a high enough temperature to kill Listeria (145°F). Happily, you can cook away bacterial risk in a piping-hot casserole, quiche, or omelet. You can also safely serve up canned or jarred shelf-stable smoked fish and seafood, as well as fish that's cooked thoroughly to the proper temperature while it is being smoked (grilled or baked with smoke chips or on a wood plank).

Unpasteurized/Raw Cheese and Dairy Products

Pasteurization is a form of food processing that's actually good for you and your baby, safely destroying bacteria in dairy products and juice without destroying nutrients. And it comes in very handy when it comes to certain soft cheeses—fresh mozzarella, feta, brie, blue cheese (Roquefort, for instance), camembert, soft Mexican-style cheese—since these can be contaminated with Listeria, a particularly dangerous bacteria (see the box on the following page). If you see a hunk of cheese or a carton of milk that's marked "raw" or doesn't say "pasteurized" on the label, pass it by. Domestic varieties of cheese are more likely to be pasteurized than imported

Listeria Alert

What's this you hear about eating your cold cuts hot now that you're pregnant? And skipping the feta on your Greek salad (unless you're positive it's pasteurized)? And cooking your smoked fish? These pregnancy diet restrictions may seem random—and unfair—but they're actually designed to protect you and your unborn baby from Listeria, a harmful bacteria that can cause listeriosis. This serious illness is particularly dangerous for pregnant women, for a couple of reasons. One, because expectant moms are about 20 times more likely than other healthy adults to contract listeriosis, due to the normal immune suppression of pregnancy. And two, because listeriosis can lead to premature delivery, miscarriage, or serious illness in a developing baby. And, unlike other bacteria, Listeria enters the bloodstream directly and can get to the baby quickly. Though the overall risk of contracting listeriosis is extremely low—even in pregnancy—the potential of it causing problems in pregnancy is higher, which is why you should avoid unpasteurized juice, unpasteurized dairy, raw or undercooked meat, fish, shellfish, poultry, or eggs, unheated deli meats, hot dogs, or smoked fish, and unwashed raw vegetables and salad.

For more information, visit the FDA Center for Food Safety and Applied Nutrition at foodsafety.gov or the Centers for Disease Control and Prevention at cdc.gov/foodsafety.

---

ones are, but always check the label to be certain. If you're not sure whether a soft cheese is pasteurized, don't eat it unless it's cooked until bubbling. All pasteurized dairy products are safe to eat when you're expecting—including mozzarella, feta, blue, or brie (again, just look for the "pasteurized" label). Processed cheeses, cream cheese, cottage cheese, and yogurt are also safe bets, as long as they're not made from raw milk. What about hard cheeses, like parmesan? Due to their much lower moisture content, hard cheeses are far less likely to be contaminated with Listeria, even if they're made with raw milk. Still, with so many pasteurized cheeses available, why take any risk?

Raw Eggs

Overly uneasy about your over-easy eggs? Wondering whether it's safe to poach a taste of your partner's eggs Benedict at brunch? You're wise to be wary. Raw and undercooked eggs may be contaminated with salmonella, which means it's best to avoid raw eggs and runny eggs in all forms—soft poached, sunny-side up with runny yolks, soft boiled. Skip raw eggs in salad dressings (try one of the Caesar salad dressing recipes on page 263 instead of a traditional one). Don't eat homemade foods that contain raw eggs, including ice cream, mayonnaise, hollandaise, eggnog, cookie dough, and cake batter—even if it's finger-licking good. Same for whipped-up desserts that won't be cooked (like mousse). Store-bought versions of these foods are usually safe to eat, since they're typically made with pasteurized eggs, but when in doubt, pass it up. Pasteurized eggs (and egg whites) can also be bought for home use, and are safe to use raw in prepared foods (including that classic Caesar) or to serve undercooked. Restaurants may use these in their recipes, too—but also may

Try These Instead

What happens if your pregnancy cravings get in the way of sensible and safe eating? Not to worry. There are many ways to safely satisfy those yearnings—even when they're for foods you're supposed to be steering clear of. Try these sensible substitutions:

INSTEAD OF	TRY
Sushi with raw fish	Rolls made with cooked fish or vegetables
Raw shellfish	Steamed or boiled shellfish
Swordfish	Roasted or grilled halibut
Deli turkey	Fresh roasted turkey
Salad dressing with raw eggs	Substitute mayo or avocado or use pasteurized eggs in the dressing
Raw sprouts	Shaved carrots or cucumbers
Store-bought fresh-squeezed juice (unpasteurized)	Juice squeezed or juiced at home

not. Get the all clear from the kitchen before sampling the house Caesar or hollandaise.

Raw or Rare Meats

Sorry, rare-meat lovers—it's time to change your order to medium (at a minimum). That's because undercooked meats can harbor microorganisms that can make you sick. Any raw meat, including tartare and carpaccio, is considered unsafe during pregnancy. Smoked meat is also considered unsafe (see below). See page 183 for more info on safe meat prep.

Deli Meat

Ready-to-eat doesn't always mean safe-to-eat when you're expecting. Case in point: All deli meat, salami, sausages, prosciutto, pepperoni, chorizo, and paté, and other charcuterie should be heated until steaming. That's to protect against the dangerous bacteria Listeria. Same goes for ready-to-eat hot dogs (they're not ready for you to eat until you heat them up) and all types of smoked or cured (not cooked) meats. Even meat jerky may expose you to harmful bacteria unless it's heated first. Not loving the idea of hot cold cuts or steaming jerky? Nobody does—but it's safer than going cold (smoked) turkey and risking infection. Fresh roasted meat (like that fresh roasted turkey, fresh roast beef, or pork loin) is safe to eat cold.

Another reason to steer clear of smoked or cured meats such as bacon, ham, cured pork, sausage, dried beef, luncheon meats, salami, and hot dogs (as well as smoked fish): They often contain nitrates. Nitrates are used as a preservative in processed meats (actually keeping the amount of bacteria down).

Now You Tell Me

Does this chapter have you stressed about all the things you'd have done differently if only you'd known? Like sucking down that sake (and that huge plate of sashimi) 2 days before the pregnancy test came back positive? Ordering a cold sub before reading the section on deli meat risks? Tossing down a Caesar salad before realizing the dressing was made with raw eggs?

Relax. Most women have at least a few expectant encounters with food or drink that isn't considered fit for pregnant consumption (especially before they find out they're expecting)—some have many. In the vast (very, very vast) majority of cases, there's no harm done. For instance, sushi and sashimi only rarely contain organisms that cause illness, ditto deli meat. So use this chapter as a guide to making your pregnancy diet as safe as you can make it from now on—but don't use it to drive yourself crazy about the food and drink that's already behind you.

But they can be converted in your stomach to nitrites or nitrosamines, powerful carcinogens—something you don't want at any time during your life, and especially not when you're pregnant.

Raw Sprouts

Raw sprouts (including alfalfa, clover, radish, and mung bean sprouts) may look pretty (and pretty healthy) on top of your salad or stuffed into your wrap, but what's not pretty is the bacteria they may harbor. Sprouts have sometimes been linked to outbreaks of E. coli, Listeria, and salmonella and, unfortunately, should be avoided when you're pregnant. So, no sprouts for your little sprout when you're expecting. That is, unless you cook them through (and from a taste and texture perspective, hot sprouts aren't so hot). And while you're playing it safe on your salad or sandwich, it makes sense to stay away from microgreens, too, which may be cross-contaminated.

Raw Juice

Before you belly up to the juice bar or apple cider stand—consider this: Raw (unpasteurized) juice or drinks or smoothies made from it can be contaminated with bacteria like Listeria (see the box on page 82) and should be off the menu when you're expecting. Make sure all the juice you drink is pasteurized, unless you squeeze it or juice it yourself from washed produce.

Kombucha

Seems like everybody's sipping kombucha these days, but it's probably best for pregnant women to take a pass on this health food trend. Kombucha, a fermented drink made with tea, sugar, bacteria, and yeast, can cause stomach upset in some new drinkers, something no mom-to-be needs more of. Unpasteurized kombucha (particularly home-brewed varieties) can be contaminated with harmful bacteria. What's more, some kombuchas contain alcohol (clearly a no-go when you're expecting).

CHAPTER 6

Gaining for Two: Baby and You

....

Maybe you've spent half your life trying to lose weight—chasing a goal that you've never managed to reach. Or you've been happily hovering at about the same weight for years, give or take a few holiday pounds. Or you've yo-yoed your way up and down the scales, and have a closet full of jean sizes to prove it. Or maybe you've always wished you could add a little more to your bottom line, especially around your bottom. Maybe you're at peace with your weight, maybe you fluctuate between embracing it and battling it.

Whatever your relationship with your weight, there's one thing for sure: It's time for change. Your weight, wherever it is, will likely be on the upswing now that you're expecting. A healthy weight gain is a key ingredient in the making of a healthy pregnancy and a healthy baby. So get ready to get gaining for two . . . baby and you.

How Much to Gain?

Are you fully over the moon at finally having a fully legit reason to pile on the pounds (you're pregnant!)? Or are you a bit unnerved at the thought of watching the numbers on the scale creep upward, even though you know they're supposed to? Or maybe you've never been a scale watcher, and plan to take pregnancy weight gain equally in stride. You're probably still wondering just how much weight you should plan on gaining over the next 9 months. After all, you've heard of women gaining as few as 20 pounds and as many as 70 . . . or even more. What's the right gain plan for you?

Calculating Your BMI

Weight alone doesn't tell the whole story—for a better bottom line assessment, your practitioner will also take a look at body mass index, or BMI. Your BMI is a calculation of your weight in relation to your height. Though when used alone it doesn't necessarily give a full picture of your actual body fat amount or overall fitness, BMI is often used as a starting point for determining whether a person is underweight, average weight, overweight, or obese. Doctors and midwives typically use the measurement as the basis for weight-gain recommendations during pregnancy.

You can easily calculate (at least, using a calculator) your BMI using the following formula: [Weight (in pounds) ÷ height (in inches squared)^2] × 703.

For example, a woman who is 5 feet 5 inches tall and weighs 145 pounds will have a BMI of 24.1, based on the following equation:

First, figure out the inches:
5 feet 5 inches = 65 inches

Next, square 65 (multiply it by itself):
65 × 65 = 4,225 inches

Then divide the weight by the inches:
145 ÷ 4,225 = 0.0343

BMI (kg/m^2)	18	19	20	21	22	23	24	25	26	27	
Height (in.)						Weight (lb.)					
58	87	91	96	100	105	110	115	119	124	129	
59	90	94	99	104	109	114	119	124	128	133	
60	93	97	102	107	112	118	123	128	133	138	
61	96	100	106	111	116	122	127	132	137	143	
62	99	104	109	115	120	126	131	136	142	147	
63	102	107	113	118	124	130	135	141	146	152	
64	105	110	116	122	128	134	140	145	151	157	
65	109	114	120	126	132	138	144	150	156	162	
66	112	118	124	130	136	142	148	155	161	167	
67	115	121	127	134	140	146	153	159	166	172	
68	119	125	131	138	144	151	158	164	171	177	
69	122	128	135	142	149	155	162	169	176	182	
70	126	132	139	146	153	160	167	174	181	188	
71	130	136	143	150	157	165	172	179	186	193	
72	133	140	147	154	162	169	177	184	191	199	
73	137	144	151	159	166	174	182	189	197	204	
74	141	148	155	163	171	179	186	194	202	210	
75	145	152	160	168	176	184	192	200	208	216	
76	148	156	164	172	180	189	197	205	213	221	

And multiply the result by 703:
0.0343 × 703 = 24.1

Once you've calculated your BMI (or, if you don't want to do the math, just check the chart below), you can determine the category you fall into:

- If your BMI is less than 18.5, you're considered underweight.
- If your BMI is between 18.5 and 24.9, you're considered average weight.
- If your BMI is between 25 and 29.9, you're considered overweight.
- If your BMI is greater than 30, you're considered obese.

28	29	30	35	40
134	138	143	167	191
138	143	148	173	198
143	148	153	179	204
148	153	158	185	211
153	158	164	191	218
158	163	169	197	225
163	169	174	204	232
168	174	180	210	240
173	179	186	216	247
178	185	191	223	255
184	190	197	230	262
189	196	203	236	270
195	202	207	243	278
200	208	215	250	286
206	213	221	258	294
212	219	227	265	302
218	225	233	272	311
224	232	240	279	319
230	238	246	287	328

Since every pregnant woman—and every pregnancy—is different, one answer to that question doesn't fit all. Just how many pounds you should put on during pregnancy depends on a number of factors, including your height and your weight before you conceived. Your practitioner will probably recommend an ideal weight gain, possibly based on your body mass index (BMI, see the box on these pages).

- If your BMI is average—or close enough—you'll probably be advised to gain between 25 and 35 pounds (the weight-gain total recommended for an average-weight pregnant woman).

- If your BMI is well below average, meaning that you're considerably underweight, you may be advised to gain a little—or a lot—extra, about 28 to 40 pounds, which will compensate for the fat stores you don't have.

- If your BMI classifies you as overweight, you may be advised to gain between 15 and 25 pounds (because you'll have some extra fat stores to tap into).

- If you're obese, you may be told to limit your gain to about 11 to 20 pounds, or perhaps less. This may help you prevent some of the pregnancy complications related to obesity, such as gestational diabetes or having a too-big baby.

- Got twins (or more) on board? The weight recommendations differ for you. See page 101 for more.

Ideal recommendations aside, how much you actually gain—and how quickly you gain it—will depend on your metabolism, a little bit of genetics, your level of activity, and, of course, how many calories you consume. Take in more calories than your body needs to fuel baby making and other activities (like exercise), and you'll likely gain more than recommended. Take in too few calories (or burn too many through exercise), and you'll gain less weight than you should. More about those weight-gain equations—and how to help get yours to add up in your favor and your baby's—later.

Gaining Weight at the Right Rate

Now you know about how much weight you should plan to gain over the next 9 months. But how quickly should you plan to gain it? A little at a time? In bigger chunks? Does it really matter how fast or slowly you pack on the pounds if you end up packing on just the right number?

Actually, it does matter. Slow and steady wins the pregnancy weight-gain race hands down, and here's why. For your baby, who's constantly growing, a continuous supply of nutrients and energy guarantees the fuel necessary for that epic growth. Not surprisingly, the bigger baby gets, the more fuel your baby-making factory will require. So while a skimpy first trimester weight gain (or even a loss, if mom's having trouble eating or keeping food down) won't slow down a still teensy-tiny baby's growth, gaining too little weight in the second and third trimesters might leave a bigger baby's growing needs unmet.

But it's not just your baby who stands to gain from a well-paced weight gain—you do, too. Your body will have an easier time adjusting to the extra pounds if they're added gradually—which could mean, among other perks, less strain, fewer aches and pains, and possibly even fewer stretch marks (after

Recommended Rate of Weight Gain

BMI	Average Weekly Weight Gain per Week During Second and Third Trimester	Total Weight Gain
Underweight (BMI less than 18.5)	Slightly more than 1 pound per week	28 to 40 pounds
Normal weight (BMI 18.5 to 24.9)	Approximately 1 pound per week	25 to 35 pounds
Overweight (BMI 25 to 29.9)	Approximately ⅔ pound per week	15 to 25 pounds
Obese (BMI greater than 30)	Approximately ½ pound per week	11 to 20 pounds

Weight Check Do's and Don'ts

DO follow your practitioner's recommendation for weight gain. It'll be tailored to your individual needs.

DO check with your practitioner if you gain more than 3 pounds in any single week in the second trimester or if you gain more than 2 pounds in any week in the third trimester, especially if it doesn't seem related to overeating. Too much sudden and unexplained weight gain can indicate a pregnancy problem, such as preeclampsia.

DO check with your practitioner if you gain no weight for more than 2 weeks in a row during months 4 through 8. Also check in if you lose a significant amount of weight at any time during your pregnancy (don't worry if it's just a few pounds). While a little weight loss isn't uncommon in the first trimester (especially if you've been throwing up a lot), a greater than 5 percent weight loss can signal hyperemesis gravidarum (severe nausea and vomiting during pregnancy) or other pregnancy complication.

DON'T try to lose weight or try to keep yourself from gaining weight (unless your doctor has advised you to), either by undercutting needed calories or overdoing exercise. A healthy pregnancy and a healthy baby require a healthy weight gain.

DON'T obsess about the numbers. Keep an eye on your weight gain to make sure you're hitting your practitioner-recommended weight-gain goal, but don't lose sight of your most important goal: nourishing your growing baby. Remember, if your doctor or midwife is content with your weight gain, you should be, too.

---

all, gradual weight gain allows skin to keep pace, so that stretching is gradual and less likely to leave as many marks). A slow and steady gain may also lead to a somewhat speedier postdelivery return to your prepregnancy shape.

Keep in mind that a steady pace doesn't mean spreading your recommended weight gain evenly over 40 weeks of pregnancy. Early on in the pregnancy game, with baby as light as a grain of rice, weight gain can be light, too—about 2 to 4 pounds in the first trimester usually gets the job done. In fact, gaining nothing at all (or even losing some pounds because of nagging nausea and frequent vomiting) won't impact baby's development or eventual bottom line. But as baby's (and pregnancy's) needs grow, so should mom. In the average pregnancy, weight gain should pick up to a rate of about 1 to 1½ pounds per week in months 4 through 6 (for a total of about 12 to 14 pounds), then drop off again in the last 3 months to a pound or even less per week (for a total of about 8 to 10 pounds). In the home stretch of the ninth month, however, mom's weight gain typically tapers off. Some moms gain only a pound or two during the entire last month, while others even lose weight during the final weeks of pregnancy.

Will every mom-to-be follow this model formula precisely? Far from it. Some moms start off with a bang (adding 10 or more pounds in the first trimester, instead of just a few), then slow down to a more reasonable weight-gain rate as the weeks pass (and as they realize that they might be taking the phrase "eating for two" just a little too literally). Others may be too queasy to add an ounce, but do a good job of catching up once meals start staying down. Even a woman who eats with an eye on the scale right from the start will find the numbers fluctuating a little (maybe it's a ½-pound gain one week in the second trimester, 1½ pounds the next week). As long as your overall gain stays approximately on target, and your rate of gain averages out pretty close to the model formula (without any long lulls, huge dips, or giant jumps), you're in good shape. Literally.

One reason why weight gain tends to fluctuate so much during pregnancy is that appetite fluctuates, too. Your hunger will come in peaks, valleys, and plateaus, and so will your food intake. You'll have periods of below-average appetite (most common in the first few months, when nausea nips hunger in the bud, and again in the last month or two, when heartburn rules and tummy room starts to run out). And you'll have periods of above-average appetite (typically spurred on by baby's growth spurts). Moms-to-be often enter the "hunger zone" somewhere around weeks 12 to 14 as the queasy cloud lifts, aversions clear up, and appetite starts to soar. Follow those hunger pangs to the fridge—they're nature's way of ensuring you're eating enough to fuel your growing baby's needs.

Carrying more than one baby? You'll need to pack on more total pounds, and your rate of gain will reflect that. See page 101 for more.

The Downside of Too Little Weight Gain

Many moms-to-be sweat the numbers when the pounds are adding up too fast. But what if the numbers on the scale aren't moving up at all, or are even creeping down—is that cause for concern, too? It's not a worry in the first trimester, when it's common to lose weight (or not gain any at all). But weight loss or lack of weight gain that continues into the second and third trimesters is a red flag. In fact, the risks of gaining too little weight can outweigh the risks of gaining too much weight, and for an average-weight woman, there can be a significant downside to continued below-average weight gain. The risks include:

Preterm delivery. Moms-to-be who don't gain enough weight throughout pregnancy are at an increased risk of delivering too soon, especially if they came into pregnancy underweight or even average weight. Full-term babies are more likely to arrive healthy than preemies, so gaining enough weight during pregnancy can pay dividends not only in a more safely timed delivery, but in a healthier bundle at birth.

Low birthweight for baby. Gaining too little weight during pregnancy can keep your baby from gaining enough, restricting growth and sometimes resulting in a low birthweight (aka small for gestational age, or SGA). Very small babies are at an increased risk of complications and health problems at birth and beyond. Keep in mind, however, that not all cases of SGA are caused by a mom-to-be gaining too little weight—there are also genetic, environmental, fetal, and health factors that can contribute to a low birthweight.

Working Through Weighty Issues

Does the thought of gaining weight during pregnancy (even if it's for the benefit of your baby-to-be) make you shudder—and then reach for the celery sticks instead of the cheese and crackers? You're not alone. Many women—especially those who've experienced eating disorders (see the box on page 102) and/or body image issues, even mild ones—become unsettled, unnerved, anxious, even panicked at the thought of adding any pounds, anywhere, anytime. But now's the time to work through weight phobia (and any persistent body image issues)—before it can have a negative impact on your pregnancy and your growing baby. Remind yourself often: Pregnancy weight is both healthy and beautiful. Also, remember: You're not losing your body—you're gaining a healthy baby (and besides, your body is still yours, even as it's being used for the awesome purpose of nourishing a pregnancy, and later, to breastfeed). And most important, remember who you're gaining weight for. Your gain is baby's gain—literally. As long as you stick pretty close to the recommended weight-gain guidelines, each and every ounce you put on has a purpose in pregnancy—nourishing that beautiful baby of yours. And that's something to celebrate.

The Downside of Too Much Weight Gain

It's clear why gaining too little weight while you're pregnant can hamper your baby's growth and development, as well as the health of your pregnancy. But piling on far too many pounds may present its own set of problems. Many of the problems are mommy-centric, affecting the mom-to-be, her health, and her comfort (make that, her discomfort), while putting her pregnancy at greater risk. Expectant moms who gain much more than the recommended amount of weight during pregnancy may be at risk for:

An uncomfortable pregnancy. Pregnancy complaints multiply with the pounds. Excessive weight gain can be a contributing factor to just about every discomfort of pregnancy, from backaches to fatigue, leg pain to varicose veins, heartburn to hemorrhoids, breathlessness to joint pain.

Labor and delivery complications. As a general (if not inevitable) rule, the heavier mom is before pregnancy and the heavier she gets during pregnancy, the heavier baby gets. Not surprisingly, bigger babies have a harder time exiting the traditional way than do ones of average size, increasing the chance that a cesarean delivery may be necessary and increasing the chances of labor complications (such as excessive bleeding).

Weight that lasts. A woman who gains more weight than recommended during pregnancy tends to hold on to more

Where Does All the Weight Go?

With the average bundle of joy weighing in at about 7 to 8 pounds, there's definitely more to pregnancy weight gain than baby's weight. In fact, a lot more—for an average-weight woman, upward of 28 pounds more. All of these extra pounds (even the ones slated for places you may wish they weren't headed) serve one of two important purposes: baby making (during pregnancy) or baby feeding (after delivery). Adding to that final bottom line will be pounds allocated to baby-making materials (including the growing placenta), maternal fat stores (these are the ones your body will use to fuel baby's growth during pregnancy and produce breast milk after delivery), extra breast tissue (clearly, earmarked for milk production), and the expanded blood volume pregnancy requires. And while baby will be a lightweight through most of the action, he or she will double in size during the last trimester (happily, you won't).

Although the numbers vary from mom to mom, this is how those pounds may add up:

Baby:	7 to 8 pounds
Breast enlargement:	1 to 3 pounds
Placenta:	1½ pounds
Enlargement of uterus:	2 pounds
Amniotic fluid:	2 pounds
Your extra blood:	3 to 4 pounds
Your body's extra fat:	6 to 8 pounds
Your body's extra fluids:	2 to 3 pounds
Average total weight:	30 pounds

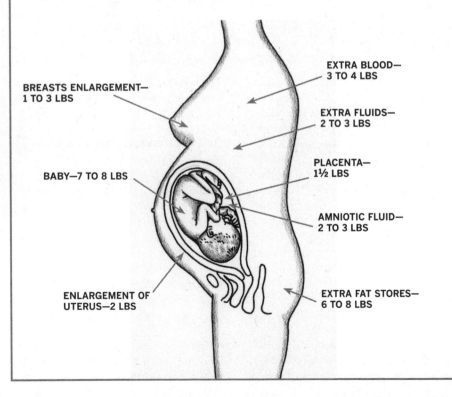

EXTRA BLOOD—
3 TO 4 LBS

BREASTS ENLARGEMENT—
1 TO 3 LBS

EXTRA FLUIDS—
2 TO 3 LBS

BABY—7 TO 8 LBS

PLACENTA—
1½ LBS

AMNIOTIC FLUID—
2 TO 3 LBS

ENLARGEMENT OF
UTERUS—2 LBS

EXTRA FAT STORES—
6 TO 8 LBS

weight afterward—an average of 10 to 20 pounds that she's not likely to end up shedding. That extra weight may set her up for a variety of potential health problems later in life, including hypertension, diabetes, stroke, and heart disease.

Complications in future pregnancies. You may not be thinking ahead to another pregnancy, but here's something to think about during this one. Gaining too much weight in a first pregnancy ups the chances of gaining too much weight in a subsequent pregnancy—again increasing the risks of complications. Another minus to adding on too many pounds in this pregnancy: Data shows women in general are statistically likely to gain weight between pregnancies—a factor that adds risks (of gestational diabetes, pregnancy-induced hypertension, preeclampsia, cesarean delivery, preterm birth, and more) to a next pregnancy.

When a mom who has already accumulated extra pounds from her previous pregnancy gains more weight between pregnancies, she's further increasing her risks of a complicated next pregnancy.

Complications for baby. Babies born to moms who have gained too much weight during pregnancy are at a higher risk of being born overweight (LGA, or large for gestational age). Having a bigger bundle of joy sounds like a good thing—but LGA puts a baby at risk for birth injuries such as shoulder dystocia (when baby's shoulders get stuck inside mom's pelvis during delivery) and collarbone fractures (from having a hard time making it out of the birth canal), hypoglycemia (low blood sugar), respiratory distress, and low Apgar scores. Extra-large babies are also at increased risk of being overweight or obese and/or developing diabetes during childhood and beyond.

Weighing In

Let's face it. Many women have a complicated relationship with the scale—whether it's love/hate, all hate, or can't live with/can't live without. While some end up making peace with their scale (or at least de-escalating to something of a frenemy status), few become besties with it. Even fewer actually look forward to stepping on a scale, whether in the privacy of their bathroom or in front of a health care professional. And for some women, the scale represents painful, very real struggles with body image and eating issues that can bubble up big-time during pregnancy, when vital weight gain has the numbers on the scale edging up.

Fortunately, weighing yourself daily during pregnancy isn't necessary—or even the most effective way of tracking your pregnancy weight gain. Your weight can fluctuate too much from day to day, depending on how much you've eaten, how much water you've retained (from that pickle juice chaser, for instance), and whether you've moved your bowels (or how long it's been since you've pooped). And if you have a really uneasy relationship with your scale, stepping on it too often can sabotage your best intentions to gain the weight you should.

On the other hand, waiting too long between weigh-ins can also undermine

Plot Your Weight Gain

As you'll find out, keeping track of anything when you're expecting becomes a challenge. That's why it may help to write down your weight gain as you go (or input it digitally on the What to Expect app weight-gain tracker). Weigh yourself every week or two if you have a scale at home (or use your monthly weight check from your prenatal appointment). Then plot your gain using this graph. First, locate the number of weeks along you are in your pregnancy at the bottom of the graph. Then find your weight gain in pounds along the left side of the graph. Make a dot where the pounds meet the weeks. Play "connect the dots" to watch your curve as you add those beautiful pregnancy curves. Or let the What to Expect app do the tracking for you.

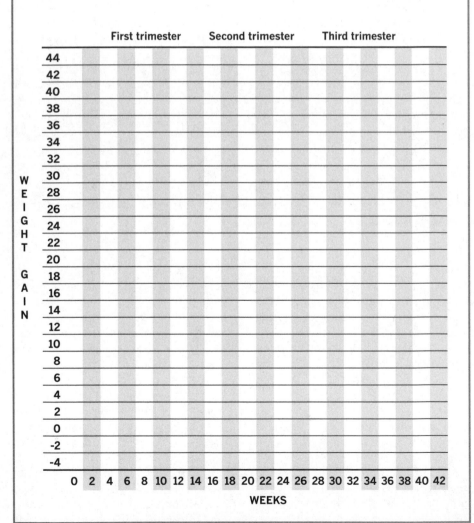

Eating for Two After Weight-Loss Surgery

Lost a lot of weight after bariatric surgery—and now you're gaining a baby? That's plenty of good news already, and there's even more to celebrate: Your weight loss has increased your chances of having a healthy pregnancy and a healthy baby, plus decreased your risk for gestational diabetes, preeclampsia, and having a too-big baby.

Still, there are some extra precautions you'll have to take as a mom-to-be who's had weight-loss surgery:

- Watch your weight. Keeping an eye on the scale is nothing new to you—but since your weight-loss surgery, you've likely become accustomed to (and proud of!) watching the numbers go down. Now that you're growing a baby, those numbers will have to start inching up so you can reach (without overshooting) the weight-gain goal recommended by your practitioner. Keep in mind that there's an increased chance of having a too-small baby after bariatric surgery, but that gaining the right number of pounds can help ensure a healthy bottom line for your baby at birth. On the flip side, gaining too few pounds or too many can add unnecessary risks.

- Get those vital vitamins. Something else you're used to since your bariatric surgery: taking vitamin supplements to fill in nutritional blanks left by restricted food intake and post-surgery malabsorption issues. Your prenatal vitamin is a good place to start when filling in those blanks, but you'll probably need even more iron, calcium, folic acid, vitamin A, and especially vitamin B_{12} than a standard pregnancy formula can provide. Be sure to discuss your specific supplement needs with both your prenatal practitioner and your surgeon.

- Focus on high-quality eating. Your stomach space has been downsized by your weight-loss surgery, making eating for two already somewhat more challenging—and more challenging still when your uterus and baby start to grow, crowding out your already small stomach. Since the quantity of food you can comfortably eat is limited, you'll need to focus on quality: foods that efficiently pack the most nutrients into the smallest volume (see page 27 for more).

those best weight-gain intentions. Step on the scale just once a month at your regular prenatal visits and you might find you've lost a pound when you should have gained 4—or that you've gained 10 pounds instead of 4. Either scenario could throw your total off target, but could also spell extra risks if it's a trend that's not reversed.

That's why, at least for most pregnant women, a once-a-week (or once-every-other-week) weigh-in is the best way to go—so you can keep your eye on your weight gain without obsessing over it. If you feel compelled to step on the scale every day, record a week's worth of weigh-ins, then add them up and divide by 7 to calculate your average weight for the week. Compare that number to last week's bottom line to see how much you've gained week to week. This figure will give you a more accurate picture of your progress. And no matter how often you weigh yourself, make sure you

Look the Other Way

If you're the type to obsess about your weight gain (and you know who you are), make a conscious effort not to. Don't weigh yourself every week. Don't plot your weight gain on the graph in this chapter or on an app. Don't even peek at the scale at your practitioner's visits—and ask the nurse not to say the number out loud. If your doctor or midwife is satisfied with your weight progress, you should be, too.

do it at about the same time and under approximately the same conditions each day (before breakfast, for instance—naked, or with the same amount of clothing). Also, remember: Your results (from scale to scale) may vary—so comparing your weight on your bathroom scale against your weight on the doctor's scale won't be helpful, and it could add up to unnecessary stress. Compare weights only on the same scale.

Keep in mind, too, that even weight gain that's right on target rarely comes in precisely packaged installments (⅐ of a pound a day, 1 pound a week, 4 pounds a month, 8 pounds over 2 months). Instead, it'll average out over time: 2 pounds one week, ½ pound the next week, 1 pound the following, and so on. Three pounds in month 5, 5 pounds in month 6. Don't forget, either, that there's a pretty wide range to aim for (in the case of average-weight women, a 10-pound spread of 25 to 35 pounds), which allows even more weight-gain wiggle room.

If You're Gaining Too Fast

How can you tell if you're gaining too much or too fast? Some research suggests that the first trimester gain is key: If you find you've piled on more than 3 pounds at that 12-week milestone (2 pounds if you're overweight, 5 pounds if you're underweight), you may need to watch your eating (and your scale) more closely to keep those numbers from rising out of the recommended range. But even a mom-to-be who ends her first trimester with a considerably higher net—and many women do, often because nausea leads them to reach for box after box, bag after bag, and carton after carton of comforting carbs—can finish up her pregnancy well within healthy weight-gain limits. Which is why most practitioners won't sweat a slightly greater weight gain in the first trimester, especially if a mom-to-be is generally eating well.

If you and your practitioner do decide it's smart to slow down a weight gain that's been on the fast track, these tips can help:

- Curb your calories. Okay, you've probably heard this one before: too many calories in, too many pounds on. Though cutting calories to lose weight is never a good idea when you're pregnant, curbing calories to curb excess weight gain may be—particularly if your practitioner has recommended that you slow down your rate of gain. Apply some simple, calorie-cutting strategies, aimed at delivering the most nutrition for the fewest calories. Sub fat-free milk,

Already Reached Your Limit?

Nowhere near the pregnancy finish line, but you've already reached your pregnancy weight-gain goal—and don't want to exceed it? Unfortunately, slamming the brakes on your weight gain now may not be a smart strategy. You may feel like you're finished growing, but your little one still has lots of growing to do—and needs a steady supply of calories and other nutrients to keep that growing going all the way to delivery day, courtesy of your womb service. Keep in mind, too, that while you're winding down pregnancy-wise (or at least, starting to feel like you're over it), baby has plenty more to do to get ready for birth. Calcium is being laid down in those baby bones (which means you need to keep drinking that milk or eating that cheese and yogurt).

Baby's developing brain, eyes, and nerves are working overtime—work that requires plenty of healthy fats, especially omega-3 fatty acids. Baby also has a number of pounds to add to his or her bottom line—which means you do, too. Cut back too much on calories in the last weeks of pregnancy, and you could cut into baby's growth potential.

But that doesn't mean you can't slow down your weight gain some, especially since it's been on the fast track up until now. Check with your practitioner to come up with a revised weight-gain goal. And as you close in on the end of pregnancy, eat as efficiently as you can to ensure you're getting the most nutrients for the calories you take in (and follow the other tips on page 27).

yogurt, and cottage cheese for whole or reduced-fat, bake your fries, dole out ¼ cup of pistachios instead of munching straight from the bag (and possibly polishing off the bag), add fresh or freeze-dried strawberries to your cereal instead of raisins, take the skin off your chicken.

■ Cut that fat. Some fat is essential in your pregnancy diet, but too much can add those pounds faster than you can say "Extra Value Meal." Try eating one less serving (1 tablespoon) of fat to see if that puts the brakes on your runaway gain. If it doesn't, trim another serving. Keep in mind that fat takes a variety of forms besides straight-up oil, mayo, butter, and nondairy butter alternatives. Pay attention to sources that may slip by unnoticed (those in the salad dressing, the sautéed scampi, the fried eggs). One easy way

to reduce fat in cooking? Use nonstick cooking oil sprays or a sprayer filled with oil to spritz instead of pouring. Another way: Choose low-fat preparations whenever you can (roast, bake, poach, steam, or grill instead of fry).

■ Be a mindful eater. Can't figure out where all the pounds are coming from? Paying close attention to your eating may help you solve that weight-gain mystery. Eating while distracted (when you're working, catching up on social media, watching TV) can lead to eating more than you should, intended to, or even end up noticing. Like that bowl of M&M's you went deep into while you were deep in a client presentation (wait, wasn't everyone eating them?). Or that whole bag of chips you polished off while checking your WTE app (when you really meant to stop at a handful). Instead of

Fighting the Fat with Fact

Myth: Foods that are labeled "fat-free" are a better choice when you're trying not to gain too much weight.

Fact: Do fat-free cookies sound too good to be true? That's because they often are. That fat-free banner may seem like an invitation to reach the bottom of the box or bag, but eater beware: Being free of fat doesn't make a product free of calories. In fact, manufacturing a palatable product while taking out the fat typically requires adding other ingredients that can add up in calories but usually don't add up nutritionally. In fact, these products can score extra low on the nutrition scale. So watch portion size, and for a moderate weight gain, eat any processed foods—even the "fat-free" ones—in moderation. Incidentally, the same can be said for many "sugar-free" foods: What's free of sugar may be full of calories from a variety of other sources.

Myth: "Low-carb" foods aren't fattening, so you can eat as many as you like.

Fact: Turns out there really is no such thing as a free lunch—or, in this case, a free bag of chips, candy bar, or cheesecake. Truth is, many products labeled "low-carb" are highly processed, high in fat, and high in calories—definitely not a dieter's dream come true. What's more, low-carb products aren't designed for pregnant women, who need carbs in their diet. Another reason to step away from the low-carb section of your market: Many of the ingredients that stand in for carbs aren't pregnancy-friendly (like sugar alcohols). So (low) carb your enthusiasm. Favor foods that are naturally low in carbs, not ones that are processed to fit that formula, and balance them with plenty of healthy carbs (like whole grains and legumes) and healthy fats.

distracted eating, try putting mindfulness on the menu—eyes on your meal (or your dining partner) instead of on a screen. And because eating on the run can also lead to overeating, brake for meals. Take a seat at the table (or the breakfast bar, or your desk) even at snack time. Slowly savor your food (taking the time to actually taste what you're chewing—and while you're at it, taking your time with chewing), and you'll feel full and fully satisfied before you've overdone it.

- Get active. There's more to the calories-in, pounds-on equation—that is, if you add exercise. Getting a minimum of 30 minutes a day of moderate exercise—as recommended for most

pregnant women—will allow you to eat more calories while keeping your weight gain in check (that's the calories-out part of the equation). Plus, fitting in fitness is good for your body, your mood, your sleep, and your overall pregnancy health. Your workout even offers baby benefits, especially in the brain development department, research shows. Ask your practitioner for exercise guidelines, and then consider hitting the gym or the pool, joining a pregnancy exercise class, tuning in to the *What to Expect When You're Expecting Pregnancy Workout*—or just taking several brisk 10-minute walks a day. You'll find more fitness facts and workout ideas in *What to Expect When You're Expecting*.

Myth: Eating foods that are "gluten-free" will keep you from gaining too much weight.

Fact: Hoping to catch the gluten-free express to avoid excess weight gain? Don't hop on just yet. Products labeled "gluten-free" are a must for people with celiac disease or gluten intolerance. But if you don't have either one, ditching gluten in an effort to keep your weight from escalating too fast isn't the best move. Sure, if you replace your lunchtime cheeseburger with a gluten-free grilled chicken salad, you'll be piling on fewer pounds—but that's because the salad is lower in calories than the cheeseburger, not because there's no gluten in the salad. If, on the other hand, you swap something healthy for a gluten-free version of the same—say, a bowl of whole grain cereal for a bowl of processed gluten-free cereal—you're probably not saving yourself calories, but you probably are inadvertently skimping on nutrients. That's because processed gluten-free foods are often full of fillers (including fat, sugar, and starches) added to compensate for loss of taste and texture when whole grains are swapped out.

Processed gluten-free foods tend to have less fiber, fewer B vitamins, and lower amounts of minerals than their gluten-containing counterparts. Which means that if you're cutting out gluten, you're also losing all the nutritional benefits found in foods with gluten—all without cutting any calories. Bottom line: If you're going to go gluten-free (or need to because of a health condition), stick to nonprocessed GF foods. Bake your own GF bread and desserts using healthy gluten-free grains, focus on vitamin- and mineral-packed high-fiber, naturally gluten-free substitutes (brown rice, quinoa, buckwheat), and keep your diet high in healthy foods. For more on gluten-free diets, see page 150.

■ Check in with your practitioner. If you're eating sensibly, getting plenty of exercise, and still packing pounds on too quickly, it's possible there may be a medical reason to consider (such as a hormonal imbalance). Sudden rapid weight gain (more than 3 pounds in a single week in the second trimester or 2 pounds in a single a week in the third trimester), especially when accompanied by swelling of hands and face, headaches, blurring of vision, or any combination of these, could be a sign of the serious pregnancy complication preeclampsia and should be reported to your practitioner right away.

If You're Gaining Too Slowly

Nagging nausea. Annoying aversions. Metal mouth that makes everything you eat taste like loose change, and bloat that leaves you feeling full when you're actually running on empty. There are plenty of reasons why your first trimester appetite might have taken a hit, or even a nosedive—and why gaining enough

When a Big Weight Loss Can Lead to a Big Weight Gain

Are you gaining too much weight, but can't figure out why? Unfair as it seems, overweight women who are chronic dieters or who lost a substantial amount of weight just before becoming pregnant may be prone to gaining too much weight during pregnancy, even if they don't overeat. Experts speculate that a body that's been through a recent major weight loss may feel "starved" and overcompensate during pregnancy for that earlier loss of fat by piling on more pounds. Tell your practitioner or check in with a dietitian about any significant prepregnancy weight loss, and discuss a game plan for keeping your pregnancy weight gain on target.

weight may have become an unexpected struggle. (Wasn't that supposed to be the easy part of pregnancy?) Happily, there's nothing to worry about if your weight gain is still at a standstill as you end your first trimester, or even if it has dipped into the negative zone—after all, your baby (and baby's needs) are still relatively tiny. Once you graduate to the second trimester, though, it's time to start putting on the pounds. To get your weight gain going:

- Fatten up your diet. Since pure fat is the most concentrated source of food energy (aka calories), adding fat to your diet is usually the easiest way to pack on pounds. While any fat will get the job done from a calorie perspective, choosing healthy fats will help get it done nutritiously, too. So butter up your toast, by all means, but also try spreading peanut butter on your apple slices, adding nuts to your yogurt (make it whole-milk yogurt while you're at it), adding avocado to everything, and saying "cheese" often.

- Don't be too efficient. For an expectant mom who's gaining weight too quickly, efficient eating is often the answer—filling up on foods that supply the most nutrients for the fewest calories (those veggies, that salad). Gaining too slowly? Just flip the equation. Focus on foods that are dense in nutrients and calories, supplying more of both with every bite: nuts and seeds, avocados, cheese, beans, hearty whole grains.

- Sneak in snacks. Snacking is a smart strategy for every mom-to-be, but it's wiser still if you're looking to jumpstart your weight gain. Build snack breaks (one midmorning, one midafternoon, and one before bedtime) into your schedule. Make the snack substantial in calories (go nuts!), but not so filling that you end up sabotaging your appetite for your next meal.

- Slow down the burn. If you're working out too much or too hard, you may be burning calories you need to nourish your body and your baby—and to gain those pregnancy pounds. So cut back on strenuous workouts, and don't forget to replace calories you do burn so you're not running at a deficit. And speaking of slowing down, if a high-stress job plus a fast-paced

Boys Will Be Boys

Are you eating like a teenage boy? It could be you're carrying one— or at least, a baby boy on his way to becoming a teenage boy. According to researchers, women pregnant with boys tend to eat 10 percent more calories (approximately 200 calories), 8 percent more protein, and more carbohydrates and fat per day than those carrying girls. And a boy bonus: Piling on those extra calories doesn't necessarily mean you'll be piling on extra pounds. Boy-carrying moms-to-be don't gain more weight, on average, than girl-carrying ones do. These findings may explain, in part, why boys are typically heavier than girls at birth. It also suggests a fascinating prenatal premise: That the fetus sends signals to its mother that drive her appetite during pregnancy (as in "Feed me, Mom— I'm hungry again!"). In other words, male fetuses require more calories for their optimal in-utero growth, so they send their moms to the refrigerator more often. Interesting science and, perhaps, a glimpse of refrigerator raids to come during those teenage years?

schedule has you missing breakfast or working through lunch, schedule eating into your daily calendar (even if it means setting reminders).

- Check with your practitioner. This is important, especially if your slow weight gain doesn't seem related to undereating or doesn't change after you add extra calories. A thyroid condition or some other undiagnosed medical problem may be keeping you from achieving your weight-gain goals and needs prompt attention.

If You're Gaining for Multiples

More than one baby on board? Then your goal will be to gain weight faster than the typical expectant mom, right from the start—not only because you're housing two (or more) growing babies, but also because you're toting two placentas (unless your identical twins are sharing a large one). You'll also be carrying additional blood and fluid supplies, a larger (and heavier) uterus, and more amniotic fluid.

Your recommended weight gain will, not surprisingly, be substantially higher than that for a singleton pregnancy.

If you're carrying twins and your pre-pregnancy weight (and BMI) was normal, it's recommended that you gain 37 to 54 pounds. If you started pregnancy overweight, aim to gain between 31 and 50 pounds. If you have triplets on board, your weight gain recommendations will be a little higher (your ob will give you a target number).

Problem is, gaining enough weight isn't always as easy as it seems when you've got two or more on board. That's especially true during the first trimester, when double the hormones can spell

Eating Disorders and Pregnancy

There isn't much research in the area of eating disorders and pregnancy, mostly because few women suffering from anorexia or bulimia become pregnant in the first place (these disorders often disrupt the menstrual cycle). But the studies that have been done suggest that having an active eating disorder during pregnancy can increase the risk of many complications, including miscarriage, preeclampsia, premature birth, cesarean delivery, and postpartum depression. Taking laxatives, diuretics, appetite suppressants, and other drugs during pregnancy is harmful, too, leading to multiple serious problems, including possible birth defects, if used regularly. Happily, the studies also suggest that moms-to-be who once suffered from eating disorders but have put those unhealthy habits behind them are just as likely to have a healthy baby as anyone else.

But what if you're no longer anorexic or bulimic, yet the thought of pregnancy weight gain has brought back some of those old feelings about your body image that you'd fought hard to overcome—and thought you'd shed forever? What if you're having trouble eating normally now that you're eating for two? Or if you're having a hard time distinguishing between morning sickness and bulimia? Or if you're hiding a return of your bulimia under the cover of morning sickness? Or you have signs of disordered eating: anxiety around specific foods, meal skipping, feelings of guilt and shame when you eat, a rigid approach to eating, self-esteem that's based on body shape and weight, preoccupation with food and weight, and/or using exercise to make up for bingeing?

First, make sure you get the help you need as soon as possible. Start by telling your prenatal practitioner about your eating disorder—not only so he or she can help make sure it doesn't affect your baby or your pregnancy, but also so you'll get the supportive care you need to get healthy and stay healthy. Then ask for a referral to a therapist who is experienced in treating eating disorders. Professional counseling is always smart when you've been

double the morning sickness, making it difficult to get food down—and then keep it down. Eating tiny amounts of comforting (and, hopefully, sometimes nutritious) food throughout the day can help get you through those extra-queasy months. Aim for a pound-a-week gain through the first trimester, but if you find you can't gain that much, or have trouble gaining any at all, relax. You can have fun catching up later (or not—read on). Just be sure to take your prenatal vitamin and stay doubly hydrated.

Your second trimester will probably be your most comfortable and the easiest for you to do some serious chowing down in, so use it as an opportunity to load up on the nutrition your babies need to grow. If you didn't gain any weight during the first trimester (or if you lost weight because of severe nausea and vomiting), your practitioner may want you to gain an average of 1½ to 2 pounds per week starting now. If you've been gaining steadily through the first trimester, you can aim a little lower. Either way, that may seem like a lot of weight in a short time, and you're right—it is. But it's weight that's doubly important to gain. Supercharge your eating plan with

battling anorexia or bulimia, but it's really essential when you're trying to eat well for two. Seeing a registered dietitian may also be helpful in coming up with a healthy pregnancy eating plan you can feel good about. And look toward support groups, too—made up of pregnant women and moms who are currently facing the same struggles or have faced them before. Check online, or ask your practitioner or therapist for a recommendation.

Second, try to put the dynamics of pregnancy weight gain and the normal body changes that go along with it in perspective (something your therapist and a support group can also help you do). Pregnancy curves and a healthy weight gain are healthy and beautiful— signs that you're growing a baby. And the right amount of weight (as recommended by your practitioner), gained at the right rate, on the right foods is vital to your baby's growth and wellbeing in utero and beyond (some of the extra fat you lay down during pregnancy will be used after delivery to help you breast-feed your baby). Be prepared for—and talk to your therapist about—the reality

of what a healthy new-mom body looks like and feels like after pregnancy and delivery: That you won't lose all the pregnancy pounds or inches overnight. That it takes 9 months to gain pregnancy weight, and it can take at least that long to lose it. That the weight you'll still be wearing postpartum is not only normal, but necessary to fuel your recovery and to feed your baby. Don't try to minimize weight gain during pregnancy in an effort to avoid the postpartum body image struggles you may be anticipating (there's no reason to struggle if you know you're supposed to look that way postpartum). The most important thing to keep in mind: Your baby's wellbeing depends on your wellbeing during pregnancy. If you're not well nourished, your baby won't be, either.

If you can't seem to stop bingeing, inducing vomiting, using diuretics or laxatives, or practicing semistarvation during pregnancy, discuss with your practitioner the possibility of hospitalization until you get your disorder under control—which, with the right care and support, you absolutely can.

extra servings of protein, calcium, whole grains, and healthy fats. Heartburn and indigestion (again, both more likely to be more miserable in a mom-to-be of multiples) starting to cramp your eating style? Spread your nutrients out over 6 (or more) mini-meals.

As you head into the home stretch (the third trimester), you'll still need to continue your steady rate of gain. By 32 weeks, your babies may be just under 4 pounds each on average, which won't leave much room for food in your crowded tummy. Still, even though you'll be feeling plenty bulky already,

The Long Road Back

Gaining the weight is (usually) the easy part. It's losing all that weight after the baby is born that's often hard. Keep in mind that it takes time—and that there shouldn't be too many shortcuts on that long road back, especially if you're breast-feeding. Check out Chapter 10 for tips on how to shed the pounds sensibly postpartum.

CHEW ON THIS. Going for a baby surprise? Or know your baby's sex but not yet telling—or not sharing with random strangers at the mall? Then you've probably been treated to any number of predictions based on any number of pregnancy legends, including this one: If the weight you've gained has headed straight to your belly, you're having a boy. If it's spread out all over your body (with special mention to those X-chromosome favorites: hips, buttocks, and thighs), you're carrying a girl, destined for curves of her own.

Guessing this isn't the most reliable way to predict your baby's sex? You're right. The fact is, how you carry has far more to do with a variety of other factors (including your size, shape, genetics, diet, and rate of weight gain) than it does with the sex of your unborn baby. Like all unscientific methods of predicting a baby's sex, this one has just about a 50 percent chance of being correct.

your babies will have to bulk up quite a bit more—and they'll appreciate the nutrition a healthy diet provides. So focus on quality over quantity, and expect to taper down to a pound a week or less in month 8 and just a pound or so total in month 9. (This makes more sense when you remember that most multiple pregnancies don't make it to 40 weeks.)

CHAPTER 7

Eating Well When You're Feeling Lousy

Oh, the irony: The reason you want to eat healthy is that you're pregnant—and the reason you're having a hard time eating healthy is . . . that you're pregnant. Let's face it—between morning sickness, food aversions, constipation, and indigestion, there are plenty of appetite-cramping pregnancy complaints that can come between a mom and her broccoli. Or that can push her buttons at breakfast time—and have her pushing the buttons on the vending machine 2 hours later. Or that can have her gagging over a glimpse of a raw chicken breast or a sniff of steamed spinach (at 20 feet).

A few lucky moms-to-be may breeze through pregnancy with healthy appetites for healthy foods for a full 9 months. But most find that their tastes change and their tummies take a hit when they're expecting—especially in the first trimester (when cravings, aversions, and morning sickness peak) and in the last trimester (when heartburn fires up and a growing baby encroaches on stomach space).

So, it's completely understandable if on some days (or most days) you're far more interested in feeling well than eating well—reaching for what helps ease the quease instead of what fills your calcium quota. Happily, however, many of the pregnancy symptoms that can dampen your appetite for healthy foods can actually be minimized by eating healthy foods—it's just a matter of finding the right ones. That way, everyone wins—you feel better and your body and your baby score the nutrients they need.

Morning Sickness

Do you heave at the sight of hamburger meat? Are you queasy just contemplating a bowl of your formerly favorite cereal (or even seeing the box on your pantry shelf)? Are you looking greener than that salad you were planning to eat? Welcome to the first trimester of pregnancy, a time when, if you're like about 75 percent of all pregnant women, morning sickness will change the way you look at food (not to mention the way you smell it, taste it, even think about it), taking a toll on both your tummy and your ability to fill it. Or, at least, to keep it filled.

As just about every veteran of morning sickness knows, the joker who coined this pregnancy symptom's name clearly never experienced it. Morning sickness isn't just for mornings—it's a round-the-clock, 24/7 sickness. Which is one reason why some experts have tried (with minimal success) to get a more accurate name trending: NVP, or nausea and vomiting of pregnancy.

Whatever you call it (besides miserable), there's no such thing as a textbook case. Morning sickness symptoms vary from mom to mom—and sometimes, from pregnancy to pregnancy in the same mom. Some may experience only occasional queasiness. Others may suffer through constant nausea and frequent bouts of vomiting, especially during the early weeks. While symptoms typically taper off by the end of the third or fourth month, a small percentage of women find the misery lingers—at least to some extent—into the ninth month. And even those who sail through that second trimester without a queasy moment may find it returns with a vengeance during the third trimester. It can even make its pregnancy debut in the third trimester (though late-pregnancy nausea and vomiting should always be checked with your practitioner, to rule out a complication).

Those who have spent weeks hovering over the toilet, avoiding onions (and people who eat them) like the plague, and subsisting on ginger ale and saltines may find it hard to believe that there's a silver lining to the cloud of morning sickness. But actually, there is. Since it's pregnancy hormones that trigger the nausea and vomiting of early pregnancy, morning sickness usually means that those hormones—which also help protect a pregnancy—are in good supply. Which is definitely not to say that morning sickness is a must-do for a healthy pregnancy (plenty of moms never have a queasy moment), just that morning sickness is usually a sign that pregnancy is proceeding normally. What's more, while you're certainly suffering, your baby almost certainly isn't. Even if you have a hard time keeping much of anything down, and even if you lose a little weight during the first trimester, your baby is able to weather morning sickness far better than you.

Of course, while all this good news about morning sickness probably makes you feel better about having it—it won't make you feel better while you have it. But, queasy fingers crossed, some of these tips will:

- Follow your nose. Your pregnant nose knows—everything. What your coworker had for dinner last night. What your partner had for lunch. What your neighbors are cooking for breakfast (sausage, again?). That's because the hormones of pregnancy sharpen the sense of smell, making for

The Six-Meal Solution

When heartburn, nausea, gassiness, and other pregnancy symptoms make eating (and digesting) 3 meals a day seem like too much hard work, turn to the Six-Meal Solution instead. Eating half as much twice as often will keep your blood sugar steady, your appetite appeased, and your digestive tract running more smoothly, providing relief from pregnancy tummy troubles. Dividing your meals will also help you conquer your nutritional requirements more easily.

There are two ways to tap into the Six-Meal Solution. One is to cut your usual 3 squares in half, so you're eating half of each meal every 2 to 3 hours. Or put traditional meals out to pasture for now (at least until you're feeling less green), and try grazing your way through your day. Opting for 6 mini-meals or 6 maxi-snacks will not only be gentler on your overtaxed tummy, but sustaining to your blood sugar—boosting energy, minimizing mood swings and headaches, and helping you get a better night's sleep, among other benefits.

Here are some mini-meal suggestions (see page 138 for some snack ideas):

- A cup of soup sprinkled with grated cheese, whole-grain saltines
- Half a peanut butter sandwich, a snack bag of freeze-dried fruit
- A muffin, a cheese wedge, a clementine
- Half a bagel and a scrambled egg
- Egg in a hole, made crispy with a sprinkle of parmesan
- A baked potato filled with cheddar and broccoli
- A small bowl of whole-grain cereal with milk, half a banana
- A small salad topped with sunflower seeds and shredded cheese

- A yogurt-and-fruit smoothie
- Sliced tomato and Swiss cheese melted in a small whole-wheat pita pocket
- Half a grilled chicken breast wrapped in a whole-grain tortilla
- A cup of yogurt topped with granola and blueberries
- A cup of Greek yogurt with chopped cucumber, scallions, cherry tomatoes, and a sprinkle of salt
- Two hard-boiled eggs, sliced in half and topped with flaky salt and cracked pepper or with "everything bagel" seasoning
- Baked sweet potato with butter and hot sauce
- Pasteurized mini mozzarella balls and jarred roasted peppers on toothpick skewers
- Sliced ripe tomato, lightly salted, on lightly buttered multigrain toast
- Bowl of oatmeal with strawberries and milk
- Whole-grain toaster waffle with peanut butter and chopped strawberries (or blueberries)
- Quick quesadillas with shredded cheese, beans, and salsa, heated for a few minutes in a skillet or microwave
- Avocado toast (sliced avocado, lemon, and olive oil on whole-grain toast)
- English muffin pizza (whole-wheat English muffin, tomato sauce, shredded mozzarella, melted, black olives or another favorite topping optional)
- Vanilla Greek yogurt, dark chocolate chips, salted almonds
- Cottage cheese, sliced almonds, a drizzle of honey

a super-sensitive sniffer that's easily offended, heightening nausea. So go out of your way to avoid those now sickening smells, at least as much as you can. Steer clear of stovetop cooking when the ingredients will make a stink as they're sautéed—say, onions, garlic, peppers. Or nix those ingredients altogether (substitute garlic powder for minced fresh garlic, or leave the onions out of the recipe). Favor microwave cooking, which minimizes odors (especially if you cook in parchment packets that enclose the aromas). Be mindful of odors when you pack a lunch so that opening it up later won't knock you off your feet. Choose restaurants with outdoor dining, weather allowing, and opt out of those where you can smell what's on the menu before you even walk in the door.

- Eat often. Empty tummies can brew up trouble. That's because when there's no food around to break down, digestive acids are left with only stomach lining to munch on—a process that produces nausea. To keep your tummy from running on empty, eat 6 mini-meals a day (see the box on the previous page. And sneak in plenty of between-meal snacks, like freeze-dried fruit, crunchy freeze-dried cheese, nuts, or crackers.

- But don't eat too much. An overfilled tummy is just as likely to cry queasy as an empty one. During pregnancy, food travels at a snail's pace through your digestive tract so that nutrients are better absorbed. Cram in the chow, and you'll end up with more than your tummy can digest—something you'll end up regretting (and possibly, upchucking).

- Eat in bed. Before you settle down for the night, snuggle up with a snack that's high in both protein and carbs, such as a fruit and nut bar with milk, cheese and crackers, or half a PB&J on whole wheat. A sustaining bedtime snack will sustain your blood-sugar levels during the night—helping you not only sleep better, but (hopefully) wake up feeling better. Does morning sickness tend to creep in with dawn's early light? Open a bedside snack stand, stashed with crackers, dry cereal, freeze-dried fruit and cheese, or nuts, and get in the habit of having a nibble before you even swing your legs over the side of the bed. Let that early morning snack settle in before you attempt to start your day, and hopefully you won't start your day as sick as you were the day before.

- Stay ahead of the game. To kick morning sickness in the butt, nip it in the bud. Stay ahead of the nausea game by eating before those queasy waves hit (if your nausea is on a schedule), when food is more likely to go down and stay down. And, if you're really lucky, filling up (a little) before an attack may actually help to ward it off. Caught

---

CHEW ON THIS. B.C. (before crackers), there were a variety of other morning sickness cures far more exotic than the humble saltine. For centuries, healers (and those who play them at home) have suggested ways for moms-to-be to combat morning sickness through diet. From wild yam to papaya, many of these cures have been passed down from generation to queasy generation as supposedly effective weapons in the fight against morning sickness. Ginger and fresh lemons are among those that have survived the test of time—and in the case of ginger, even some medical testing.

Thinking Outside the Cracker Box

Sick of choking down dry crackers every morning to combat your queasies? You've discovered, as so many morning-sick moms-to-be eventually do, that crackers aren't always all they're cracked up to be—especially once you've crunched your way through cartons of them. While some moms find crackers comforting throughout their queasy weeks (or months), others find them tummy-turning from day one. Still others may find that comfort can turn to discomfort once crackers (or any food) become deeply associated with nausea and vomiting—and even the sight of a dry saltine starts the dry heaves. That's just sometimes how the cracker crumbles—and if that's the case, it's time to kick those crackers out of bed once and for all.

Where can you turn when you're thinking outside the box of crackers for bedside relief (or relief at your desk, or in your car)? Think of other foods that you can reach for and munch on easily—without having to drag yourself to the kitchen or the office fridge: dry cereal (no need to bring the box to bed—just keep a container handy), snack bags of popcorn or popcorn chips, pretzels, salted or unsalted nuts, trail mix, all-fruit fruit snacks, freeze-dried fruit, freeze-dried cheese. Can't contemplate chewing anything? Keep pouches or individual cups of applesauce stashed within reach. And of course, don't forget the ginger— whether it's a ginger drink that doesn't need refrigerating, some gingersnaps, or ginger chews.

in a vicious morning-sickness cycle (you're too queasy to eat, but when you don't eat, you get more queasy— making it hard to eat)? The best way to break out is to remember the three S's: slow, small, steady. Even if you're hungry, or in a hurry to get something in your stomach before you start feeling super-sick again, don't gulp or gobble. Too much, too soon, and you'll pay the queasy cost. Instead, have a few sips of lemon water, ginger tea, cold smoothie, or whatever liquid your tummy can tolerate. Alternate sips with a nibble of a solid you can stand—whether that's a chunk of cheese or a chunk of watermelon, a few almonds or a few pretzels . . . or yes, even a few of those crackers. Once you've let those sips and nibbles settle and coat your stomach, gradually move on to your mini-meal or maxi-snack (hopefully one that contains

the quease-easing combo of complex carbs and protein; keep reading). Or if that proves too tummy taxing, just keep the grazing going for now. And don't forget the steady part. To prevent that cycle from starting all over again, keep your blood sugar up and your tummy just a little bit full all day long (including just before you head to bed and as soon as you wake up in the morning).

- Concentrate on carbs. From the cliché cracker to the driest of dry toast, carbs often bring comfort to the queasy. When you can (that is, when your tender taste buds will cooperate), go for the grain when satisfying your craving for the bland and starchy—opt for whole-grain toast, pretzels, saltines, and graham crackers. Another carb that's complex yet easy to get down: fruit. Many moms find relief in

Soothing Smoothies

Need something in your stomach besides water but can't stomach solids? Try a liquid that eats like a solid: a smoothie. Hydrating, soothing, and packed with nutrients (more than many solid meals have, depending on which ingredients you're blending together), a fruit smoothie can be tummy coating without being tummy overloading. Use frozen fruit (berries, bananas, mangoes) instead of fresh, and you'll make your smoothie extra icy—and extra easy going down (the colder a food or drink, the less pronounced the smell or taste, usually a plus for sensitive pregnant palates). Experiment with the milk you use (coconut and almond make great nondairy options), or blend with Greek yogurt (high in protein, a proven quease-reliever, especially when teamed with the complex carbs found in fruit). And don't pack away your blender after your morning sickness (hopefully) passes. Smoothies make a perfect energy-boosting pick-me-up or a power-packed breakfast-on-the-go anytime during your pregnancy and beyond (new moms, you may have heard, are always on the go). Ready to get blending? You'll find some smoothie ideas starting on page 345.

Not near a blender but need a little something smooth and refreshing? Chilled applesauce, fruit, or yogurt pouches designed for little ones are also super-convenient and potentially comforting mom snacks, too.

---

fresh fruit, particularly when it's juicy (nature's way of ensuring fluid intake) and icy cold: watermelon, oranges (or those cute easy-peel seedless clementines), grapefruit, frozen grapes, frozen bananas, frozen mango chunks. Others prefer a chewy or crunchy approach to their fruit—raisins and dried apricots, or freeze-dried strawberries and bananas.

- **Think protein.** Though carbs are the first food group moms-to-be usually turn to when they're queasy, adding a little cheese (or another protein food, like almond butter) to those crackers can fight nausea even more effectively. Studies show that pregnant women experience less nausea when eating high-protein snacks—and that eating them in combo with complex carbs brings even more relief. So reach for any protein your tummy finds tolerable (a cheese stick or some crunchy freeze-dried cheese, some almonds, a container of Greek yogurt, for instance). Packets of peanut or almond butter (ready to pull out and spread on crackers or apple slices) may be an especially handy protein source.

- **Stay off the fat track.** If it's greasy and/or fried, your stomach will have a harder time digesting it. Those oils can also send your nervous system into overdrive, activating more nausea.

- **Let your tastes take the wheel.** If the sight, smell, or even suggestion of a food makes you sick, don't eat it—no matter how healthy it is. Veer, instead, for foods that you find appealing, or at least, inoffensive—even if they're not the healthiest food since sliced whole-wheat bread. And remember what they say about variety being the key to good nutrition? Forget about it for now if only a few foods make the quease-easing cut. Once the morning sickness cloud has lifted, you'll be able to lift yourself out of your food rut.

- Be dense. In your food selections, that is. If half of everything you eat comes up, the half that stays down should (as much as possible) provide you with as many nutrients as possible. So choose foods that are packed densely with high-quality nutrients. Think whole grains, nuts, peanut or almond butter, cheese, beans, avocados, sweet potatoes, dried or freeze-dried fruit, mangoes, melon.

- Take a fluid approach. Fluids are more important in the short term (aka your first trimester) than solids are, and they'll be more important still if you've been doing a lot of vomiting. So do your best to drink up and stay hydrated (you'll know you're lagging on liquids when your urine is dark—it should be clear). If even the thought of drinking glass after glass of water makes you gag, quench your quota with icy cold watermelon (1 cup of watermelon cubes equals half a cup of water), suck on ice chips, slurp some frozen juice pops, chew on some cold, crunchy cucumber or celery. Flavoring your water with cucumber, lemon, or watermelon slices, or a squeeze of lemon or lime juice (and sticking it in the freezer for a few minutes to get it as cold as possible) may make it more palatable, too. Switch to electrolyte water, which may replenish better than regular—or sip cold coconut water, which may be extra soothing and hydrating. Or icy almond milk. And if solids are not your friend, take a fluid approach to those, too, in the form of a fruit smoothie or a soup. Check out the smoothie recipes starting on page 345 and the soup recipes starting on page 222.

Whatever Gets You Through the Day (and Night)

Morning sickness has cut your can-eat list to 2 foods? Or maybe just 1? No worries. For now your only objectives are staying hydrated and keeping your head out of the toilet, at least as much as possible. So, eat whatever gets you through the day (or night)—even if it's breakfast served for breakfast, lunch, and dinner. Once morning sickness has passed, you'll have plenty of time to add variety back into your diet.

- Freeze the quease. Many women find that icy-cold or frozen fluids and foods are easier to get down. Try frozen grapes or bananas or mango, well-chilled fruit cups, applesauce cups, or fruit pouches (they may be marketed for tots—but they also hit the spot for those growing a tot). Or try sipping on icy-cold almond milk, also touted for its stomach-settling benefits (it works on heartburn, too). Another reason why you may want to chill out: Cold foods don't come with as much of a smell or taste.

- Snap out of it with ginger. Score one for the ages—and an age-old solution to the age-old problem of tummy troubles. Ginger has been used for generations to settle stomachs, ease cramps, combat indigestion, nix nausea—and as it turns out, this is one remedy that has made it out of the home and into the medical books. Already scientifically proven to alleviate motion sickness, ginger can also be good for what ails a queasy mom, according to research.

Take it in capsule form (sold in the supplement aisle, but ask your practitioner to recommend a safe dose, and screen for other ingredients), make ginger tea by infusing gingerroot in boiling water or using ginger tea bags (again screen for added ingredients that might not be pregnancy-safe), cook with ginger (in those snaps, muffins, or a soup) or turn to prepared ginger-based foods and beverages: ginger biscuits, crystallized ginger, ginger sucking candy, soft chews, and lollipops, and real ginger ale. Even the smell of fresh ginger (cut open a knob and take a whiff) may quell the queasies.

■ Find the power in sour. You can also try another trick of the queasy trade: lemons. Many women find both the smell and taste of super tart and sour foods super comforting. So when life gives you morning sickness, try making lemon- or limeade (or a lemonade slushie). Or reaching for a grapefruit—the more mouth puckering, the better. Or a jar of sauerkraut—or a bowl of hot and sour soup. Wondering if there's really any cred behind the pregnancy cliché of pickles? Pickles (or really, anything pickled in vinegar, from mushrooms to carrots to pepperoncini) do comfort many queasy moms. And while the pickle jar is open, consider that some moms-to-be actually find sipping pickle juice incredibly (and surprisingly) soothing—and some swear by cubes of frozen pickle juice (freeze the juice in ice cube trays). Sour or peppermint-flavored sucking candies spell relief for others.

■ Take your vitamins. In general, women who get enough vitamins and minerals before they get pregnant (say, from taking a prenatal vitamin preconception) experience less morning sickness misery than those who come into

pregnancy vitamin deficient. The train has already left the preconception station? Taking your one-a-day prenatal supplement can decrease nausea symptoms once you're pregnant.

■ And keep them down. Wondering how that daily prenatal is supposed to relieve your morning sickness when you can't choke it down (or keep it from coming back up)? The pharmacy shelves are lined with prenatal supplements, and one's bound to be better tolerated by your tummy. Your practitioner can recommend some good options, such as a coated one, or one that has a slow release formula, or one that adds ginger. Ask about ones that come in powder form (you can sprinkle it into your smoothies or mix with water—just remember you'll have to drink up the whole dose) or as gummies. Minimize the tummy troubles a prenatal may trigger by taking it with a meal or substantial snack. Taking it with dinner or with a bedtime snack may provide the perfect timing, since you might be able to sleep through any queasiness it causes. If you find your prenatal vitamin doesn't agree with you no matter what time of day you take it and no matter what form or brand you use, ask your practitioner about prescribing one that has a greater amount of vitamin B_6 than a standard prenatal vitamin. (Research has shown that vitamin B_6 in moderate dosages—30 to 75 mg per day—successfully relieves nausea for many moms-to-be.) Bonus if it also has a controlled formula that releases the vitamins in your body evenly throughout the day and contains no iron, which can upset the stomach. You probably won't need the added iron until midpregnancy, when moms start running low on stores—and by that time, you'll hopefully be out of the morning sickness woods. If not, your practitioner can recommend a formula that's easier on the stomach.

- For a tough case, try a tough approach. Is your morning sickness significant enough that dietary changes aren't changing a thing? It's time to ask your practitioner about medication options. For information on prescription and OTC meds that can help combat your morning sickness, check out *What to Expect When You're Expecting*.

If your nausea and vomiting are severe and unrelenting, you may be experiencing hyperemesis gravidarum, a pregnancy complication that requires prompt treatment. Treatment for HG will include IV fluids as needed to combat dehydration, medications, and sometimes hospitalization. Check in with your practitioner and see more about HG in *What to Expect When You're Expecting*.

Food Cravings

Was that you foraging in the freezer for the slow-churned vanilla ice cream, and in the fridge for the sliced pepperoncini to sprinkle over it? Spending your whole lunch hour searching for a deli that would make you a peanut butter and pickle sandwich on raisin bread (then adding a layer of chocolate chips while no one was looking)? Embarrassing your partner at the buffet table during last week's cocktail party by dipping the grapes into mustard? Wishing you could find a pizza place that served chocolate pudding—not for dessert, but to spread on your black-olive-and-anchovy pie? Or a lunch place that serves breakfast all day—because it's the only meal you can stomach?

Welcome to the cravings club. More than three-quarters of all women experience food cravings at some point in their pregnancy, usually in the first trimester. The most commonly reported cravings (not surprisingly, many women prefer to keep their cravings to themselves rather than report them) are for sweet, sour, salty, and spicy foods—often in combination, sometimes in unlikely combinations. Carbs top the cravings chart

(again, no surprise), as does fruit. But few moms-to-be actually go by the book when it comes to their pregnancy cravings, which can range from the peculiar (French fries layered between waffles, topped with equal amounts of hot sauce and maple syrup) to the particular (a brand of salt-and-vinegar potato chips available only within a 2-state radius, dipped in an egg salad made only at a certain deli, topped with a salsa available only at a single market that's 30 miles away), from the unexpected (raw red onion, eaten like an apple, or pumpkin pie topped with ketchup) to the obvious (a whole box of donut holes), from the downright healthy (citrus fruit by the crateful, cheese by the wheel) to the downright dangerous (such as dirt or clay; see the box on page 116).

Can you blame your pregnancy cravings on pregnancy hormones? Of course you can—just as you can (justifiably) blame those monthly hormone-charged visits from Aunt Flo for your monthly visits to the House of Fudge. Except, supercharged, since the hormonal changes of pregnancy are far more dramatic than the premenstrual variety.

Craving That? Try This Instead

From salty to sweet, starchy to crunchy, hot to cold, there's a nutritious yin for just about every food you have a yen for during pregnancy. Will it be easy to convince your inner chocoholic that fruit is just as sweet as fudge? To fill that donut hole in your heart with a bran muffin instead of a Bavarian cream? Realistically, not always. But with a little creativity—and some willpower—you may sometimes be able to secure a substitute that truly satisfies both body and soul. Accept substitutes often, and you may be surprised to find your tastes—and your cravings—adjusting accordingly, ultimately making that slice of melon as tempting as that slice of cake. Well, almost.

INSTEAD OF	TRY
Chocolate bar	Low-fat chocolate milk or hot chocolate
Frozen chocolate bars	Frozen bananas, dipped in chocolate
Cinnamon roll	Whole-grain cinnamon toast
Jelly donut	Grilled PB&J sandwich
Chocolate donut	Grilled peanut butter and chocolate sandwich
Cake	Any of the nutritious and delicious cookies and muffins in this book (recipes begin on page 352)
Candy	Trail mix (made with dark chocolate chips) Dried or freeze-dried fruit, frozen grapes
Apple pie	Baked apple Apples slices spread with peanut butter, sprinkled with brown sugar, raisins and cinnamon, microwaved until gooey
Gummies	All-fruit snacks
Slushie	Applesauce, frozen until slushy; an icy smoothie (recipes start on page 345)
Ice cream	Frozen yogurt
Potato chips	Soy, vegetable, grain, kale, or bean chips or crisps, baked cheese puffs or veggie puffs, whole-grain tortilla chips, air-popped popcorn (tossed with grated parmesan cheese for extra flavor), pretzels, salted edamame, seaweed snacks, lentil snacks, toasted chickpea snacks
French fries	Baked sweet potato fries
Soda	Fruit juice mixed with sparkling water
Sour cream on everything	Greek yogurt on everything

CHEW ON THIS. Old wives, not surprisingly, have their share of theories about pregnancy food cravings. Check out these tales:

- If you crave sweets, you're having a girl.

- If you crave meat or cheese, salt or spice, you're having a boy.

- If you crave something during pregnancy and don't get it, the baby will have a birthmark in the shape of the craving. (A good reason to give in to that chocolate-dipped dill pickle?)

Possibly intensifying those cravings are a mom-to-be's intensified senses, especially a keener sense of taste and smell, also triggered by hormonal surges—which drive her away from some foods and have her (or her partner) driving at 2 a.m. to the nearest convenience store for others.

Another popular explanation for pregnancy cravings: You crave what your body needs. Crave salty foods? It may be your body's signal that it needs more sodium as it pumps up your blood volume. Or more fluid (if you listen to your body and break out the salted nuts, you'll get thirstier, sending you to the fridge for a bottle of water). Can't get enough grapefruit? Maybe it's your body's way of sending an SOS for vitamin C. Cheese on everything? Your body might be campaigning for calcium.

Can you bet on your body delivering accurate messages through your cravings? Sometimes probably yes, sometimes maybe not. This biological messaging system probably worked best before humans started departing from the food chain and relying so much on fast-food chains—and, of course, before the invention of fast fast-food delivery

(your cravings, delivered). With no apps and limited food choices, a pregnant cavewoman's craving for something sweet sent her foraging for berries full of vitamin C or picking fruit packed with vitamin A—a sign that she and her body had communicated well. Today, it's too easy for your body's signals to become scrambled—having you scrambling for the nearest pint of cookies-and-cream instead of the nearest pint of berries. Far from a nutritional disaster, but definitely a disconnect.

Most likely, food cravings are a complex mix of physiological, psychological, behavioral, and cultural factors—with a down-home component tossed in (you crave the comforting foods of your childhood when you need that comfort most). Handling them, however, doesn't have to be so complicated. Here are some tips that might make your cravings easier (and healthier) for you to deal with:

- Cave when you crave. Pregnancy cravings are a powerful force of nature, and fending them off around the clock could take everything you've got—maybe more than you've got. So don't feel compelled to fight them, at least not all of the time. Remember, they're not likely to last—they're usually at their peak in the first trimester, when hormonal changes are also at their peak, and even when they do linger, they usually ease up in intensity. Caving to cravings occasionally (or even regularly) won't wreak nutritional havoc during that first trimester, when your baby's nutritional needs (like your baby) are tiny. Especially if you add a side of good sense (you submit to a single brownie, but not the whole pan). Plus, if you're trying to battle your cravings while you're battling morning sickness, nobody's going to end up a winner—catering to your cravings may be the only way

Don't Eat This at Home (or Anywhere)

Most pregnancy cravings can be satisfied safely—even if they're for foods that aren't exactly nutritious. But sometimes pregnancy cravings take a turn for the inedible and the dangerous. Women who experience the eating disorder called pica crave the taste, smell, and textures of nonfood items such as dirt, clay, soap, chalk, tar, or ashes. Giving in to these (sometimes uncontrollable) cravings can be harmful to both mom and baby, and can even be fatal.

What triggers such a risky compulsion? It's believed that pica may be linked to an extreme deficiency in minerals, such as iron or calcium, or to general malnutrition. No matter what

the cause, if you find yourself craving anything that isn't edible, don't give in (and if you have trouble controlling the urge to eat it or drink it, make sure you don't keep the substance in your home or anywhere you can access it). Call your practitioner for advice.

Another compulsion that might signal a nutritional deficiency (but that isn't harmful, except to your teeth) is ice chewing. Research has shown that ice-cravers are more likely to be suffering from iron-deficiency anemia. Though sucking ice chips to relieve nausea is perfectly fine (and a good way to stay hydrated if you've been vomiting) check with your practitioner if you're constantly craving that icy crunch.

you can get or keep anything down at all. And if you're craving something healthy—like mounds of melon—by all means, yield to your yearnings, without limit. Go for the gusto—and that third serving of cantaloupe. Or that bowl of cereal for breakfast, lunch, dinner, and snacks. Craving something that isn't a food at all, like dirt or laundry detergent? Don't give in, and do check out the box above.

- Eat before you crave. You're more likely to give in to a less wholesome craving when you're running on empty, so (when possible) try to preempt cravings with sustaining meals and snacks. Chowing down on breakfast Cheerios can avert a midmorning cruller crisis, while breaking for a sensible sandwich can keep you from braking for an afternoon brownie binge.

- Seek substitutes. When you can, try to find (somewhat) nutritious foods that

can pinch-hit for the less wholesome ones you crave. If you're longing for potato chips, reach for bean or whole-grain tortilla chips instead, which offer protein and fiber along with that salty crunch. Focused on fries? See if sweet potato will get the job done, but with a vitamin A bonus. Satisfy your sweet tooth with chocolate-dipped strawberries instead of chocolate-dipped cookies—or at least give a nod to nutrition with a dark chocolate bar that's packed with nuts. (See the box on page 114 for more substitution ideas.)

- Think small. If you're craving chocolate, go for a snack-size bar instead of a king-size one (freeze it first, and it'll satisfy even longer). If ice cream is what your heart desires, follow your heart to the freezer aisle, but choose a variety that builds in portion control (like single-serving ice-cream cups or pops), so that a scoop doesn't lead to a half gallon.

Food Aversions

So, maybe it's the sight of chicken that suddenly has you running scared—and gagging to the nearest bathroom. Or your morning must-have eggs-over-easy are now making you unexpectedly queasy. Or the taste of that foamy, hot latte (the one that you could never start your day without) that's inexplicably leaving you cold. Or the smell of melting cheese (the smell that always melted your resolve to stop at 2 slices of pizza!) that's currently giving your tummy a meltdown.

If pregnancy has you loathing the foods and drinks you've always loved, you've discovered the flip side of food cravings: food aversions. And, as with food cravings, you're in plentiful pregnant company—in fact, up to 85 percent of expectant moms experience at least a single food aversion (many have multiple ones). Thought cravings were a compelling force of pregnant nature? Aversions can be even stronger. Confusing, too, since they can have you heaving over the sight, smell, or even suggestion of foods you've always favored.

Some researchers say that food aversions, like cravings, are related to your hormone levels: They peak when your hormones are in their greatest period of flux, during the first trimester (which explains why most—though not all—food aversions pass by the time you're midway through your pregnancy). They can also be closely tied to morning sickness—the sicker you are, the more likely you are to have aversions . . . and in turn, the sicker the aversions will probably make you feel.

Another popular premise parallels the your-body-craves-what-it-needs theory of food cravings, but in reverse: Food aversions are nature's way of steering you away from foods that might be harmful to your pregnancy or your baby. Which makes a lot of sense when you consider that 2 of the most common early pregnancy aversions are to alcohol and coffee—beverages that don't mix well with pregnancy (at all, in the case of alcohol, and in large quantities, in the case of coffee). Or when you think of other foods that newly expectant moms often shun, like chicken, meat, fish, and eggs. Nutritious, for sure—but in the days before refrigeration (and meat thermometers) made these animal-sourced foods a mostly safe bet, they were a risky proposition, a potential breeding ground for the kinds of parasites and microorganisms that could make anyone sick (particularly pregnant women, whose immune systems are naturally suppressed). Another wise (if outdated) example of how nature may have had mom's back, and her baby's, when coming up with food aversions.

Broccoli's turning you green? Kale has you cringing? Some scientists suggest that these common pregnancy aversions also have their roots in ancient times—when vegetables were foraged for, not shopped for in produce departments. The very plausible theory: An aversion to bitter, pungent flavors was nature's way of steering moms-to-be clear of toxic plants that might poison their babies. These days, it's a lot safer to eat green—and foraging for them doesn't get any easier than going to your local market or pulling up an app. And while vegetable aversions have clearly outlived any protective purpose, the instinct to step away from the salad bar lingers on, especially in the first trimester.

Because food aversions are so closely connected with nausea and

Metal Mouth

Do even your favorite foods taste tinny these days? You can thank your pregnancy hormones for giving everything you eat or drink that distinctly flinty flavor. This metallic taste is actually pretty common among newly minted moms-to-be. As with the morning sickness it often accompanies (doesn't misery love company?), metal mouth should taper off—or, if you're lucky, disappear altogether—in your second trimester, when those hormones begin to settle down. Until then, attack it with acid. Assertive acidic foods—like citrus juices, lemonade, sour sucking candy, and even pickles and other foods marinated in vinegar (often pregnant crowd-pleasers, anyway)—can dial down that metallic taste. Those acids will also step up saliva production, which will help wash that tinny taste away (hey, what's a little more saliva when your mouth's already flooded with the stuff?). Since the heavy metals in your prenatal vitamins, like copper, zinc, chromium, or iron, can (no surprise) leave a metallic aftertaste, ask your practitioner whether a switch to a more easily absorbed formula might help. Brushing your tongue (or using a tongue scraper) each time you brush your teeth can help minimize the metal, and rinsing with a baking soda solution (¼ teaspoon baking soda to 1 cup water), which neutralizes pH levels in your mouth, can also provide relief.

vomiting, some of the tips for dealing with morning sickness (beginning on page 106) can help with aversions as well. Here are a few other things to keep in mind if you've lost that loving feeling for foods you've always been fond of:

If the aversion is to something you're better off without . . . embrace your aversion. Consider yourself lucky if you suddenly can't stand coffee, or wine smells sour, or beer tastes bitter. It'll never be easier to give them up than when they're turning your stomach.

If the aversion is to something you feel you should eat, but just can't . . . just say no for now. Even if it's the healthiest food on the planet—or several of the healthiest foods on the planet, or seemingly all of the healthy foods on the planet—don't force yourself to eat it. Try, when possible, to find a substitute that's acceptable to your tender tummy and taste buds but approximates the nutrients in the food you can't handle (maybe it's peanut butter instead of chicken, or almond milk instead of cow's milk, or a mango smoothie instead of a salad). Are meat, fish, chicken, eggs, and other animal proteins off your menu for now? Happily, protein comes in all kinds of packages, not just in the standard steak-house favorites. Instead of the meat or seafood counter, head to the dairy case, where you'll find cottage cheese (1 cup easily subs for a 4-ounce chicken breast, protein-wise), yogurt (Greek or Icelandic are especially protein packed), as well as eggs.

Dairy's too close for comfort to cows, and eggs make you think too much of chickens? If the carb card is the only one you can easily play right now, play away. You can net that carby comfort plus a protein punch with a spin down the bread, cereal, and pasta aisles—where high-protein grains, seeds, nuts, and legumes have found their way into a carb-lover's variety of meat-free products. Remember, too, that a small hill of beans can stand in for a mound of meatballs (that is, if your tummy can handle the gassy side effects). And don't forget that peanut butter (and almond butter) can spread a little protein on your toast, your apple slices . . . or even your pickles, if that's where your cravings have been taking you.

Not ready to give up on meat? Consider that it might be the sight of that slab that offends, in which case you might try hiding the meat rather than headlining it. Ground beef that's lost in a sauce, or soup, or stew—instead of front and center as a burger. Chicken that's minced up and camouflaged in a casserole instead of confronted on the bone (or as a boneless cutlet). Diced shrimp that's barely recognizable in that sea of pasta.

Can't look at anything green? Until this aversion passes (as it likely will by the end of your first trimester, or soon afterward), take a break from the salad bar—or from any vegetables that turn you into a Kermit look-alike. Take a walk on the sweeter side of the produce aisle, where you'll find mellow yellow and orange veggies, like carrots and sweet potatoes, which offer the same beta-carotene benefits without the bitter taste. Or trade in your vegetables entirely for now and turn to fruit that can fill your need for those nutrients,

> ### Beyond Eating Well
>
> Non-diet-related tips for fighting all of the pregnancy symptoms discussed in this chapter can be found in *What to Expect When You're Expecting*.

like cantaloupe, mango, papaya, nectarines, peaches, and apricots.

Can't sublimate or substitute? Not to worry. Though occasionally an aversion to a healthy food (or foods) plays for keeps during pregnancy (or new ones keep popping up), it doesn't typically outlast the first trimester. Which means you'll probably be back on the egg (or spinach, or beef) express before you know it—and before your still-teeny baby could possibly miss the nutrients in the foods you're skipping. You may find, in fact, that nutrient-packed foods you can't look in the face (or wing, or drumstick, or fillet) now become foods you can't get enough of later. For example: You couldn't eat meat in the first half of pregnancy, but by the time you reach week 20, you can't get enough of it—perhaps nature's way of reminding you that it's time to step up your iron intake.

Constipation

As if getting food down (or keeping food down) weren't challenging enough these days, maybe you've discovered that getting it out can also be a struggle when you're expecting. The real bottom line: Constipation clogs up the works for at least half of all expectant moms.

As with so many pregnancy discomforts, constipation is a crappy symptom that's around for a good reason. Here's why it happens: During pregnancy,

The Poop Scoop

Assume you're constipated because you're not having a daily bowel movement? That's a popular assumption, but not an accurate one. Constipation is defined as the passage of small amounts of hard, dry bowel movements, usually fewer than 3 times a week, and often with difficulty and pain. It's usually accompanied by gas, bloating, and that "sluggish" feeling (cue the laxative commercial).

Not pooping daily but eliminating with ease—and without discomfort—when you do? Having infrequent bowel movements, by itself, isn't a sign of constipation—in fact, there is no "right" number of daily or weekly bowel movements. Normal is what's normal for you—whether that's 3 times a day or 3 times a week.

progesterone (one of the hormones responsible for a healthy pregnancy) relaxes the muscles of the bowels and causes the digestive tract to move at a much slower pace. The positive result of this digestive relaxation: better absorption of nutrients earmarked for baby making. The not-so-positive result: stool that sticks around too long becomes harder (often literally) to eliminate. As pregnancy progresses, mounting pressure on the bowels from a growing uterus often compounds constipation.

How do you combat constipation without interfering with intestinal best (for baby) intentions?

■ Focus on fiber. Of course you've heard that fiber helps fight constipation—but do you really know how? It's easy: Foods high in fiber absorb water, softening stool and expediting and easing its passage, essentially preventing or clearing up clogs in your digestive pipes. Not a bran flake fan? Think seniors when you think prunes? There are plenty of other fiber foods to focus on: Whole grains of all kinds (grains that are "whole" include the bran, so no need to go all-bran—you'll get plenty in a bowl of any whole-grain cereal, a

slice of whole-grain bread, or a plate of whole-grain or legume pasta). Vegetables (especially raw or lightly cooked). And fruit (fresh, dried, or freeze-dried). You should aim for about 25 to 35 grams of fiber a day, but there's no need to count. You'll know you're fitting in enough fiber when your stools are large and easy to pass, not hard or pelletlike (poop frequency is less important than poop consistency). But also know when enough of a good thing becomes too much. An excess of fiber in your diet can loosen stools up too much, and pass them through the digestive process too quickly, leading to diarrhea and a loss of needed nutrients.

■ Don't clog up the works. So now you know why getting plenty of fiber is the key to keeping your pipes clean and running smoothly. But just as important is knowing which foods can clog you up. Common constipators: white rice, white bread, cereal that's made from refined grains (like cornflakes), baked goods made with refined grains (especially if they're also packed with sugar), white pasta. Bananas may be the only fruit that's constipating instead of regulating, but they still come with nutritional benefits and are soothing for many queasy moms. So while it's smart not to go bananas with bananas if you're super-constipated, there's no need to ban them from your diet, either.

- Drink up. Fluids keep digestive by-products moving efficiently through your system, so keep your water bottle handy. Experts recommend aiming for about 80 ounces of fluid a day—and you can reach your share with water and other drinks as well as with fluid-rich foods, like melon, citrus, lettuce, cucumbers, smoothies, and soups. Stepping up your fiber? You'll need to step up your fluids, too (the fiber needs to absorb water to soften stool—otherwise, the fiber itself can constipate you). Another time-honored way to get things moving: Turn to warm liquids, including that spa staple, hot water and lemon. It'll help stimulate peristalsis, those intestinal contractions that help you go.

- Befriend bacteria. The good kind, that is. Probiotics (aka good bacteria) are pro-digestion—they'll stimulate the friendly bacteria that's already in your digestive tract to break down food more efficiently, keeping it moving more effectively. Enjoy probiotics in yogurt and yogurt drinks (like kefir) that contain active cultures. You can also ask your practitioner to recommend a good probiotic supplement—in capsules, chewables, or a powder form that can be added to smoothies.

- Make use of magnesium. It's a pregnancy nutrient touted for easing leg cramps. But did you know that an adequate intake of magnesium may also help kick constipation in the butt? It works by relaxing the muscles in your bowels and drawing water into

Fine Fuzzy Friend

Eating prunes is definitely one way to combat constipation, but if you like your fruit fresh—and not too sweet—look no further than the kiwi to get things moving. Besides providing that prunelike laxative effect (with no stewing required), this diminutive fruit packs plenty of nutrition within its fuzzy skin. In fact, ounce for ounce, the juicy kiwi provides more vitamins C and E than any of its produce peers. Peel kiwis, then slice them into salads, into yogurt, on top of cottage cheese, or into cereal (they pair especially well with strawberries)—or simply split one in half and scoop out that yumminess with a spoon.

the intestines, allowing smooth passage of poop. Definitely check with your practitioner before you consider popping supplementary magnesium (you'll probably get the go-ahead at a safe dosage), but there's no need to check before adding plenty of magnesium-rich foods to your diet. Many of them are also high in fiber, including beans, dried fruit, brown rice, bran cereal, nuts, peanut butter, spinach and other green leafies, and oatmeal. One dietary source of magnesium that's almost sure to put a smile on your face: dark chocolate.

- Be supplement savvy. Sometimes, supplemental iron can contribute to constipation, as well as other tummy troubles. Talk to your practitioner about whether a switch in your prenatal supplement (or your iron supplement, if you've been prescribed one) may help relieve your constipation. And though they may be a mom's best friend when heartburn strikes, popping too many antacids may also be constipating—so limit those if you're feeling stopped up.

Looking for overnight relief? Consult your practitioner before using over-the-counter laxatives or herbal or home remedies.

Gas and Bloating

Wondering how that bulge around your belly can be so big when your baby is still so small? Chances are that's gas, baby. Gassiness—and its uncomfortable buddy, bloating—often appears early in pregnancy, keeping your pants from buttoning even while baby's still pea-size. For some expectant moms, it's happily short-lived. For others, it can linger through the entire 9 months.

And, once again, you can blame your pregnancy-relaxed digestive system. As the system that processes your food slows down, gas production (resulting in flatulence) steps up. Constipation (and bowel distention) compounds the bloating problem by keeping both stool and gas trapped inside the digestive tract.

Gas production isn't harmful to you or your baby, of course. But it can be endlessly annoying and, let's face it, potentially embarrassing. To diminish the discomfort and beat the bloat, try the following:

- Go slow. A slow digestive system calls for slower eating. Taking meals on the run (one hand filled with a breakfast burrito, the other with car keys as you dash out the door), tossing down snacks (trying to beat nausea to the punch by gobbling up an extra-large tray of watermelon chunks while you're racing through the market on the way home from work), or mixing business with food

pleasure (negotiating a crucial deal on a conference call while simultaneously negotiating a chicken sub) can lead to air swallowing. The gulped air forms pockets in the intestines that cause pressure, fueling more gas pains. Instead, make time for your meals and snacks (even if that means getting up 10 minutes earlier in the morning to build in breakfast or signing out for an actual lunch break) and take them sitting down. As hungry as you are, or as eager as you are to get a little something in your stomach, chew on this: Chewing is the first part of digestion, and breaking food down thoroughly with your teeth gives your sluggish system a much-needed head start on the process. And then, to avoid extra air, swallow with care (instead of inhaling your food).

- Avoid overload. Stuffing yourself will—obviously—only make you feel fuller and more bloated while leaving your digestive system with too much to tackle at once. Again, even if you're feeling like a bottomless pregnant pit, try not to fill your stomach to capacity. Eat enough to sustain and satisfy yourself but not to bloat yourself— grazing on 6 small, closely spaced meals and snacks a day instead of 2 or 3 gut bombs.

- Keep it moving. The more trouble you have passing stool, the more gas you'll accumulate—and the more gas you'll pass. So take steps to combat constipation.

- Phase in fiber. Does your battle to beat constipation have you going crazy for kale and bananas for bran cereal (without the bananas you were afraid might clog you up)? Doing too much too soon in the fiber department can overtax your digestive system before it has a chance to adjust. Take your fiber intake down a notch or two and then, as your tummy acclimates, gradually step it up again.

- Bypass the beans. They're a great source of fiber, protein, vitamins, and minerals—but they're also a notorious source of flatulence. So until gas eases, consider limiting the amount of beans you eat (or even banning beans altogether for now), along with other common gas producers, such as onions, broccoli, cabbage, brussels sprouts, cauliflower, green pepper, and greasy, fried foods.

- Be less bubbly. For now, favor flat water if sparkling water (or other carbonated drinks) gets your tummy bubbling, too.

Heartburn

What do pregnancy and pepperoni pizza have in common? That's easy—they both deliver heartburn, and lots of it. In fact, no one does heartburn like a pregnant woman (except, of course, for a pepperoni-pizza-eating pregnant woman).

Despite its name, heartburn has nothing to do with your heart—though that's approximately the area where you'll feel that burning sensation when acid from the stomach leaks up into the esophagus. Normally, the esophagus acts as a one-way valve—allowing food to enter the stomach, but not letting anything back up. During pregnancy, however, the muscle at the top of the stomach that usually prevents digestive acids from splashing up relaxes (like all those other muscles in the digestive tract), causing heartburn and indigestion. Even if you order in a grilled chicken salad, instead of that pepperoni pizza.

More than 1 in 4 women experience heartburn at one time or another during pregnancy (or all the time), but it usually worsens in the third trimester. That's because as the baby grows, the uterus puts pressure on the stomach, crowding the digestive tract and making it even easier for those acids to back up where they don't belong.

Reflux Redux

If you have GERD (gastroesophageal reflux disease), heartburn's nothing new, but treating it during pregnancy might be. Many of the dietary tips for fighting heartburn can also help with your reflux, but be sure to ask your practitioner about whether the prescription meds you're used to taking are still okay to pop. Some are not recommended for use during pregnancy, but most are safe.

Heartburn, like so many other pregnancy symptoms that bug you, will not bother your baby. And as with so many other pregnancy symptoms, the best cure for heartburn is prevention. Taking these steps can help cool the burn:

- Take it slow. Eating quickly may save you time, but you'll pay in heartburn. So take a tip from your digestive system, and relax. Don't rush through your meals, and chew thoroughly (so that your stomach doesn't have to work so hard digesting food).

- Take it early. Try to eat dinner at least 2 hours before going to bed at night so your body has time to digest the meal. An easy-to-digest bedtime snack (as recommended for a better night's sleep, anyway) is fine, though.

- Take it easy. Though heartburn is technically caused by a relaxed digestive tract, it's often related to stress—especially if you're stress-eating or eating while stressed. To prevent the burn, try to chill out while you eat. Avoid checking messages or emails or news apps that are likely to aggravate you, and try not to talk or think about stressful topics. Make mealtimes as zen as you can, and don't eat on the run if you can manage to sit.

- Keep it small. Large meals will stuff up your stomach, making it more likely that some of the food (and accompanying stomach acid) will find its way back up the esophagus. Yet another reason to eat small meals more frequently.

- Keep fluids separate. There's a place for fluids and a place for solids, but when you're suffering from pregnancy heartburn, there may not be a place for both at the same sitting. Drink before and after meals instead of with them, or just drink a little. Too much fluid mixed with too much food will distend the stomach, aggravating heartburn.

- Keep your head up. Sit in an upright position when you're eating, and avoid lying down, slumping, slouching, or bending over immediately after meals.

- Keep your weight on track. The heavier a load you're carrying, the more pressure you place on your esophageal sphincter, the gatekeeper of the stomach. So try to gain your pregnancy pounds at the recommended pace (see Chapter 6).

- Don't pull the heartburn triggers. It doesn't take long to figure out which foods fire up the worst burn—once you do, you can eliminate them (at least temporarily) from your diet. Though your offenders may vary, common culprits include tomato-based foods, highly seasoned, spicy foods (that pepperoni pizza comes to mind, as do those hot wings), caffeinated drinks (because they also relax the esophageal sphincter), mint (particularly peppermint), and citrus. A diet high in fat can also contribute to heartburn, so ease up on the greasy foods (another strike against the pizza and hot wings). Some moms even find that cold water can lead to heartburn, and sadly, that chocolate can get high heartburn marks.

- Chew it away. Chew some sugarless gum for a half hour after meals to increase saliva production. Naturally alkaline, saliva helps neutralize the acid in the esophagus. If peppermint is a trigger for you, try switching to cinnamon or fruit-flavored gum.

- Go on an almond offensive. These tasty nuts neutralize stomach juices, relieving or even preventing heart-burn. Grab a few almonds for an after-meal chaser, or soothe the burn with an icy glass of almond milk (you'll get a calcium bonus).

■ Search for other soothers. Some moms-to-be find sweet relief by eating fresh, dried, or freeze-dried papaya (which scores vitamins A and C, too). Others find comfort in warm milk mixed with a tablespoon of honey (or even honey straight up)—especially taken just before bed, to prevent nighttime heartburn. Some say milk or yogurt can soothe, but your results may vary (you may actually find that dairy gives you heartburn). Some moms-to-be swear by small amounts of baking soda or apple cider vinegar in water, and others say bubbly sodas work for them. Experiment to see what spells relief for you (or at least, what doesn't make your heartburn worse).

■ If you can't prevent, try popping. An over-the-counter antacid that contains calcium (such as Tums or Rolaids) is safe to take during pregnancy and may keep the burn at bay while boosting your intake of that important mineral. If your heartburn is severe, check with your practitioner to get a prescription for a safe medication that might help.

Fatigue

Used to be, you could hit the gym before you hit the morning com-mute—now you're hitting the snooze button . . . over and over again. You could top off a client lunch with an after-noon of meetings before capping it off with a client dinner—now your shoul-ders are sagging, your feet are dragging, and your eyelids are drooping by 3 p.m. Your weekends were always packed with activities—now they're packed with naps. And like most pregnant women, especially in the first and last trimester, you're wondering where your "get-up-and-go" has gotten up and gone.

The answer is simple. The energy you used to take for granted is now being taken up with the monumental physical challenge of making a baby. Your body is currently working harder at rest (the rest you're always yearning for) than it used to work when you were on the run—yes, even during those 5-mile runs you once had the energy for. In addition to nurturing and nourishing a baby, you're fueling its factory. Your heart rate and metabolism are up. You're producing more blood. You're using up more water and nutrients. And if that's not enough to knock you down, higher levels of the hormone progesterone are circulating in your system, making you feel fatigued when your day's just starting, and sleepy hours before bedtime.

Looking to put more pep in your pregnancy step? Clearly, giving your body the sleep it needs and the rest it craves will help relieve some of your fatigue. But how you eat can also make a difference. To eat your way to more energy:

■ Cash in on those extra calories. Your baby-making factory will need extra fuel as it kicks into high gear, which means you'll need extra calories (about 300 extra calories each day during the second and third trimesters, fewer in the first trimester). Undercutting this

The Flip Side of Fatigue

Could this be another pregnant para-dox? You're so tired all day, you can hardly keep your eyes open . . . and then you fall into bed and can't sleep? Here's how to eat well to ease expectant insomnia:

- Have your morning joe in the morning. It can take 8 hours for caffeine to leave your system—and that can leave you buzzing at bedtime if you don't time your intake wisely. The better-sleep takeaway: Avoid caffeine in any form (coffee, tea, caffeinated soda) in the afternoon and evening so you're not all wound up when you're trying to wind down. Ditto for dark chocolate—have your fix earlier in the day.

- Snack before you snooze. Remember milk and cookies? It's time to revisit your childhood bedtime snack routine, with maybe a few modifications. The right bedtime snack will not only help you fall asleep, but stay asleep. Milk (warmed for those fuzzy slipper feelings) plus a whole-grain muffin or graham crackers will provide the protein and complex carbs you need to keep your blood sugar on an even keel all night long. So will cheese and whole grain crackers. Or a banana and a yogurt. And presto, you're getting sleepier . . . and sleepier . . .

- Limit fluids after 6 p.m. so you aren't kept awake by (even more) frequent bathroom runs. Get your fluid fill, but get it early. (Of course, if you're thirsty, drink up no matter what time it is.)

- If your practitioner has prescribed a magnesium supplement for constipation, take it before bed. Magnesium has relaxing properties that can help you drift off (while warding off the leg cramps that can stand between you and a good night's sleep). Plus that laxative effect you may be seeking will kick in just when you need it to . . . in the morning.

amount will undercut your body's already overtaxed energy reserves.

- Pack in extra nutrition. It may sound obvious, but a healthy diet provides higher-grade fuel for your body as it tackles not only the demanding job of baby growing, but also the other demands of your busy life. Simply put: More nutrients equal more energy. Another reason to be faithful about taking your prenatal vitamin, too.

- Breakfast like a champion. After a food-less night, your body needs to refuel before you start your engine—so start your day with a healthy breakfast that would make your own parents proud.

Stay away from quick fixes that don't last (like sugar and caffeine), and stick to the dynamic duo of protein and complex carbs that will stick with you all morning long (or at least, until your midmorning snack), keeping your blood-sugar level up and your body revved: oatmeal with walnuts and raisins, almond butter and sliced banana on a whole-grain bagel, a cheese-and-tomato melt on whole wheat.

- Eat extra often—and extra sensibly. That's right: The early-and-often approach to pregnancy eating applies to fighting fatigue, too. You'll keep your energy up by keeping your blood sugar up—and you'll keep your blood sugar up by eating small amounts of healthy food throughout the day (aka the Six-Meal Solution). Eat too much at a time, on the other hand, and the energy your body needs to get through the day will be shifted to digestive duties—after all, it's hard work to process a meatball sub. Also, try to eat for long-term energy as you graze through your day. Though candy bar commercials may promise an energy boost to help you through those afternoon slumps, there's little truth in that advertising. You may get a quick lift from that Snickers bar, but it'll likely be followed by a blood-sugar crash that will leave you lagging. Caffeine will give you an energy rush, but it will do nothing to sustain your blood sugar. And because that jolt will trick your body into thinking it doesn't need rest when it really does, it may keep you from falling asleep and staying asleep, especially if you suck down that espresso drink late in the afternoon. For a lift that lasts, turn instead to snacks that combine protein and complex carbs: peanut butter on apple slices, a slice of cheese and whole-grain toast, a smoothie blended from Greek yogurt and fruit. Be sure, however, to get most of your calories during the day, instead of saving them up for a supersize dinner. Your body needs the most energy (and so, the most food) when you're on the go, not when you're about to head to bed. Stocking up on food when you're most active will give your body energy when it most needs it. Plus, you'll sleep better if you're not stuffed. (Do make a bedtime snack part of your bedtime routine, however; see the box on the facing page.)

■ Add extra fluids. Your body doesn't just need extra fuel when you're pregnant—it also needs extra fluids. Not getting your fill of those fluids can lead to fatigue.

■ Pump extra iron. Occasionally, extreme fatigue (as opposed to run-of-the-mill pregnancy fatigue) is related to iron-deficiency anemia. Since iron reserves typically start dipping midway through pregnancy, your practitioner may run a routine check of your iron levels at about 20 weeks to see if you're starting to run low—and may prescribe an iron supplement as needed (many practitioners routinely advise an iron supplement in the second half of pregnancy as a precaution). Don't take extra iron beyond what's in your prenatal without your practitioner's go-ahead (it could constipate you), but do try to include iron-rich foods (such as red meat, spinach, and iron-fortified cereal) in your diet. Still inexplicably exhausted? Check in with your practitioner.

Other Pregnancy Symptoms

Eating well isn't the answer to every pregnancy complaint (if only!), but it can have a positive effect on a surprising number of aches, pains, and more pains. Here's a sampling of additional pregnancy symptoms that you may encounter during your 9 months and how diet can help:

Tooth and gum problems. Besides the obvious (see your dentist, brush your teeth at least twice a day, and floss regularly), making sure you get enough calcium and vitamin C foods will strengthen your own teeth and gums, and ultimately, your baby's as well. When you're nowhere near a brush, munching on some cheese or nuts, or chewing on some sugarless gum, can do a good stand-in cleanup. Crisp fruits and raw vegetables, like apples, carrots, and celery, can also help clean plaque from teeth.

Dizziness. Running on empty for long stretches (something you're more liable to do in the afternoon, when many dizzy spells strike) can cause your blood sugar to dip, leaving your knees weak and your head spinning. So can being dehydrated. Snacking and drinking regularly to boost your blood sugar and keep yourself hydrated can ward off those woozy moments—especially if pregnancy nausea and vomiting are making it hard to stay well hydrated.

Leg cramps. Nothing cramps a good night's sleep like leg cramps, which keep many moms-to-be tossing and turning in the second and third trimesters. Hormones play a role, but some say diet can contribute, too. One theory suggests that an excess of phosphorus and a shortage of calcium circulating in the blood trigger leg cramps. Another implicates a shortage of magnesium or potassium (usually due to dehydration). To get a leg up on leg cramps, be sure your diet includes adequate calcium, magnesium, potassium, and fluids.

Swelling. Nobody thinks puffy ankles are swell, but a certain amount of swelling (also called edema) is normal and healthy during pregnancy. And it's common, too: About three-quarters of all expectant moms experience some. But excess water retention, especially when your shoes don't fit by the end of each day and you can barely stand on those swollen dogs, can make pregnancy (especially the second half of pregnancy) a pain. Not surprisingly, excesses of salt (say, that whole jar of pickles) can increase water retention. But in a less intuitive twist, drinking extra water can keep you from retaining too much, by helping you flush out waste products. And, of course, saltier foods can make you thirstier, making you reach for more water (so maybe those pickles aren't such a bad idea after all).

Headaches. Pregnancy can sometimes be a headache . . . and for some expectant moms, headaches can strike more often during pregnancy. The number one culprit: those pregnancy hormones. But headaches (especially the migraine kinds of headaches) can also be triggered by diet. To keep headaches at bay as best you can, steer clear of your headache triggers (caffeine or chocolate, for instance) and be sure to eat regularly. A grazing approach keeps your blood sugar level, so you'll avoid those headaches brought on by low blood sugar. Keep a supply of high-energy snacks (such as lentil chips, fruit-and-nut bars, peanut butter packets and crackers) at hand (in your bag, at home, in your office) so those headaches never even get off the ground in the first place. Also, drink lots of water, since dehydration can lead to headaches. Since going cold turkey on coffee can also trigger headaches (these from caffeine withdrawal), it's smart to cut down on a hefty coffee habit gradually.

Mood swings. As with headaches, mood swings can be brought on by low blood-sugar levels—and that's yet another compelling reason to ditch your usual 3-meals-a-day eating routine and switch to the Six-Meal Solution. Keep complex carbs and protein front and center in your mini-meals so that your blood sugar—and mood—stay stable. And keep sugar and caffeine consumption to a minimum, since both can give your blood sugar a quick spike—followed soon after by a downward spiral that can take your mood down with it. Getting plenty of omega-3 fatty acids in your diet (from walnuts, fish, and enriched eggs) may also help with mood moderating. And here's some news that's sure to keep you in a good mood: A daily dose of dark chocolate can help boost your mood.

Skin and hair troubles. So your complexion didn't get the glow memo? That's actually true for many moms-to-be. But no matter what's wrong with the pregnancy skin you're in, it's possible that a healthy diet can help make it right. Dry, flaky, itchy skin? Try upping your fluids and adding some healthy fats (like walnuts and avocados). Skin discoloration? Some blotchiness comes with the pregnant territory, but too much may be linked to a folic-acid deficit—so make sure you're taking your prenatal supplement faithfully, as well as eating plenty of green vegetables and whole grain breads and cereals.

Teenage-style breakouts, and bacne? Hormones are the culprit (as they were when you were 15), and a practitioner-prescribed vitamin B$_6$ supplement—which seems to help treat hormonally induced skin problems—may be the answer. But since some research also links acne to inflammation (possibly triggered by a diet that's high in sugar and other simple carbs), cutting back on refined foods may get you in the clear. Skin and nail beds that are paler than usual? You may be low on iron. Ask your practitioner whether you might need a supplement, and make sure you're getting enough iron-rich foods.

Spider veins and varicose veins starting to spin their unsightly webs? Turn to sources of vitamin C, known to promote elasticity. Ditto for all-over skin blahs—see the vitamin C light, and you may actually see the glow you've been looking for in the mirror.

Flaky scalp issues? Some research suggests that getting enough B vitamins from your diet can help reduce dandruff. Dry scalp, like dry skin, may benefit from a healthy dose of healthy fat. If your dandruff is caused by yeast overgrowth, eating a diet low in yeast-friendly foods (sugar, refined carbs and bread, dried fruit, vinegar, soy sauce, peanuts, and mushrooms) may starve that funky fungus and feed a healthier scalp.

CHAPTER 8

Eating Well Whenever, Wherever, Whatever

Y ou count your Daily Dozen at night, instead of sheep. You've become a nutritious-food foodie and a serious label reader. You're completely committed to eating well while you're expecting. And then, real life gets in the way. Your budget is blown by your first trip through the organic produce section, before you even picked up that grass-fed steak. You have to work through lunch, again, and push "select" on the vending machine, again. You have to work late, again, and end up at the drive-through on your way home, again. Business dinners challenge your resolve—and your ability to simultaneously feed your clients and your baby what they're hungry for (client: sushi and sake . . . baby: roasted salmon and steamed broccoli). The airline you've chosen for a 3-hour flight tosses a bag of snack mix your way and calls it lunch. The destination you've chosen for a babymoon is known less for its green leafies and more for its white gravy. The holiday buffet tables are covered with red flags (from the raw oysters to smoked salmon to the possibly unpasteurized brie and eggnog). Not to worry—you can eat well whenever, wherever, whatever pregnant life throws at you.

On the Job

Mixing business with baby growing is always challenging (what you really need is an afternoon nap but what you really have is an afternoon presentation), but never more so than at meal and snack times. You packed a well-balanced brown bag (good for you!), but left it at your front door. Your morning meeting puts you face-to-frosting with the pastry tray. Your stomach's been growling since 11, but you're not on break until 2. Here's how to make sure that your 9-to-5 job doesn't conflict with your 24/7 job of feeding baby.

Stock up on supplies. Fill your desk drawer, your locker, your briefcase, and your handbag with a selection of healthy snacks and quick bites to ward off hunger pangs between meals. A convenient fridge makes snack-stashing easier, but isn't a necessity. For great snack ideas, see page 138. Also good to stock up on: containers for lunches and snacks. Be the cool mom with the bento box lunch—or the layered salad in a jar (see the box on page 267). Grab a thermos while you're at it, for hot lunch options.

Pack it. Leaving your next meal up to chance is never a good idea when you're trying to eat well, but especially when you're trying to eat well on the job. So unless you know where your lunch will be coming from (and you're afraid it may end up coming from the vending machine), don't leave home empty-handed. Pack up a healthy lunch (and a healthy breakfast, too, if you don't have time to eat before you run; see the recipes starting on page 191). See the box on page 132 for some lunch suggestions. See the recipes starting on page 210 for sandwich ideas.

Serve it hot. Cold sandwiches for lunch every day starting to leave you cold? Think hot instead. Bring a thermos of chili or hearty soup. Use the office microwave to warm up a chicken breast and some pasta, brown rice and steamed vegetables, or a tuna melt on seven-grain bread.

Keep it cold. Take advantage of the office refrigerator (if there is one) and put any perishable foods you've brought from home in it. Or, pack your lunch in an insulated bag with an ice pack to keep it cold.

Think drink. You're not just eating for two—you're staying hydrated for two, too. Which can be extra challenging when you're on the job instead of within steps of your kitchen fridge. Stay hydrated by keeping a tall glass or a water bottle at your desk and refilling it often (giving you a chance to stretch your legs and catch up on the watercooler gossip). And though it's hard not to think coffee when you're thinking drink on the job, it's smart to limit your caffeine consumption (see page 69 for the reasons why).

Stick to a schedule. Never find time for meals when you're at work? Start thinking of baby's next meal as a clock you

---

CHEW ON THIS. In Chinese culture, a pregnant woman is expected and encouraged to continue working throughout her pregnancy because it's believed that pregnancy "labor" eases delivery. And if you have to work anyway—wouldn't that be nice to believe?

What's for Lunch?

Here are some lunch-in-a-box suggestions:

- Any of the sandwiches starting on page 210

- A thermos of hot or cold soup (see the recipes starting on page 222), a cheese stick, whole-grain tortilla chips

- Leftovers from last night's dinner

- Layered salad in a jar. A great way to bring your salad to go. See the box on page 267 for tips on creating a salad in a mason jar.

- A bento box lunch—perfectly portioned meals separated into distinct compartments

- A baked potato stuffed with leftover steamed broccoli and cheese (heated up in the office microwave)

- Cottage cheese, cut-up fruit, whole-grain muffin

- Greek yogurt, nuts, a granola bar, a peach

- A hearty salad, whole-grain roll

- Fresh roasted turkey breast and cheese wrapped in a whole-wheat tortilla

- Turkey, beef, or vegetarian chili topped with cheese and chopped tomato, side salad

---

must punch, a deadline you must meet, or an appointment you've got to keep. Plan for a lunch break at the same time each day, and follow through as though your job (of baby feeding) depended on it. If your work takes you out to late lunches or dinners, have a healthy snack at your regular lunch or dinner hour to tide you (and baby) over until you and the clients can stop talking turkey and start eating it.

Make it easy. Feeding baby on the job doesn't have to be complicated, stressful, or time consuming. Whenever possible, take the easy way out. Cook dinners with leftover lunches in mind. Toss juice or milk boxes (the kind that don't need refrigeration) into your bag so you won't have to run to the nearest deli for a drink. Let someone else do the peeling and chopping, and visit a nearby salad bar for lunch.

On a Budget

Watching your wallet? A tight belt may not be the most comfortable accessory when you're expecting—especially when you're always being advised to reach for the pricier organic produce or spring for the grass-fed lamb. Still, there are plenty of ways to

squeeze in good nutrition when you're feeling the financial pinch:

Bag your lunch. Need another reason to bring your own lunch? It'll save you big bucks. Instead of paying a premium for a take-out lunch, lay out for less a delicious layered salad (see the box on page 267), dinner leftovers (that extra grilled chicken breast and brown rice you wisely made), a thermos of hearty soup and some whole-grain chips, or any sandwich on whole-wheat. Bag it (better still, pack it in reusable containers), and you'll save a bundle by the time your baby bundle arrives. See the recipes starting on page 210 for savvy sandwich ideas.

Tap into savings. You can save money multiple times a day—each time you reach for a glass of water instead of a soft drink or fruit drink. It's not only free, but it's the healthiest drink in the house. And in most houses (and offices, and restaurants), it's safe to drink straight from the tap. So instead of pouring money down the drain by buying bottled water (many brands are sourced from the tap, not from a spring, anyway), invest in a refillable water jug (with a filter as needed)—it'll pay for itself in no time. Bring a refillable water bottle to work, too.

Be a planner. Impulse shopping can cost you plenty. Use a menu planning/grocery shopping app to keep you on the straight and narrow shopping list.

Go generic. While the packaging on store-brand foods isn't usually as pretty to look at, it's what's inside that counts. And generally, what's inside is of comparable quality and nutritional value to pricier name-brand products. Happily, most packaged foods are available in generic form—and more and more often, there are organic options in that no-name space as well. And here's something the food-industry giants might not like you to know: In many instances, the store brand is actually a name brand with a store label.

Stay seasonal. Buying fruits and vegetables in season isn't healthier just for you and baby, it's also healthier for your bank account. For instance, peaches and strawberries may be available year-round, but they're most nutritious and cheapest in the summer months. When the season is over for a certain fruit or vegetable, head to the frozen foods aisle, where the price and the nutrition are right year-round.

Pick and choose organic. No need to shell out the big bucks for all organic products—just the ones where it'll make a difference. See the box on page 66 for the details on when it pays to pay for organic produce.

Eat a hill of beans. Or bean pasta. Or quinoa. Or eggs. Or canned salmon. Lean sources of baby-building protein don't always have to come in pricy packages, like steak or fresh fish. So explore lower-cost protein options. (Who says you can't have an omelet for dinner?)

Keep it simple. Sauces add extra price—and extra calories. So choose simpler preparations: steaming, roasting, grilling, broiling.

Consider whether convenience is worth the price. Time is money, sure. But are the couple of minutes you save when you buy your carrots already peeled and cut or your cheese already shredded worth the extra money you'll pay for these convenience foods? Sometimes they will be, sometimes they won't.

Buy in bulk. Bigger is almost always better when it comes to budget grocery shopping. So buy economy sizes of nearly everything you can—from chicken breasts to oatmeal. Stock up on sale items, too, if they're not perishable and you're sure you'll be able to use them. (That case of grapefruit might look like a good deal, until you realize

Planning Ahead

The best way to ensure that your next snack or meal will be a healthy one—and that you'll have it when you're hungry for it? Plan ahead. That way, you'll have healthy eating in the bag (and your fridge, and your car, and your desk) whenever you're in the market for something to eat. Another perk to planning ahead? You'll often save time (in the long run) and money. Here are some realistic plan-ahead strategies:

- Plan for between-meal hunger. If healthy snacks are always within arm's reach, you'll never have to make a trip to the vending machine (for a pack of cookies) or to the corner convenience store (for a bag of chips) when hunger strikes. Bag some crunchy freeze-dried peaches and toasted almonds to toss in your work tote, stash some kale chips in your desk drawer and some fruit-and-nut bars in your car, and keep the fridge filled with ready-to-munch hard-cooked eggs, cheese sticks or individual wedges, cut-up raw vegetables, and fresh fruit. Prepping ahead will help: Boil a big batch of eggs in advance (they'll stay fresh in their shells for a week). Cut up those fruits and veggies twice a week, and keep them stashed in plastic containers. Or buy them precut.

- Plan for shopping. Don't just stop and shop with some vague idea of what you'll be eating. Take a few minutes to draw up a weekly (or daily, if you shop that often) menu and arm yourself with a shopping list (on paper or an app) that covers it all. If that's too much prep work for the spontaneous you, at least make sure your cupboards, fridge, and freezer are filled with healthy choices you can build meals from. If grocery delivery's your deal, place those carefully planned orders ahead.

- Plan for real life. Don't plan for meals you don't have time to make. The Beef Stew with Wild Mushrooms (45 minutes prep time; 1½ hours to braise) may have looked fabulous on your favorite food blog, but if you're likely to get home from work at 7 p.m. to an empty pot and an empty stomach, it wasn't the wisest choice for dinner (unless, of course, you're a slow cooker; keep reading).

you can't fit them all in your fridge—or eat them before they've gone soft.)

Get loyal. Download or sign up for grocery store loyalty programs, where you'll get weekly items at lower prices and be eligible for special coupons to bring the cost of your trip to the market down.

Shop online and with apps. Online supermarkets and consolidators have sales on every type of food—from cereal to bananas, whole-grain bread to oranges, healthy soup to nuts. Take advantage when you see online sales, and then multiply your savings by using rebate sites and/or apps.

Grow your own. Whether it's fresh herbs on your windowsill, a small crop of tomatoes on your terrace, or a full-on garden of seasonal produce, cultivating a green thumb can save you green.

- Plan on taking it slow (cooker). A small investment of time in the morning can pay delicious dividends in the evening when you come home to a ready-to-eat meal, thanks to your slow cooker. Sure, you can go all traditional with slow-cooked soups and stews, but you don't have to limit yourself to just those dishes. The slow cooker is plenty versatile, allowing you to whip up chili, pulled beef, sweet-and-spicy chicken, lasagna, meatballs, sweet potato casserole, and even dessert with minimal prep and little kitchen mess.

- Plan for leftovers. There's no rule that says you have to cook from scratch every single day. But when you do cook, consider doubling the recipe and freezing the extra portion for a different day. Or make just enough extra one night so that the leftovers can do double duty for a delicious meal the next day. The leftovers from your grilled chicken and broccoli dinner can turn into a leafy green salad with chicken strips and broccoli the next day, for instance. Baked salmon can be eaten hot and fresh from the oven one night, with the extra saved to be shredded and turned into salmon-and-quinoa patties for later in the week.

- Plan for tomorrow, tonight. If mornings are rushed for you, there's a good chance you'll dash out the door without breakfast. And as for packing a brown bag when you're already running late? Forget about it—it'll never happen. So instead of leaving tomorrow's meals up to chance—and up to the twists, turns, and snooze buttons of real life—spend a few minutes before you turn in at night doing some advance work. Combine the yogurt and fruit and refrigerate it in the blender jar, so you can crush your morning smoothie, or pile some fresh spinach and cheese on a whole-grain tortilla and roll it up, ready for the morning microwave. When you're done prepping tomorrow's breakfast, pack tomorrow's snacks, bag (or box) tomorrow's lunch—and hey (why not?), fill up tomorrow's slow cooker dinner so all you have to do in the morning is set it and forget it. (And don't forget to make an extra batch of that stew to freeze—one less thing to plan for next week.)

When Time Is Tight

Feel like you barely have time to eat, never mind eat well? Not to worry. Even if time isn't on your side, good nutrition can be. Following these time-saving tips will help:

Stock up. No time to stop at the market after work? No problem—as long as your kitchen's well stocked. Keep your pantry, fridge, and freezer filled with all the ingredients you'll need to make quick, healthy meals all week long.

Shop once. With a good shopping plan and list in hand (or on your phone), do a week's worth of shopping for staples at once, supplemented, if necessary, by quick trips to the fish market for fresh

Microwave Smarts

It cooks, reheats, defrosts—and saves time. That is, if you know how to use it. Armed with the following tips, you might really be able to turn your microwave into the little appliance that could:

- Start with microwave-safe containers. Use only cookware that is specifically manufactured for use in the microwave (look for a microwave-safe BPA-free container), and don't let plastic wrap touch foods during microwaving. Better still, use a paper towel or paper plate to cover your food before you zap it.

- To maximize the retention of nutrients when cooking vegetables in the microwave, add only a few drops of water. Too much water, and the nutrients will be washed away. Even better, keep your vegetables on top of the water (with a microwave-safe rack) so you're steaming, rather than boiling. Be sure, too, to keep your microwaving time to a minimum, so that your broccoli ends up crisp and green, not soggy and gray. Three minutes (for 2 cups) should be the ticket to crisp-tender. Easiest of all: Skip the water entirely (and the washing and cutting up) by choosing microwave-in-the-bag vegetables. (Those steam-in-the-bags don't contain BPA or other chemicals and are safe to use in the microwave as directed by the instructions.)

- Use your microwave for all it's worth. Sure, it's great for reheating those leftovers from last night. But there are plenty of other ways to work microwave magic. Here are a few:

  ◆ Before squeezing an orange, lemon, or lime for its juice, microwave the fruit on high for 20 seconds. You'll get more juice flowing.

  ◆ Toast nuts in a flash by spreading them out on a plate and heating them on high for 2 to 3 minutes, stirring every minute.

  ◆ Make your own bread crumbs by cutting a slice of bread into cubes and microwaving on high for 1 to 2 minutes, stirring once. Then crumb in a blender, and toast as you would nuts.

  ◆ Thaw a 6-ounce can of frozen juice concentrate by removing any metal lid and microwaving on high for 30 seconds.

  ◆ For tear-free onions, trim the ends off a whole onion and heat on high for 30 seconds.

fillets. Or forget trips to the store altogether. Do all your shopping online and get your groceries delivered.

Equip yourself. So you got home from work at 7, have a class at 8—and somehow have to cook and eat dinner in between? The right kitchen equipment can shave many valuable minutes off your food-preparation time:

- A microwave. Use it to defrost frozen foods fast, reheat leftovers in no

time, and even cook a whole dinner. A microwave cookbook or online microwave-specific recipes can show you how to make zap magic happen. See the box on this page.

- A slow cooker. Despite its name, a slow cooker can save more time than practically any appliance in your home. Chances are you got at least one as a present or on a whim at some point—dust it off and get busy. Just toss some dried beans and meat or chicken, some vegetables and flavorful broth, and a few herbs into the slow cooker before leaving the house in the morning, and a delicious stew will be ready and waiting when you walk in the door. Instant dinner! And yes, some slow cookers are Bluetooth enabled.

■ An instant pot. This multitasker appliance is more than a pot—and depending on the brand you get, it could be a pressure cooker (which cooks food quickly—up to 70 percent faster than traditional cooking methods), a slow cooker (see above), a rice maker, a steamer, a sauté pan, an egg boiler, plus more . . . potentially making mealtime magic happen in one pot, in no time. It also allows prepped meals to go directly from freezer to piping hot to satisfied tummy without pausing for defrosting. An added bonus: Instant pots are extra smart—thanks to sensors, they won't overcook your food. Not smart enough? Pick one that's Bluetooth enabled.

■ An air fryer. Sure, it's another appliance, but with no need to preheat and a faster cooking time, vegetables come out perfectly crisp and proteins perfectly cooked—in less time than it would take in the oven. (An added perk: You get your foods crisped perfectly without all that extra oil.)

■ A wok (or large frying pan). The secret of really speedy—and healthy—cooking is stir-frying. Throw some chunks of chicken, broccoli, carrots, and water chestnuts into the wok—and in a matter of minutes, a delicious dinner is served.

■ A blender. You can enjoy a breakfast smoothie in 30 seconds flat.

■ A food processor. Who has time to chop? Who would bother when there's a food processor to do the work for you? These handy appliances can dice, slice, mince, and puree onions, vegetables, potatoes, fruit, or just about anything else that would otherwise take time and elbow grease.

■ A really good knife. Don't have the budget or the space on your kitchen counter for a food processor? Invest in the next best thing: a good-quality knife. A really sharp blade will chop hours off your food-preparation time.

Cook fast foods. Instead of going out for fast food, choose foods that cook up fast. A fresh fillet of fish or a boneless chicken breast can be broiled, poached, or air-fried in minutes. Thinly sliced strips of lean beef or chicken can be stir-fried in moments. Vegetables can be air-fried or steamed to just-tender more quickly than they can be boiled, and you'll have saved not only time, but the vitamins and minerals from going down the drain with the cooking water. Instant-pot dinners are ready in a flash. Many recipes in this book can be prepared in 20 minutes or less.

Or don't cook at all. Serve vegetables raw. Eat leftover grilled chicken cold on a bed of greens. Enjoy some chunks of cheese and a pear straight from the refrigerator. Open a bag of baby carrots, snack on dry cereal or freeze-dried fruit, or peel a banana and slice it into a single-serving container of cottage cheese or yogurt. All nutritious—all in no time at all.

Concentrate on convenience. When feeding yourself and your baby is going to take more than just reaching into the refrigerator and chewing, look for ways to make cooking and preparing meals easier and faster. Instead of buying heads of lettuce that need to be torn, washed, and spun dry and vegetables that need

Launch a Snack Attack

Poking around the fridge, the freezer, or your local market for some good healthy snacks to round out your day and your Daily Dozen? Give these a try:

- Hard-boiled egg (keep a supply in your refrigerator for a quick protein fix)

- Avocado toast with sliced egg (add sriracha for a kick)

- Drinkable yogurt or kefir

- Low-fat yogurt with granola, nuts, and/or berries sprinkled on top

- Freeze-dried cheese

- Parmesan crisps (see box, page 252)

- A mozzarella stick and frozen grapes

- Mango, lime, chili powder, pasteurized feta

- Babybel cheese and an apple

- Sliced tomato topped with pasteurized feta (or mozzarella) and olive oil (add some basil for a caprese salad)

- Whole-grain crackers with a cheese wedge

- Whole-grain tortilla, rolled up with shredded cheese and tomato

- Whole-grain waffle

- Whole-wheat pita chips—store-bought or homemade (add your own salty, sweet, or spicy flavorings)

- A healthy protein bar

- Carrot muffin (page 206)

- Ants on a log (peanut butter on a celery stick, studded with raisins or chocolate chips)

to be peeled and chopped, open a bag of precut, prewashed greens, a bag of pre-shredded carrots or cabbage, and a box of ready-to-pop cherry tomatoes, dump them all into a bowl, and top with oil, vinegar, dried oregano, and some pre-grated Romano cheese. Presto—you've just made a fresh salad (and that took how long?). Scan supermarket shelves for other time-saving ingredients: shredded low-fat cheese, pasta-ready tomato sauces, pre-peeled baby carrots, pre-shredded cabbage for coleslaw, bags of microwave-ready vegetables, chopped, sliced, or diced fruits and veggies, chopped garlic. Though these might cost more at the store, you'll likely find they're worth the price when time is at a premium. Look, also, to the grocer's freezer for frozen vegetables and fruit, as well as healthy frozen entrees. And don't forget the takeout aisle, where you can pick up a roast chicken to go (a healthy choice once you've removed the skin and added that 10-second salad, a microwave-baked sweet potato or a container of precooked brown rice, and quick-cooked frozen vegetables).

Cook for an army. If you cook enough for 2 or more meals at once (which takes only a few moments longer) and tuck the extras, in meal-size portions, in the freezer for future use, you'll save loads of time. (Mark the meals, so you won't be left with unidentified frozen objects.) Make a big batch of whole-wheat pancakes or waffles on Saturday and freeze, and reheat for quick weekday breakfasts. Do the same when you're simmering up a batch of chili. Broil, bake, or grill a multipack of boneless, skinless

- Almond butter spread on whole-grain graham crackers
- Peanut butter and dark chocolate between 2 apple slices
- A handful of almonds or walnuts mixed with raisins or freeze-dried blueberries or strawberries
- Dark chocolate chips with nuts or coconut flakes
- Fruit smoothie (see the recipes starting on page 345)
- Dried or freeze-dried fruit
- Frozen blueberries
- Frozen banana, spread with nut butter, sprinkled with dark chocolate chips
- Sliced banana topped with nonfat Greek yogurt and chopped walnuts
- Watermelon cubes, lime, a sprinkle of salt, a sprinkle of pistachios
- Carrot and celery sticks with hummus or guacamole
- Cucumber hollowed out and filled with hummus
- Baby cucumbers and tzatziki
- Toasted seaweed
- Broccoli crisps (homemade or store bought)
- Bean chips, lentil chips, veggie chips, soy chips, whole-grain tortilla chips, kale chips, root vegetable chips
- Crunchy freeze-dried green peas or snap pea crisps
- Air-popped popcorn, sprinkled with parmesan cheese and chili powder
- A cup of soup sprinkled with cheese
- Crunchy roasted chickpeas (see page 252)

chicken breasts and freeze them individually so you'll always have some to top a salad, fill a sandwich, or add to a veggie stir-fry or pasta dish. Cook a huge batch of brown rice or other grains, and freeze flattened in portioned-out sizes. Just remember to date your freezer stash, so you'll know which items to use first. Have an instant pot? You can use it to heat up your stash without defrosting first.

Prep for an army. Cut up fruits and vegetables twice a week, and keep them stashed for easy snacking in airtight plastic containers. Boil up a big batch of eggs so you'll have them at the ready for snacking, slicing on top of salads or on toast, chopping into egg salad. They'll stay fresh in their shells for up to a week in the fridge.

Give leftovers a new lease on life. Roast a large turkey breast on Sunday, have warm turkey leftovers on Monday (along with leftover mashed sweet potatoes), turkey salad for lunch on Tuesday, turkey stir-fry with brown rice for dinner Tuesday night, and (because you're probably sick of turkey by Wednesday) freeze the rest for turkey cacciatore (just add ready-to-eat tomato sauce and some pasta) whenever the turkey mood strikes again. Or freeze the leftover turkey in slices, ready for workweek sandwiches. Make a double batch of steamed broccoli, have it hot the first night and cold with a vinaigrette or warmed up in a pasta dish or casserole on the second.

Put time on your side with planning. See the box on page 134 for tips on planning ahead.

Ordering Up Labor

Are you over being pregnant (or even overdue)? Looking for a miracle meal to bring on those contractions sooner or help them get the job done faster? A last pregnant supper? Choose from this menu of supposedly cervix-friendly foods, some of which have become labor legends in the mom community, others of which have a side of medical evidence to back them up:

Dates. Thinking dates will be the last thing on your mind when you're pushing 9 months of pregnancy? You might want to think again—and stock up on dates. Not the kind with your sweetie (though you might as well stock up on those dates, too, while you still have the chance), but the kind you can eat—also sweet. Not because they'll bring on labor sooner, but because research shows that eating dates in the last month of pregnancy can lead to a shorter, easier labor. Date-munching moms appear less likely to have premature rupture of the membranes and appear more likely to go into labor spontaneously (avoiding labor induction), have a shorter first phase of labor, and have greater cervical dilation upon admission to the hospital or birthing center. What's in a date that makes it so labor-friendly? Besides all the nutrients that are packed into

those tiny sweets (including potassium, magnesium, vitamin K, and folate), dates have an oxytocin-like effect on the body, helping to stimulate uterine contractions. Their laxative effects (rivaling those of their dried-fruit friend the prune) also stimulate uterine contractions. How many dates will you need to pop to expedite becoming a mom? The researchers had expectant mothers eat 6 dates daily beginning at week 36 of pregnancy. Just remember that dates are very high in fruit sugar, so if you've been instructed to mind your sweets (for instance, if you have gestational diabetes), ask your practitioner before you start dating that much.

Licorice. Real black licorice (not a pack of Twizzlers) contains an ingredient called glycyrrhizin, which, when eaten in very large quantities (repeat: very large quantities), may speed up the onset of labor. The theory: Glycyrrhizin interacts with cortisol levels and/or increases prostaglandins, which brings on those contractions. But beware: That same compound can also cause potassium levels to drop, and in some people, possibly lead to heart arrhythmias. For moms with GD, there's a downside to all the sugar that licorice candy contains.

When Eating Out

Whether you're grabbing a lunch-break bite from a food truck, lingering over a leisurely brunch with friends, or stopping for a quick dinner on the way home from work because you don't have the strength to lift a

spatula, chances are you'll be eating at least some of your pregnancy meals out. Maybe most of them. But how do you make sure eating well is on the menu, even when cooking isn't? And how do you keep the pounds from piling on too

Spicy foods. In the category of no harm, no foul, and no proof: spicy foods. While there isn't any evidence that wolfing down some spicy hot wings or anything doused in sriracha will bring on contractions, plenty of moms swear they've gone straight from a spicy meal to the labor and delivery floor. Of course, if your tummy (and your heartburn) can't take the heat, you probably won't want to turn it up—especially not in the last, extra-uncomfortable weeks of pregnancy.

Pineapple. Prefer a sweeter option? Pineapple or pineapple juice contains the enzyme bromelain, which (when consumed in large quantities), some believe, can contribute to cervical ripening and uterine contractions. There is no scientific proof confirming this theory, but if you're pining for labor, it's worth giving pineapple a try.

Italian food. Some moms credit the balsamic vinegar in popular "labor salads." Others point to those tasty Mediterranean herbs, like oregano and basil, used in Italian cooking. Still others swear it's the eggplant that edged them closer to the delivery room. But scientists aren't buying it (though they may be eating it).

Castor oil. Hoping to sip your way into labor with a castor oil cocktail? Women have been passing down this yucky-tasting tradition for generations on the theory that the powerful laxative will stimulate a mom's bowels, which in turn will stimulate her uterus into contracting. The caveat for this one: Castor oil (even mixed with a more appetizing drink) affects your bowels more than it affects your uterus—causing diarrhea, severe cramping, and vomiting. Before you chugalug, check with your practitioner—and make sure you're ready to begin labor that way. A less aggressive way to get your bowels (if not your uterus) in an uproar: Have a bowl of all-bran cereal.

Herbal teas and remedies. Raspberry leaf tea, black cohosh, and evening primrose may be just what your ancestors (and Instagram buddies) ordered for the overdue, and some studies show that these herbal remedies may actually help trigger or speed up contractions. Since there's no proof of their safety or effectiveness, it's best to ask your practitioner about whether (and how much of them) you should take and how. And turn to them only once you've reached full term.

For more DIY labor-induction tricks that may (but probably won't) do the trick, see *What to Expect When You're Expecting*.

---

fast when eating out comes with your job or your lifestyle? Easy—just keep these tips in mind:

■ Choose a baby-friendly restaurant. It won't be high chairs you'll be scouting for when you're taking your baby out to dinner (at least not yet)—it'll be healthy eating options. Realistically, you won't always get to pick the restaurant, but when you do, be picky. Before you ask for a table, ask for a menu. Better still, scope it out online ahead of time, and scan it for nutritious items (most restaurants have at least some).

■ Have your order in mind. Again, you can't always plan ahead or run the dinner show. But when you can, try to have at least a general idea of what you'll order before you sit down. One, because you'll be able to order it faster, which means you'll be tucking into your meal faster (especially important if you're running on empty). Two, because it will leave less room for impulse orders (if you've mentally prepared for grilled chicken and a salad, you're less likely to end up wandering to the fried side of the menu).

- Take the hunger edge off. Whether it's a handful of almonds or a wedge of cheese, have a light snack before you head out to eat, so you won't be starving by the time your food arrives.

- Ask . . . and you will probably receive. Rare is the server (and kitchen) who won't accommodate a pregnant woman's special requests. So make them.

- Be on portion patrol. Many restaurants dish out portions that well exceed suggested serving sizes for most foods—whether it's a 12-ounce steak or 4 ounces plus of pasta. Too much food (which you may feel obligated to eat, since you're paying for it) can lead to too many calories . . . and/or too much heartburn. Especially if you eat out often, consider sharing an entree or bringing home half (bam, there's tomorrow's lunch, ready to roll). Or skip the entree and go appetizer-happy. Order 2 apps, 1 for your starter, 1 as your entree.

- Look before you leap into the bread basket. Check out the contents for whole-grain options. If none turn up there, ask your server if there are any available from the kitchen. If you're still out of luck, try to go easy on the white stuff, saving your appetite for more wholesome foods still to come.

And mind the butter and olive oil, since that fat can add up fast—and your meal's just getting started. Dip and spread with a light hand.

- Go for green. Select a salad as a first course or a side, so you're sure to score your leafy greens. Ask for the dressing on the side so you can choose how much you want to spoon on or dip in. Not feeling like a salad? Start with some grilled vegetables instead.

- Seek soup. In many restaurants, some of the most nutritious dishes come in bowls (or cups). Look to lentil, bean, or vegetable soups (from minestrone to tomato, sweet potato to winter squash), and don't forget to consider cold ones, too (gazpacho, for instance, is a veritable salad-in-a-soup-bowl). Clamoring for clam chowder? Take Manhattan when you have the chance, since New England chowder and other cream-based soups are typically heavy on the fat.

- Keep it simple. Stick to lean meat, poultry, fish, or seafood, and order them simply broiled, grilled, roasted, baked, steamed, or poached—"fried" and "sautéed" are often keywords for "full of fat." Ask for sauces and gravies on the side, so you can drizzle as desired.

- Be side savvy. The company your meat (or fish) keeps is important, too. Since restaurants usually offer a choice (or will allow substitutions), choose wisely: Opt for a side salad, steamed or grilled vegetables, beans, a baked potato, sweet potato, or, if it's offered, brown or wild rice or another whole grain. Since vegetable servings are often skimpy (are those orange slivers the carrots you ordered?), you might consider asking for an extra portion.

- Treat yourself with care. Is the dessert menu sweet-talking you? Try talking yourself into fresh berries, or maybe a scoop of ice cream or fruit sorbet, instead of the dulce de leche cheesecake (or other desserts that come with a hefty calorie tab). Cravings are calling? Give in while still being sweets-smart: Consider sharing with the table, instead of attacking it all by yourself.

While Traveling

Never again will it be so easy to travel with baby on board. (No diapers! No car seats! No childproofing hotel rooms!) Still, whether you're flying from Phoenix to Fargo, driving from Detroit to Denver, or on the road for business, pleasure, or a little mix of both, being a pregnant traveler poses certain challenges—especially when it comes time to feed your hungry load. After all, it's easy for your eating habits to wander when you're roaming.

How do you schedule in regular meals when you're on an irregular schedule (you just lost 3 hours to a time change, or 2 hours sitting on the tarmac)? How can you handle blood-sugar dips on takeoff—or 2 hours from landing? A grumbling tummy between train stations or miles from the nearest highway rest stop? And what do you do when you can't drink the water or eat the local produce?

You won't have to stick close to home to stick close to healthy pregnancy eating. What you will have to do is include baby's nutritional needs—and yours—in your travel plans:

On a Plane

- Plan ahead. As you know if you've traveled recently, meal service on domestic flights has just about disappeared in coach (you may still find it on international flights). The best you can expect is a sandwich or snack for purchase, if that. Call ahead or check online to find out exactly what will be served and if meals are available for purchase (or for free on international flights). Sometimes a snack means nothing more than a beverage and a bag of pretzels. Takeoff delays can result in mealtime delays, food service carts can move at a maddeningly slow rate down the aisles, and special meals sometimes don't show up at all (plus, let's face it—they're not all that special).

- Pack a snack (or a meal). Even if you'll be served a meal or have the option of buying one, chances are that what you'll find on your tray table won't fill your belly. Not by a long shot. Plus, you have no control over when it will arrive or whether they'll run out of the only healthy choice by the time it's your turn to order. So don't leave meal service up to chance. Always pack a healthy meal or a substantial snack, as well as a few light snacks, in your carry-on bag. Consider a cold sandwich or salad, a cheese stick and crackers, fresh or freeze-dried fruit, a fruit-and-nut bar, a bag of trail mix, bean or vegetable chips. Check out tsa.gov to find out what you can bring along from home and what you'll have to purchase once you've passed through security (like drinks and yogurt).

- Keep the fluids flowing. Flying can be dehydrating because of the low humidity in aircraft cabins, so be sure to drink a lot before and during the flight. Besides keeping yourself from becoming dehydrated, increasing your fluids will send you to the bathroom often—a great way to stretch your legs and prevent circulation problems. But plan on picking up or filling up your own bottle of water before you board. That's because beverage service can take forever on a jumbo jet, and those tiny plastic tumblers may not satisfy your thirst. Never drink the tap water on an airplane.

In a Car

- Plan ahead. If you have many miles ahead of you, check out travel apps to see if there are frequent rest stops on the highway and what kinds of restaurants are available on the road you'll be traveling. (Keep the eating-out tips on page 140 in mind when making those pit stops.)

- Pack a bag. Wherever you're headed, don't leave home without a snack bag. Options to include: beverages, nonperishable snacks (those nuts, that freeze-dried fruit and cheese), a thermos of soup for easy sipping, and (if

---

Fill 'Er Up

Stopping to fill up your car with gas doesn't mean you'll have to fill yourself up with junk food. Most gas station markets carry frozen fruit bars, bananas, peanut butter packets, yogurt, nuts, cheese, whole-grain crackers, healthy chips, and healthy bars.

---

you're carrying a cooler) a selection of cheese sticks or wedges, hummus and cut-up vegetables, and sandwiches (pitas and wraps make for neater eating). If you're in it for the long haul, you can always pull off the interstate and restock your snack supply at a local supermarket.

On a Train

- Check to be sure there's a dining car with a full menu. If not, pack enough meals and snacks for the ride. The snack bar, most likely, won't cut it.

- If you're traveling overnight, check to see if you'll be allowed off the train at stops along the way for a quick trip to markets or restaurants in the station.

On a Ship

- Assuming you're allowed on a cruise ship (your trip will have to be completed before week 24), it's practically impossible to go hungry on an all-you-can-eat cruise. But it is pretty easy to eat more than you're hungry for—and far more calories than you actually need. Fortunately, most cruise kitchens offer healthy options, and many will honor special requests. There will be plenty of temptations for sure, but try to shop the buffet and the menus with an overall healthy big picture (and your Daily Dozen) in mind.

- Be aware of bugs on board. Outbreaks of norovirus and other gastrointestinal illnesses are not uncommon on cruise ships and may be especially dangerous when you're expecting. Check a ship's safety record before you book, and follow the safe eating tips on the pages that follow when you're cruising with a baby aboard (you).

At Your Destination

- Build meals into your itinerary. Whether you'll be sightseeing or meeting, shopping or swimming, schedule in breakfast, lunch, dinner, and snacks. Keep as close to the rhythm of your daily eating routine as you can, but when you can't (you slept through breakfast after a late hotel check-in, or the local restaurants don't open for dinner until 8 p.m. and your tummy can't wait), have a snack to tide you over until mealtime.

- Pack snacks (again). Because you never know when those hunger pangs may strike (and in case they hit when you're far from a restaurant or market—or before the dining room opens or after it has stopped serving), carrying easy-to-munch, energy-boosting snacks is a roaming-mom must.

- Request a mini-fridge. Don't be held captive to the high-priced contents of the hotel minibar (if there is one). Most hotels will provide guests with a small, empty refrigerator upon request (sometimes for a fee) or allow you to empty the stocked minibar. Ask about fridge access ahead of your arrival if you can, and stock your mini to the max with milk, juice, cheese, yogurt, fruit cups, veggie trays, and other drinks and nibbles that need refrigeration. You'll be glad you did when midnight snack attacks strike. Want to avoid the sticker shock of hotel-provided bottled water? Stock up on your own supply and keep it chilled in your mini-fridge.

- Play it even safer. Eating carefully—avoiding raw fish and shellfish, undercooked meats and eggs, unpasteurized soft cheeses—is even more important on the road, especially if the road has taken you to a foreign country. If it's a foreign country with poor sanitation, you'll have to avoid even more. Any food that hasn't been cooked could be contaminated, so steer clear of salads and raw fruits and vegetables that haven't been peeled by you (unless you've checked with the hotel to be sure sanitation protocol has been strictly followed—for instance, the kitchen washes all produce with purified water before prepping). Stay away, also, from milk and milk products (like cheese) that you're not positive have been pasteurized. Thoroughly cooked foods that are still hot are generally safe to eat, though you shouldn't eat any food (hot or otherwise) that appears to have been prepared or stored under unsanitary conditions. If food that is served to you seems questionable, send it back and order something safer. Lovingly rubbing your belly translates in any language: "I'm not trying to be difficult—I'm just watching out for my baby."

- Hydrate with care. Getting your pregnancy quota of fluids when you're traveling is important, particularly if your flights were long or your destination is hot. But before you quench your thirst with a glass of cold local water, make sure it is safe to drink. (Visit cdc.gov/healthywater/global before you visit your destination.) If you're not sure whether the tap water is safe, avoid ice cubes and reconstituted juice or milk unless they are made with bottled, boiled, or purified water. They will be in most good hotels, but always ask. Drink bottled water instead, preferably sparkling. (If the water is still carbonated, you can be sure the bottle hasn't been refilled from a tap and resealed.)

- Don't ask for tummy troubles. A case of traveler's tummy can take the fun out of any trip. But when you're pregnant, cramps, vomiting, and diarrhea can be much more than a miserable inconvenience—and if they lead to dehydration, they can become dangerous. (Besides, who needs another reason to be nauseous when you're pregnant?) To make sure you don't pick up anything but souvenirs at your destination, follow food-safety rules like a mommy maniac—especially if you're traveling in a developing country. If Montezuma does claim revenge, be wary of self-treating. Many over-the-counter diarrhea medications are not recommended for pregnant women, though electrolyte drinks and rehydration fluids are okay. Put in a call, email or text to your doctor or midwife back home for advice.

At Parties

So maybe you're not the party animal you used to be. (Those cocktail parties aren't quite as much fun without the cocktail, your eyelids can't stay open past 10, and your dancing feet are too swollen to fit into your dancing shoes.) That doesn't have to make you a pregnant party pooper. You can still kick up your heels (maybe just not those 5-inch stiletto ones) and enjoy a few rounds (just not the alcoholic kind) on the social circuit—much as you did when your little black dress was actually little. You just have to party . . . like you're pregnant. Keep these tips in mind:

Have one for the road. Because you never know what'll be on the menu when you're not the one planning it, eat a healthy snack before you leave home to take the edge off your appetite—just in case food isn't served promptly (or at all—as in, the cocktail party is cocktails only). Or the party buffet is just desserts—or simply sushi. And for the same reason, make sure you cram a snack into your evening bag, too.

Don't pass the bar. Sure, your party (or holiday) spirit will have to come from within—not from alcohol—when you're expecting. But that doesn't mean you'll need to work the room without a cocktail in your hand. Many cocktails can easily become mocktails—from a virgin Bloody Mary to a no-tequila sunrise or a rumless piña colada. Or keep it simple: An OJ spritzer with a twist, an icy cold grapefruit-and-cranberry (stirred or shaken). House punch of hot mulled cider, unspiked. The same? Definitely not—but still fun and festive.

Survey the buffet. There may be plenty of can-do canapés: Make a beeline to the veggie and fruit trays. Nibble on nuts; olives; cheese cubes, sticks, or crisps; cocktail shrimp or other cooked seafood; deviled eggs; grilled skewers (just make sure any meat you eat isn't rare); meatballs; vegetable or cooked-fish sushi; grilled vegetables. Pass on the smoked fish; raw, seared, or otherwise rare meat or fish (as tempting as you might find that tuna tartare); raw seafood (those oysters and clams); deli meat (unless you're sure it's freshly roasted and carved); soft cheese (unless you're sure it's pasteurized or steamed to bubbly). Clearly, some chafing dishes will be worth digging into (those chicken breasts, that pork loin, those grilled

Healthy Holidays

'Tis the season to be jolly? No problem—and no need to get thrown off course, even with all those extra courses of food at family feasts. Eating well all year round is as easy as pumpkin pie, if you just remember these tips:

- Make room for tradition. No need to diss traditions—just dish up more of the right ones. Pile on the turkey and brussels sprouts. Load up on the sweet potatoes. Find the medium-well end of the roast and get busy. Go on the easy side when it comes to holiday trimmings that don't exactly fit the Daily Dozen profile—enough can be a feast. Your family's traditions don't include vegetables, whole grains, or salad or fruit in any form? Start a new tradition, and bring along a tray of roasted carrots, a quinoa salad, a festive fruit medley.

- Feast but don't fast. Don't take a holiday from regular meals and snacks—even if you'd rather save up for a big Christmas dinner, you and your baby should still eat breakfast and lunch. Just make them a little lighter than usual.

- Don't be a Scrooge. Eating during pregnancy isn't about denying yourself—especially during the holidays. Instead, make moderation your motto when it comes to the treats and sweets of the season. Where there's no wiggle room because of safety concerns—the eggnog is homemade with raw eggs (and rum), as is the holiday hollandaise, there's cold smoked salmon on the canapés, and the brie isn't baked—just take a pregnant pass (see Chapter 5 for other foods to table).

- Don't invite trouble. Enjoy the holidays, but keep sensible eating tips in mind as you do. Watch your overall consumption of calories (so you don't end up with a 10-pound gain during a 2-week holiday season), try not to stuff yourself silly (so you don't pay the price in heartburn or gas pain), and while you're making merry, try to make as many healthy choices as you can.

- Look forward to next year (and years to come). If you feel a little deprived this season, keep in mind that you have more nonpregnant holidays ahead of you than pregnant ones. So take this year's holiday cheer with moderation, and look forward to being just a little jollier when next season rolls around.

shrimp, that wild rice pilaf) . . . others, not so much (that super-creamy Alfredo, those fried potatoes, that greasy sausage, or those unidentified fritters). And of course, don't forget to leave room on your plate for salad and steamed or grilled veggies.

Be selective with sweets. If you really want it, you deserve it—so have it, in moderation. That's what celebrations are for. But try not to bust your calorie bank with sweets that are just so-so—and maybe don't take the all-you-can-eat sundae bar literally. Also be wary of desserts that might have raw egg in them—like mousse. Is there fruit on the dessert table? Go to town.

CHAPTER 9

Eating Well When Eating Is Complicated

....

I t's not always easy to eat well when you're expecting, even when you can (at least in theory) eat most anything. But it's definitely more difficult to follow a healthy pregnancy eating plan when what you can eat—or should eat—is restricted by a chronic condition (like celiac disease) or a pregnancy complication (like gestational diabetes). Or if eating—or gaining enough weight—is doubly (or triply) challenging because you're expecting multiples. Or if you're in bed with a bad cold—or on bed rest—and eating's just too much like hard work. Luckily, with a little nutritional know-how, there's a way around just about any obstacle to healthy eating.

If You Can't Handle Dairy

Milk and dairy products are nature's finest sources of the calcium your body and your baby need when you're expecting. But if milk leaves you with more than a mustache (think gas, and lots of it), you may think twice before reaching for a glass. Or before pouring milk on your cereal. Or dipping into frozen yogurt. Or cheesing up your sandwich.

What's causing all your tummy troubles? It could be that you can't tolerate the lactose or that you're sensitive to one of the naturally occurring proteins in milk. But which is it, and how can you tell those conditions apart?

Lactose intolerance results from a lack of (or inadequate supply of) lactase, the enzyme needed to digest the milk sugar lactose. Those who are lactose intolerant experience a range of symptoms, including gas, bloating, indigestion, cramping that can range from mild to severely uncomfortable, and diarrhea. Wondering if you're among the seeming legions of lactose intolerant? There actually may be fewer of them around than you might think. Studies show that many people who believe they are lactose intolerant actually aren't. Keep in mind, too, that there are degrees of intolerance. While some people can take up to a cup of milk without hearing rumbles from their stomachs, a few may be so lactase deficient that even a sip of milk triggers tummy turbulence.

To tell if you're legit lactose intolerant, take this simple test: When your stomach is empty (2 to 3 hours after a meal or first thing in the morning), drink 2 glasses of milk. If you experience the symptoms associated with lactose intolerance, it's likely you are unable to digest lactose. Need even more confirmation (just to make sure pregnancy symptoms aren't confusing the picture)? Steer clear of dairy products for 2 weeks. If all symptoms disappear, you have a pretty definite diagnosis. If you find your tummy's still acting up, you'll have to blame something else for your gastrointestinal unrest.

Want a more definitive diagnosis? Ask your doctor about a breath test that measures the amount of hydrogen your body produces in the gut after drinking a lactose-containing drink. The presence of hydrogen in your breath indicates improper digestion of lactose in your colon.

Fortunately, there's no need to torture your tummy—not even during pregnancy, when you need to increase your calcium intake. If you're lactose intolerant, there are plenty of ways to get the calcium you need without the stomach upset you certainly don't want:

- Take it slow. Try drinking only ½ cup of milk at a time, eating a small dish of cottage cheese, a thin slice of cheese. In general, small quantities of the offending dairy products spread out during the day may cause less digestive disruption than a couple of large doses.

- Go lactose-free. Shop for lactose-free milk, cottage cheese, cheese, frozen yogurt, and other dairy products. All the calcium gain, without the gas pain. For bonus calcium, look for lactose-free milk that's also calcium fortified.

- Take it with food. Lactose is easier to digest when mixed with other foods (particularly whole grains). So pour your milk into your bran flakes, or melt your cheese on whole wheat.

- Take two. Take lactase in pill form (it comes in chewables or tablets) with your first bite or sip. Or add lactase drops to your next dose of dairy.

- Say cheese. Since milk itself is usually the major culprit, the closer a dairy product is to milk, the more likely it is to offend. Aged cheeses (such as cheddar, Swiss, and parmesan) may be easier on your stomach because more than half the lactose is removed during processing.

- Get active. Active cultures, that is—the kind found in yogurt, yogurt drinks, and kefir. These active bacterial cultures (usually acidophilus) may help break down lactose. And though there's no hard evidence that shows taking a probiotic supplement will ease lactose intolerance, it could help with other tummy troubles (and there's no harm in trying one).

Don't have a problem with lactose but still end up with tummy troubles after drinking milk? You may have difficulty digesting one of the proteins in cow's milk (the A1 protein). Drinking A2 milk, which comes from cows that naturally produce only the A2 protein and not the A1 protein, could be the answer you're looking for—allowing you to drink milk without the accompanying bloating, gas, and discomfort. Not sure if your tummy turbulence is a reaction to the lactose in milk or the A1 protein? Try each type of milk for a week or two and see if your troubles subside on one or the other.

Still can't handle dairy? There's no need to force the issue, or force down that glass of milk or cup of yogurt and face the gastrointestinal music (and pain). But you will need to make up the nutritional shortfall if you're not doing dairy at all. Here's how:

- Look elsewhere. There are plenty of other sources of calcium, including fortified juice, tofu, calcium-enriched nut, soy, and other plant milks, canned salmon and sardines (bones included, but you'll never notice if you mash them up), and leafy greens.

- Don't be D-ficient. Calcium isn't the only nutrient milk provides. Milk is one of the major sources of dietary vitamin D, so if you're not getting milk, you'll need to find alternatives. Taking a prenatal supplement that contains vitamin D (which you're probably already doing), eating enriched cereals and breads, or drinking vitamin D–enriched milk alternatives or juice can help fill the gap.

- Supplement. Ask your practitioner about prescribing a calcium supplement if you're not getting enough through your diet. If your pregnant tummy gives you plenty of trouble with or without dairy, you might want to consider taking the supplement in the form of a calcium-containing antacid, such as Tums or Rolaids.

If You Have Celiac Disease (or Gluten Sensitivity)

If you have celiac disease, you already know that a strict gluten-free diet is a must. You also likely already know why: When someone with celiac disease ingests gluten (a protein found in wheat and certain other grains), the body triggers an immune response that causes damage to the small intestines, resulting in the malabsorption of nutrients and other problems, from diarrhea to bloating. Something else that's not news to you: Staying on a gluten-free diet is difficult, but it's definitely worth the effort. And that goes doubly when you're expecting. Untreated celiac disease can cause pregnancy problems, from miscarriage to premature birth and low birthweight. But staying completely gluten-free before, during, and after those 9 months can prevent all of those increased risks.

Here's how to eat well for two without gluten:

- Make your gastroenterologist part of your ob team. Adding a registered dietitian with expertise in both pregnancy and celiac disease can help, too, as you formulate your pregnancy eating plan.

- Stay gluten-free, of course. You know the drill. Strictly avoid wheat and wheat varieties (like kamut, spelt, farro, couscous, and bulgur), rye, barley, and triticale and all foods with even trace amounts of those grains. Seeking baby-nourishing whole grains that are free of gluten? There are plenty to pick from, including brown, black, and wild rice, corn (just check to be sure no other grains have been added to the corn products you choose), quinoa, millet, teff, buckwheat, and amaranth. Oats are iffy; see below.

- Consider oats carefully. Pure oats are gluten-free, but while most people with celiac disease can eat them safely, a small percentage may experience a glutenlike reaction to them. If you're not sure whether you're in that percentage and you've always avoided oats, check with your gastroenterologist before adding them into your pregnancy diet. If you do reach for oats, reach only for those that are certified gluten-free. Oats and oat products are more likely than most grains to have contact with gluten-containing grains before making it to store shelves.

- Be a label reader. The FDA's Food Allergen Labeling and Consumer Protection Act mandates that companies list allergens—including wheat—on labels of packaged foods that contain such allergens. But (and again, this likely isn't news to you) don't assume that wheat-free means gluten-free. Other grains besides wheat contain gluten and plenty of gluten-containing ingredients that might not be obvious ("natural flavoring" or added "seasonings" may contain gluten). Screening ingredients lists carefully is always a good start—if you really know your gluten and all the forms it can come in—but it doesn't protect against the possibility of cross-contact during processing or manufacturing. That's why your safest bet is to look for foods that are labeled "certified gluten-free," or "GF." That indicates that a product has undergone a stringent review process and contains less than 20ppm (parts per million) of gluten.

- Look for hidden gluten. Another reason to reach for products that are labeled "GF"? Gluten lurks in products you might never associate with it (unless you've been a gluten detective for years): soy sauce, salad dressings, sauces—even chocolate or potato chips. Nuts, seeds, and peanuts are naturally gluten-free, but always reach for ones carrying the GF label, since some may have been processed with or near gluten-containing ingredients. Check for a GF label, too, when looking for vitamins and other supplements—the FDA covers these under current regulations.

- Keep an eye on your kitchen. Cross-contact (between gluten-containing and gluten-free foods) can happen anywhere there are gluten eaters. You probably know what to look for, but look anyway: Double dipping in the peanut butter jar (the knife leaves errant crumbs of wheat bread), or dipping a wheat-containing tortilla chip into the salsa. Dishing out the gluten-free salad dressing with a spoon that has touched the regular salad dressing. Reusing the pot that cooked the regular pasta to cook the gluten-free one. Experts suggest it's safest to use separate cutting boards, toasters, strainers, and other utensils when possible (unless everyone who lives with you goes completely gluten-free, too).

- Be a wary diner. Something else you almost certainly already know: According to the FDA, restaurants that label certain menu items gluten-free should be adhering to the same strict standards as manufacturers of food products. Will the kitchen in a restaurant always be that careful? That's hard to know for sure. So always ask the waiter to check with the chef about the gluten status of menu items. Ask not only about the ingredients used, but the preparation and cooking standards. (Do they use separate pots, pans, fryers, prep spaces, and kitchen utensils for gluten-free menu items?) If you have celiac disease (as opposed to a sensitivity), be clear that your health depends on staying gluten-free. It might be easier to say that you have a "severe allergy to gluten"—the kitchen may be more likely to take your request seriously.

- Skip the gluten without skipping the nutrients. Since many processed gluten-free products are made from nutritionally meaningless starches (white rice flour, tapioca starch, cornstarch, potato starch), they may be nutritionally poor performers, lacking in (or low in) iron, B vitamins, and fiber. Select healthier gluten-free products by looking for those that are enriched and contain nutritious gluten-free whole grains and seeds.

- Keep out the gluten, keep up the vitamins and minerals. Straying from a completely gluten-free diet can result not only in intestinal damage, but also in vitamin and mineral deficiencies caused by malabsorption of nutrients (especially zinc, selenium, iron, vitamin D, and folic acid). With pregnancy's increased nutritional need for these and other vitamins and minerals, that's a doubly significant risk. Besides staying on a strict gluten-free diet when you're expecting (which can be a rich supply of vitamins and minerals that come from naturally gluten-free foods like fruits and vegetables), it's especially important to take your daily prenatal vitamin and any additional supplemental vitamins and minerals as directed by your practitioner (just make sure that all your supplements are labeled "GF").

Don't have celiac disease, but do have a suspected or diagnosed case of non-celiac gluten sensitivity—one that triggers significant tummy troubles when you eat gluten, if not serious health risks? Check with your practitioner to discuss a pregnancy diet protocol—and make sure that if you're avoiding gluten entirely, you're getting your fair share of nutrients from the foods you do eat.

If You Have Irritable Bowel Syndrome

Whether it's constipation, gas, bloating, nausea, vomiting, or all (or a combination) of the above, most moms-to-be can expect their tummies to take a hit during pregnancy. Add irritable bowel syndrome to the mix, and the normal digestive pains of pregnancy can multiply. (A few moms with chronic IBS find their symptoms ease during pregnancy, but they're the lucky exception.) Since a diet that's free of foods that trigger IBS symptoms can also be low on nutrients that are important during pregnancy, eating well while still feeling well can be extra challenging. Here are some tips to keep your symptoms in check while checking off your Daily Dozen of nutrients:

- Stick to the old tricks. A lot of the strategies you probably already use to keep your IBS symptoms under control are actually smart strategies for every pregnant woman: Eat small, more frequent meals, stay well hydrated, avoid excess stress, and, of course, steer clear of foods or drinks that make your IBS symptoms (and likely, your pregnancy symptoms) worse, like anything fried or extra-gas producing.

- Slowly step up your fiber intake. If you're used to avoiding fruits, veggies, and whole grains to avoid diarrhea, increase your fiber intake gradually. Too much too soon can tax your tummy as it adjusts.

- Enlist a professional. Following a low-FODMAP diet to manage your IBS? This diet eliminates foods containing short-chain carbohydrates that, if poorly digested, ferment in the lower part of your large intestine. The problem is it can also eliminate a lot of healthy foods that can normally do a pregnant body (and a baby) good, like dairy, certain fruits and vegetables, nuts, and some grains. To make sure you manage your IBS and your nutritional needs during pregnancy, enlist your gastroenterologist, your practitioner, and a registered dietitian to help create an eating plan that does both.

- Get cultured. Adding some probiotics to your diet (in the form of yogurt or yogurt drinks, if you can handle them, or in the form of a supplement) can be surprisingly effective in regulating bowel function, and they're safe during pregnancy. Check with your practitioner for a recommendation.

If You Have Food Allergies

Whether you developed a food allergy early in life or later in the eating game, you probably already know how to avoid the triggers in your diet, and depending on how serious the allergy is, you may already be used to playing food detective—and being extra assertive about giving strict orders with your restaurant orders. Pregnancy is definitely not a time to play around with serious food allergies, but it's also not a time to shortchange yourself on nutrients. Here's how to work around both challenges:

- Always remember to read food labels extra carefully, and always alert restaurants to your allergy before ordering.

- Find substitutes where you can, to fill in the missing nutrient gaps.

- Keep your practitioner in the loop. He or she can determine if additional supplements beyond a prenatal vitamin are necessary.

- It goes without saying, but: If your allergy is severe, make sure to carry an EpiPen with you at all times in case of emergencies.

Wondering if your history of food allergies (or your family's, or your partner's) should keep you from eating foods that are considered highly allergenic (like wheat, soy, milk, fish, shellfish, peanuts, tree nuts, and eggs) during pregnancy and breastfeeding, to avoid exposing your baby and increasing his or her risk for developing food allergies? Actually, research has confirmed that the reverse is true: Not only is there no reason to avoid allergenic foods during pregnancy and breastfeeding (assuming you're not allergic to them yourself), but eating them may reduce your baby's future risk of food allergies. Check with your practitioner about specifics in your case.

If You Have Gestational Diabetes

If you've been given a diagnosis of gestational diabetes (GD), you have plenty of company—and it's growing. It's estimated that up to 10 percent of moms-to-be develop this pregnancy-related condition, which occurs when the body becomes more resistant to insulin (the hormone that lets the body turn blood sugar into energy) and isn't able to produce enough insulin to keep blood sugar under control. Unlike other types of diabetes, GD is temporary—blood-sugar levels usually return to normal after delivery (though moms with gestational diabetes are at much greater risk for Type 2 diabetes later in life). But for a pregnant woman who is suddenly faced with major restrictions to her diet, it can seem to stretch on and on. That's the bad news. The good news is that gestational diabetes can usually be controlled by those dietary restrictions (as tough as it may seem to follow them, at least at first). Other measures can help manage gestational diabetes (like getting regular exercise; see *What to Expect When You're Expecting* for much more), but eating well when you have GD will mean:

Diet changes. There's really no way around it: Managing gestational diabetes usually takes plenty of diet changes—changes you may not be super happy about, especially if you have a sweet tooth or you're a carb-craver. Your practitioner will tell you to follow a special diet, which probably won't be all that different from the Pregnancy Diet. Working with a registered dietitian who has experience with GD (ask your practitioner for a referral) will make figuring out the best eating plan—and sticking to it—a little easier. There's no one-size-fits-all food plan for every mom-to-be with GD because everybody tolerates carbs differently, but in general, it's recommended that women with GD do the following:

- Be carb conscious. You'll likely be told to limit the amount of refined carbs you eat (white rice, white potatoes, white bread, white pasta) because they turn quickly to sugar when digested, raising blood-glucose levels. Focus, instead, on high-fiber complex carbs that have a low glycemic load, such as whole grains, beans, peas, lentils, and vegetables. So-called low glycemic index foods release sugar into the blood more slowly, helping to keep blood-sugar levels stable and within normal range. You'll find that they offer more long-lasting energy boosts, too. Chances are that fruit (another complex carb) may be limited but won't be off the menu (fruit juice may be; keep reading). Some women are told to count and curb even complex carbs, or at least to limit the amount taken at one sitting—but again, take your dietary marching orders from your doctor.

■ Unfriend fruit juice. Even fruit sugar can raise your blood sugar, which means that naturally sweet 100 percent fruit juices will have to be restricted, too. Your doctor or dietitian may (or may not) give you the green light on occasional small amounts of juice (up to 4 ounces, taken with meals). Mixing the juice with sparkling water will dilute the fruit sugar while making your treat last longer.

■ Be choosy with fruit. Can you still be besties with fruit? Unlike juice, fruit contains fiber, which slows the absorption of sugar into the blood. Still, don't get too friendly with fruit. Depending on how your body processes carbs and sugars, you might be told to eat fresh or fresh-frozen fruit in moderation, limit it to ½ or 1 cup at a time, or (less likely) to strictly avoid fruit altogether. Some fruits contain more sugar than others—you might be told to avoid only those that do, like grapes, cherries, pineapple, mango, and banana. Dried fruit contains more sugar than fresh, so it's more likely to be restricted.

■ Stay low-fat. Fat is an essential nutrient—especially during pregnancy. But fat lingers in your bloodstream, causing sugars to stay elevated and insulin to be less efficient, which means your body will need more insulin to keep blood-sugar levels within normal range. Choose lean sources of protein

and calcium, and stick to healthy fats, such as those in nuts, seeds, and avocado.

■ Skip sugar. Chances are, your sweet tooth won't get much wiggle room. To keep your blood-sugar levels from rising to unsafe levels, you'll need to stay away from foods that increase them. Not surprisingly, foods (and drinks) that contain added sugar in any form and by any name (white sugar, brown sugar, raw sugar, turbinado sugar, high-fructose corn syrup, corn syrup, honey, maple syrup, molasses, agave, coconut sugar, and so on) top that list. You may be allowed to eat small amounts of sugar-sweetened foods and drinks in moderation (or they may be officially off-limits), but try to steer clear of high-sugar standards, such as cakes, pies, cookies, ice cream, candy, and soft drinks. Check out page 74 for a list of sugar substitutes. Watch out, too, for added sugar in places you might not expect to see it, like ketchup and other condiments.

Meal control. The grazing approach to eating works best for most pregnant women, but is especially important for those trying to regulate their blood sugar. Aim for 3 meals and 2 to 4 snacks each day—spaced as evenly as possible (so that you're eating a small amount every 2 to 3 hours). Another rule that applies to all pregnant women but must be more strictly stuck to by those with GD: no meal skipping. Regularly skipping meals (or snacks) can result in hypoglycemia (low blood sugar), which can make you feel miserable—irritable, shaky, headachy.

In general, try to combine a protein and carb at each meal and snack—especially at breakfast, when blood sugar tends to be higher. A bedtime snack will be super-important, too, since it will help ward off the lower-than-normal blood-sugar levels that are common during the night in women with gestational diabetes. Before turning in, eat a snack that contains protein (such as low-fat cheese) and complex carbohydrates (such as whole-wheat bread). The carbohydrates will stabilize your blood-sugar level early in the night, while the protein acts as a long-acting stabilizer.

Weight control. Since too many pounds can send blood-sugar levels soaring, you'll have to pay even more attention to your weight gain than other moms-to-be. You'll also need to pay extra attention to the rate of gain. Gaining too much weight too quickly (2 or more pounds per week) results in extra body fat, which, in turn, can produce an insulin-resistant effect. See Chapter 6 for ways to help you gain the right number of pounds at the right rate during pregnancy.

If You're Carrying Multiples

Expecting twins (or more)? Then you'll need to pay at least twice as much attention to your diet as a mom with only one baby on board. As it turns out, good nutrition during a multiple pregnancy has an even greater impact on baby birthweight than it does during a singleton pregnancy. And quality alone won't do it—you'll also need to add some quantity. For each extra baby you have on board, you'll have extra requirements above and beyond those of an expectant mom-of-one. Fortunately for you (and your belly, which will be stretched to capacity anyway during your multiple pregnancy), that doesn't mean you'll have to consume twice as many calories or vitamins for twins, or three times as much protein for triplets. Just keep in mind the extras you'll need when you're eating for three or more:

Extra weight. Not surprisingly, toting an extra baby means you'll have to tote around extra weight. Also not surprisingly, the healthier your weight gain (and your diet), the healthier your babies' weight gain is likely to be. Most experts say that women of normal pre-pregnancy weight who are pregnant with twins should gain between 37 and 54 pounds—roughly 50 percent more than the recommended weight gain for a single pregnancy (for triplets, 50 to 60 pounds). And because you can expect your babies to arrive somewhat earlier than single babies (full term for twins is usually considered 37 to 38 weeks), you'll need to pack in that weight gain (and all those extra nutritional needs) in a shorter period of time. Challenging? You bet, especially because you're also likely to experience more nausea and vomiting in your first trimester and beyond than a mom expecting a single baby. But with a little extra efficiency, it can be done.

Extra calories. So how do you gain all that extra weight? The usual way—by piling on extra calories, about 150 to 300 extra per fetus per day. If you're carrying twins, that's an extra 300 to 600 calories, and if you're carrying triplets, that's an extra 450 to 900 calories per day (check with your practitioner to determine your magic number). A food dream come true? Depending on what your food dreams are made of, maybe (peanut butter on everything!), maybe not (fries with everything!). Most of those extra calories should come from nutrient-dense foods that best nourish your babies and your pregnancy. Studies show that a high-calorie diet that's also high in nutrients significantly improves your chances of having healthy, full-term babies.

So get ready to eat more—but to eat well. Use the Pregnancy Diet in Chapter 3 as your guide, and then add more nutrient-dense food, keeping an eye on the scale to ensure your weight gain is on target (no calorie counting necessary). With your bigger goals in mind, efficiency will be extra important. Instead of trying to squeeze the extra calories and nutrients into only 3 meals, try eating 5 or 6 small meals and several light snacks throughout the day. Another reason to eat more frequently: Research has suggested that women who eat at least 5 meals plus snacks a day are more likely to carry to term. Plus, you'll likely be less bothered by indigestion and heartburn—just a couple of the tummy troubles that are often doubled in twin pregnancies. (See page 107 for mini-meal tips.)

Extra iron. Being pregnant means your body's in the blood-making business big-time, since blood volume must increase significantly to nourish a developing fetus. Naturally, the more fetuses that blood volume must support, the more it must increase. Enter extra iron—the mineral that helps manufacture red blood cells. Most women end up needing more iron than their diets can provide at some point in their pregnancy—you'll need lots more, lots sooner. To fill that need, your practitioner will probably prescribe an iron supplement early in your pregnancy. Be

sure to supplement that supplement by eating iron-rich foods such as red meat and dried fruit. Take iron sources with a vitamin C–rich food to aid absorption, but avoid taking calcium supplements or eating calcium-rich foods along with iron, since that can block absorption.

Extra vitamins. More babies means a greater need for baby-building vitamins of every variety. Your one-a-day prenatal supplement will cover the basics, but you and your babies will benefit when you increase your vitamin intake the old-fashioned way—by eating vitamin-rich foods.

Extra minerals. Your prenatal vitamin is a good place to start, but it won't provide you with all the extra minerals you'll need when you're building an extra baby. Some doctors recommend, for instance, that women carrying twins supplement with magnesium and calcium—and for good reason. Magnesium may reduce the risk of preterm labor—something most multiple pregnancies are at risk of. Calcium, of course, builds strong bones and teeth, and with at least two sets of each growing inside you, you'll need plenty of help from that essential mineral.

Extra fluid. Being dehydrated can also lead to preterm labor, so step up the fluids—drinking at least 10 glasses daily. Drinking between meals (rather than attempting to sip with them) will keep the fluids from competing with the solids for coveted room in the closer and closer quarters of your stomach. Even better: Try to eat plenty of fluid-rich fruits and veggies, like watermelon and lettuce.

Extra help eating well. Your ob may refer you to a registered dietician who can help you figure out how to fit all those nutrition extras in.

When You're Sick

It doesn't seem quite fair, and yet it's true. As a mom-to-be—probably already saddled with a variety of uncomfortable pregnancy symptoms, from nausea and vomiting to heartburn and indigestion—you're actually more likely to become sick than members of the nonpregnant population. That's because your immune system is slightly lowered during pregnancy—nature's way of ensuring that your baby (who is a foreigner to your system) won't be rejected by your body. This immune suppression, as well intended as it is, leaves you particularly susceptible to infections, coughs, colds, gastrointestinal bugs, and the flu. And it's not just the glow that goes when a pregnant woman gets sick. It's often her appetite and her ability to eat a regular diet as well.

Should you find yourself sick in bed with more than just the usual pregnancy symptom suspects, be sure to check in with your practitioner for a diagnosis and a treatment plan. But also plan to eat well while you're feeling crappy. These tips should help:

When you have a cold. It's never a good idea to starve a cold, especially when you're expecting. (The same goes for the flu, but a case of flu—or suspected flu—also requires prompt medical attention during pregnancy.) Since your body needs energy (from food) to heal, you'll get better faster if you eat. Of course, that's easy to say, but not so easy to do when your nose is stuffy, your head achy, your throat sore and scratchy, and your mouth busy coughing. Still, try to push:

- Soft, soothing foods. Oatmeal, scrambled eggs, applesauce, smoothies—really, whatever is easiest for you to

swallow. And don't forget to sip on some soup—any soup, but especially chicken soup, which research shows isn't good just for the soul, but also for relieving congestion.

- Fluids. You'll need your usual quota of fluids when you're laid up with a bug, plus extra fluids to replace those lost through a runny nose, and to promote a quicker recovery. Staying hydrated loosens the mucus in your nose and sinuses, helping to reduce congestion. So keep a bottle or thermos next to your bed (or at your desk if you've brought your cold to work) and sip whatever you can, as often as you can. Water, ginger tea, and diluted juice are all good choices, and warming up the fluid (yes, even the water) will make it more soothing to sip. Soup counts, too, as do juicy fruits. And although milk has long been rumored to increase nasal congestion, there is no scientific evidence to back up that theory. So unless you find that it makes you stuffier, there's no need to miss out on milk while a cold has you down. Warm milk might be extra soothing, especially mixed with a teaspoon of honey.

- Vitamins. Getting your share of vitamins and minerals may help keep you from coming down with a cold in the first place—or, if it's too late for that, help you beat it back. So take your prenatal supplement as usual (but no extra doses of vitamins without your practitioner's go-ahead), and focus on concentrated sources of vitamin C, like citrus and melon.

Stomach bug. You finished weathering morning sickness, and thought your tummy had nothing but smooth sailing ahead. Then, those all-too-familiar rumblings began anew—this time, courtesy of a stomach virus or a mild case of food poisoning. While morning sickness can last for months (as probably nobody needs to tell a pregnant woman), symptoms of a stomach bug are usually brief, if intense—lasting no more than 24 or 48 hours. But because diarrhea and vomiting can rob your baby of vital nutrients and fluids—even in a short time—you'll need to pay as much attention as possible to your diet while you're waiting for the misery to pass. Push yourself on:

- Fluids. You've likely heard it before, but it's worth repeating: In the short term, fluids are more important than solids. Even when you can't keep as much as a crust of bread down, you'll need to prevent dehydration by getting enough fluids. Try plain water, sparkling water, or ginger tea. If you're vomiting, taking small sips every 15 minutes may give the fluids a fighting chance of staying down. If you can't stomach sipping, suck on ice chips or ice pops. If symptoms are severe or you can't manage to get enough fluids into you (or both), your practitioner may recommend a rehydration fluid (or frozen rehydration pops) as a precaution. Coconut water may be helpful, too. Once clear liquids (diluted fruit juices—particularly white grape, which is easier on the tummy—and clear broth) go down and stay down, you can add nutritious smoothies and fruits with high water concentration, like watermelon. Don't forget that ginger can also ease the quease when you're down with tummy troubles. Drink it in tea, ginger ale, or other ginger beverages (you can also suck or chew on ginger candy).

Weighing In on That Ounce of Prevention

The best kind of medicine—especially during pregnancy—is the preventive kind. Giving your immunity a shot in the arm—by keeping yourself well rested and well nourished—can keep you from coming down with mild infections in the first place, or help you recover from them faster when they do strike. Some of nature's finest immunity boosters also happen to be Daily Dozen hall-of-famers, including yogurt (the probiotics naturally found in them are excellent fighters against bad bacteria) and foods rich in vitamin C and beta-carotene.

On the other hand, you should definitely not reach for alternative remedies sometimes used (though not scientifically proven) to prevent or help treat infection—say, extra doses of vitamin C or zinc or such purported immunity-boosters as echinacea, Coldcalm, Zicam, Umcka, Kaloba, or Zucol to stop a cold in its tracks or minimize symptoms. None of these remedies are recommended for pregnancy use. It's smarter—and safer—to reach for an orange instead.

- Foods you can handle. If you can stomach solids, focus on whatever you can get down and keep in, like crackers, unbuttered toast, bananas, applesauce, oatmeal, brown rice, or pasta. No need to restrict your diet if (or when) food is appealing, even if you have diarrhea—though it makes sense to stay away from difficult-to-digest foods, like anything fried, greasy, or spicy.

- Vitamins as usual. Try to take your pregnancy supplement daily at a time it's least likely to come back up, and never on an empty stomach. But don't worry if you need to skip it for a day or two. Once the bug stops bugging you, you'll be able to make up those lost nutrients.

Urinary tract infection (UTI). UTIs are so common during pregnancy that an estimated 5 percent of pregnant women can expect to develop at least one. They're also serious business during pregnancy. Untreated, a UTI is more likely to progress to a kidney infection in pregnant women. So don't try to self-diagnose or self-treat a UTI—call your practitioner if you suspect one.

Prevention is always the best strategy, especially when you're expecting. But these preventive tips, when used in conjunction with your practitioner's prescribed treatment can also help speed recovery from an infection:

- Drink plenty of fluids. Water can help flush out any bacteria that are hanging out in your bladder. Some say that cranberry juice, which changes the alkilinity of urine, may keep bacteria from sticking to urinary tract walls, making it an especially beneficial fluid.

- Avoid coffee and tea (even decaffeinated) since they may increase irritation—the last thing your urinary tract needs right now.

- Ask your practitioner about taking probiotics to help restore the balance of beneficial bacteria. Probiotics could be especially helpful if you're taking antibiotics.

When You're on Activity Restriction

Just about everyone dreams of being able to kick off her shoes, put up her feet, plump up the pillows, and lounge the day (or even the afternoon!) away in bed or on the sofa—binge-watching favorite shows and (hey, since it's a dream anyway) popping chocolates. But for moms with complications who end up being prescribed any amount of enforced rest—whether it's bed rest (at home or even in the hospital), restricted activity, shortened work days, limited standing, or a combination of these, it can be less dream, more nightmare. And mealtimes? Not exactly the room service experience dreams are made of, either—especially when no one's around to deliver it.

Fortunately, bed rest in any form is rarely recommended anymore, primarily because most of the evidence shows that it's not only ineffective in treating or preventing complications (such as preterm labor) but that it can do far more harm than good. Still, if you've been issued no-marching orders (or periodic marches to the sofa for some lying-down time), you may be wondering how it's possible to stay off your feet and on the Pregnancy Diet at the same time. Here are some strategies if you're on activity restriction or enforced rest:

Stay hydrated. Reducing your activity may also have you reaching for your water bottle less often—after all, you may feel less thirsty if you're moving around less. Getting enough fluids will help minimize swelling and constipation, both of which may be compounded when you're often parked on the couch. Staying hydrated is especially important if you're trying to head off contractions.

Break for meals and snacks. All those rest breaks may put the brakes on your appetite (it may be hard to get hungry when you're not getting a move on)—or the time you have to break for meals and snacks. Keeping stocked up at the office and at home on healthy, easy eats and setting reminders to refuel on schedule may help. On the flip side, if you're pretty sure the couch potato in you will cry out for potato chips—and you're prone to snacking when you're prone and bored—be extra mindful of mindful eating. And make sure your nibbles are carefully curated to include more carrots than cookies. Either way, tap into healthy food delivery options to save yourself the time spent on your feet shopping and cooking.

Give yourself props. Not because enforced rest can be hard (it can). But because you'll feel the (heart)burn more when you're lying down. So prop yourself up with pillows as you rest, and especially if you're resting while eating.

Keep an eye on the scale. Limiting your activities will limit the calories you're burning—but it may also limit the number of calories you eat (if you never feel hungry). As always, the best strategy is to watch your weight gain, to be sure it's rising at the right rate. Also, ask your practitioner about exercises you can do while sitting (or even lying down), if only to boost your circulation, flexibility, and muscle strength.

For more on activity restrictions during pregnancy, see *What to Expect When You're Expecting*.

Eating Well Postpartum

....

Your baby-making days are officially over, at least for now—but your baby-care days (and nights) have only just begun. Especially if you're breastfeeding, the demands of new-mom life—and the demands of your hungry baby—will be at least as great as the demands of pregnancy were. At 3 a.m., maybe even more so.

Happily, the demands on your diet (and your eating habits) won't be nearly as heavy a lift. Postpartum eating—and drinking—allows for a lot more leeway than pregnancy eating does. Can't wait to dig into a fully runny egg (or an uncensored Caesar)? Your time has come! Love the way that wine with dinner winds you down after a hard day with baby? Uncork that cab! Having sushi withdrawal? Whip out those chopsticks and get busy, and even pass the sake!

Still, there are plenty of perks to healthy postpartum eating—and to keeping some of those healthy eating habits you picked up during pregnancy. Eating well postpartum can help you recover from those long months of pregnancy and those long hours of labor and delivery. But it can also help you put your best new-mom foot forward (and keep you on your feet after 2 solid hours of rocking). It can boost your energy (what there is of it), lift your mood, ease that postpartum constipation and those hemorrhoids, help you sensibly shed those leftover pregnancy pounds, and, if you're breastfeeding, help pump up your milk supply.

The Postpartum Diet

N ow that you're on the other side of pregnancy, continuing to eat well can help your body bounce back. And just as the Pregnancy Diet wasn't all that different from the average healthy diet, the Postpartum Diet isn't, either.

Nine Ways to Eat Healthy Postpartum— and Beyond

T he 9 basic principles that steered you through 9 months of healthy eating can continue to be your guide during the postpartum period and beyond— whether you're breastfeeding or not:

Choose calories you can still count on. Looking to lose the pregnancy love handles you're not exactly loving? It will help to remember that all calories are not created equal. The calories eaten in the form of a frosted pastry, for instance, are less likely to be burned as fuel and more likely to accumulate in those hard-to-trim areas than the calories consumed in an apple spread with almond butter. Try to take most of your calories through lean protein, fruits, vegetables, whole grains, and healthy sources of fat—you won't only have more energy to burn (something you'll need a lot of these days!), but you may also find those inches melting off faster.

Continue being an efficient eater. When you focus on foods that multi-task in nutritional categories—a cup of Greek yogurt (protein and calcium) with half a mango (vitamin A and vitamin C)—you're eating efficiently. Selecting foods that pack the most nutrition for the calories is a winning

strategy—for your overall health and for your waistline.

Feed yourself, feed your baby. Missing meals (who has time for breakfast when baby needs to be fed, burped, diapered, dressed, and repeat?) can leave you with less energy when you need it the most—and when baby most needs you to have it. And if you're breastfeeding, inadequate nutrition can, over time, compromise milk supply.

Be complex with carbs. Your postpartum body still needs the energy-sustaining vitamins and minerals that are naturally found in whole-grain breads and cereals, brown rice, beans, and other legumes. Complex carbs also pack a natural punch of fiber—something that will do a postpartum (possibly constipated) body good.

Spare the sugar. Maybe you've heard (and would like to believe) that nothing beats a candy bar for giving you the energy boost you so sorely need these days (and nights). But the truth is, sugary treats will lift you only briefly before sending you into an energy crash-and-burn. And while having the occasional sugary treat won't throw your postpartum eating plan into a tailspin, making them your most frequented food group will. Not to mention make it harder to (gradually) drop those pregnancy pounds.

Feature fruits and vegetables. Looking for a tasty, low-cal, and low-fat food to help keep weight loss on track? Something that's a powerhouse in vitamins, minerals, and phytochemicals? Something high in fiber to help keep constipation at bay? And something that will give you energy when baby's pulling an all-nighter? Look no farther than the produce aisle, where you can load up on fruits and vegetables that provide vitamins, minerals, fiber, phytochemicals, and energy-producing carbs in each delicious bite.

Choose foods that remember their roots. Foods that are highly processed have not only lost a lot of their natural nutrition and (more than likely) gained a lot of unhealthy saturated fat, sodium, and sugar in the processing plant, but may also contain chemical additives that could find their way into your milk supply (and your baby) if you're breastfeeding. Best, as always, to stick to foods that haven't ventured far from their natural roots.

Cave to the crave. Deprivation usually doesn't work when you're trying to eat well or when you're trying to lose weight—and you're trying to do both postpartum. So have your cake in moderation, and eat it without guilt. Just know your limits and stick to them (especially if a sliver of cake will inevitably lead to a slab . . . or two).

Eat well family-style. There's never been a better time to join nutritional family forces for a healthier future. After all, there's a new mouth to feed in the house. How that mouth will be fed (and how it will eventually choose to eat) will depend a lot on what fills your plate, as well as what fills your pantry, fridge, and freezer. A little one who's raised in a home where the protein is lean, the snack of choice is fruit, salad is friend not foe, sandwiches come on whole wheat, cereals aren't sweetened, and fast food isn't a first choice is likely to grow up thinking that eating well is, well, natural.

The Postpartum Diet

What makes a healthy postpartum diet? The same Daily Dozen that covered your nutritional bases during pregnancy. With just a few tweaks in the number of servings—more if you're breastfeeding, fewer if you're not:

Calories. After months of putting on weight, you're probably eager to start taking it off. But drastically slashing calories isn't the smart way to rediscover your waist. Instead, you'll need to strike a balance: enough calories to keep you on the go, not so many that the numbers on the scale don't start gradually dropping. Operative word, "gradually." Remember, it took 9 months to put those pregnancy pounds on, and it may take at least that many to take them off.

Breastfeeding actually requires more calories than pregnancy does (after all, you're still feeding baby—only baby is much bigger now). So, though you don't literally need to count them, you'll need up to 500 more calories a day when you're breastfeeding than you would need to maintain your prepregnancy weight (double that if you're exclusively breastfeeding twins, triple if you're the sole food source for triplets). Many moms find that breastfeeding helps melt the pounds away, even with the extra calories—other moms find that baby feeding makes them so hungry that losing baby weight becomes a losing battle. Either way, be careful not to restrict your calories too much, or you may end up reducing your milk supply.

If you're not breastfeeding, your extra calorie allowance has expired—at least, if you'd like to start losing the pregnancy weight. Eating about the same number of calories as you did to maintain your prepregnancy weight will get you back there sooner or later—sooner if you're more active than you

Help for the Zombie Mom

Feeling more zombie than mommy? Finding the little things in life—putting one foot in front of the other (and the right shoe on the right foot), pouring the milk into your coffee (not into your orange juice), putting the dirty clothes into the washer (not the dryer)—harder and harder to achieve in your chronically sleep-deprived state? Of course you are—that's part of the new-mom package, especially when your package includes around-the-clock breastfeeding. Still, while sleep deprivation will probably be a given for months to come, utter exhaustion doesn't have to be. Just fight fatigue with food.

In general, the same tips that helped you (sort of) deal with pregnancy fatigue can help now, too (sort of). For instance, opt for eating small amounts of energy-sustaining food frequently throughout the day instead of three hearty meals (as if you had time to sit down for even one). Mini-meals won't give you more sleep, but they will help keep your blood sugar (and thus your stamina) up. And because they don't put as much demand on your digestive tract, they won't tap into those energy stores as much as a gut bomb would. (The bigger the meal, the more energy it takes to digest, so the more tired it makes you feel.) Try, also, to include a combination of carbohydrates and protein in each mini-meal so that you get the energy-enhancing benefits of both nutrients.

Hold the simple sugars (like that Pop-Tart you're contemplating popping), which pick you up only briefly before sending you crashing. Instead, snack on some of the following (you can also revisit the snack and mini-meal ideas on pages 138 and 107).

- Trail mix. You don't need to be planning a hike to munch on a combo of dried and/or freeze-dried fruit, nuts, and seeds. It has a good balance of complex carbs and protein—plus it's high in iron, which helps combat the fatigue caused by postpartum anemia. Toss in a few dark chocolate chips for extra energy (and extra happiness).

- Whole-grain cereal with milk. Chock-full of B vitamins that help break down food into fuel, whole-grain cereal is a great way to energize your day after an all-nighter. And don't save the cereal for breakfast. It makes a high-energy lunch or snack, too.

- A real-food protein bar and a banana. Or a cheese stick and an apple.

- Half a whole-wheat bagel, topped with melted Swiss. A tasty way to combine carbs and protein, plus an energy boost with a calcium bonus.

- Half a peanut butter and banana sandwich on whole wheat, or apple slices and almond butter.

- Hummus in a whole-wheat pita—protein plus carbs, plus it doesn't get easier.

- Fruit and yogurt sprinkled with chopped walnuts or sliced almonds. Complex carbohydrates in the form of fruit provide sugar the way nature intended, supplying longer-lasting energy for your body. The nuts deliver protein and healthy, brain-boosting fats, and the yogurt adds protein (even more if you go Greek) and calcium.

Time to Shake the Salt?

No need for an all-out assault on salt—everyone needs some sodium in her diet. Still, if you picked up a pickle habit while you were expecting, it's probably wise to cut back now. After all, most Americans consume too much sodium, which is linked to a higher risk of heart disease and stroke. And too much sodium in your diet certainly isn't helpful when you're trying to lose pregnancy water weight. So as a sensible rule, limit those super-salty foods (like the ones you'll run into at the drive-through) and salt lightly at the table. But while you're holding the pickles, make sure you get enough iodine, especially if you're breastfeeding. Check to see if the salt you shake is iodized—most sea salt and kosher (coarse) salt isn't. Other great sources of iodine to tap into: seafood and seaweed (roasted seaweed makes a tasty snack that's also high in iron).

used to be, later if you're less active. But don't cut calories too drastically until you've completely recovered from pregnancy and childbirth (at least 6 weeks after giving birth)—even if you're eager to expedite weight loss. Once you've gotten your practitioner's go-ahead, you can go ahead and reduce your number of calories by 200 to 500 per day. Even then, slow is the better way to go when it comes to weight loss.

Protein: 3 servings daily if you're breastfeeding; 2 if you're not. See the list of protein choices on page 34, keeping in mind (as always) that many also double as a calcium serving. If you're breastfeeding twins or triplets, get ready to eat hearty: You'll need an extra serving of protein for each additional baby.

Calcium: At least 4 servings daily if you're breastfeeding; 3 if you're not. Whether you're making milk or not, you should still be drinking it (or taking the equivalent in other calcium sources) to strengthen your bones. Remember that many of the calcium choices on page 40 also serve up a considerable amount of protein, so take full advantage of this nutritional overlapping. If you're breastfeeding twins or triplets, you'll need an extra calcium serving for each additional baby. An important note for breastfeeders: While your baby won't suffer if you don't meet your calcium requirement, your bones might. To keep your milk calcium rich, your body will draw this essential mineral from your bones for milk production, possibly setting you up for osteoporosis later on if you don't take in enough calcium from your diet. If you find it's hard to reach your calcium quota through your diet, fill in the gaps with a calcium supplement. Choosing calcium-fortified dairy products will also help boost your intake.

Vitamin C: 2 or more servings daily whether you're breastfeeding or not. See page 40 for vitamin C choices—and remember that many vitamin C foods also fill the vitamin A bucket.

Vitamin A: 3 to 4 servings daily whether you're breastfeeding or not. See page 41 for good food sources, keeping in mind that many of these also fill the requirement for vitamin C.

Other fruits and vegetables: 1 or more servings daily whether you're breastfeeding or not. See page 45 for good choices.

Whole grains and legumes: 3 or more servings daily whether you're breastfeeding or not. See page 47 for good choices.

Iron-rich foods: some daily whether you're breastfeeding or not. You'll need iron to replenish your blood stores after delivery and to prevent fatigue caused by anemia (you'll be plenty tired without it). See page 48 for good choices. If you're low on iron stores, your practitioner may tell you to continue (or begin) taking an iron supplement.

Fat and high-fat foods: small amounts daily. Even though a breastfeeding mom needs fat (half the calories of breast milk come from fat), you don't need as much as you did when you were pregnant. If you're gaining weight (or not losing any), cut back on the amount of fat you're taking in. If you're losing too quickly, add more fat servings into your diet. See page 50 for a list of fat servings.

Omega-3 fatty acids: some daily. In your quest to drop those postpartum pounds, remember that fat isn't the enemy and that some fats are still your friends—namely, those DHA-supplying ones. DHA is just as important while you're breastfeeding as it was during pregnancy, and here's why. The DHA content of your baby's brain triples during the first 3 months of life, and getting enough of this vital nutrient through your milk (which already contains DHA) will help fuel that growth. It's recommended that breastfeeding moms—like pregnant moms—eat 8 to 12 ounces of low-mercury fish (see page 72) per week to meet their omega-3 requirement, so definitely go fish when you're breastfeeding. Your prenatal vitamin, which likely includes omega-3s, will also help you fill your quota. For other good sources of DHA see page 51.

Back on the Postpartum Menu

With your pregnancy days behind you, it's time to celebrate what is back on the menu (and hopefully, it's some of your favorites). Whether you're breastfeeding or not, you can go back to eating raw or rare fish and seafood (though restrictions on high-mercury fish still apply if you're breastfeeding or planning to become pregnant again), rare or raw meat, unpasteurized cheese, unpasteurized juice, runny eggs, raw dairy, deli meat and smoked fish that aren't heated to steaming, raw sprouts, and fermented foods. (See page 173 for breastfeeding caveats about alcohol and caffeine.)

Fluids: at least 12 8-ounce cups daily if you're breastfeeding; approximately 10 8-ounce cups daily if you're not. Here's one requirement you might expect to increase when you're in the milk production business—and it does, somewhat. The best way to tell if you're getting enough fluids is to keep an eye on your pee. If you're not getting enough, it will be darker and more scant. If you're getting enough, your urine will be clear and plentiful. Since you'll be nursing 8 to 12 times a day, one of the simplest strategies for keeping up with your fluid intake is to drink when baby drinks—keeping a bottle or glass of water close during breastfeeding sessions. As always, remember that other fluids work toward your quota (including milk, broth, and juice), as do juicy fruits and veggies. Think more of a good thing is even better? Actually, drinking way too many fluids can decrease your milk supply.

Not breastfeeding? You don't need fluids for milk production, but you do need them to help recover from childbirth and flush out extra fluids retained during pregnancy. Dehydration can also contribute to fatigue, headaches, and other postpartum symptoms you definitely don't need.

Vitamin supplements. Continue to take your prenatal vitamin or a breastfeeding supplement daily if you're breastfeeding. Though it's likely you'd make good-quality milk without it (just by eating well), taking one provides a dose of insurance, providing you with the extra vitamins and minerals you need during breastfeeding, including vitamin A, vitamin C, vitamin E, biotin, calcium, choline, chromium, copper, and iodine. Ask your practitioner for supplement advice if you're a breastfeeding vegan—you may need additional supplements, such as vitamin D and B_{12}. If you're not breastfeeding, continue taking your prenatal for at least the first 6 weeks postpartum, and then talk to your practitioner about whether you should stick with it or switch over to a standard multiple vitamin and mineral supplement (a formula with enough folic acid to keep you covered throughout your reproductive years, just in case).

Eating Well When You're Breastfeeding

All new moms (and new dads, for that matter) can benefit from eating well, especially during those early endless days and nights after a baby's arrival, particularly during the first 3 months postpartum (dubbed the fourth trimester, since this period is an integral part of the reproductive cycle). Sleep deprivation plus recovery from pregnancy and delivery can drain energy and put a strain on nutritional status. But moms who are also taking on the (literally) draining job of breastfeeding have an extra reason to eat well. Here's what you need to know.

What to Eat

Wondering if feeding your baby well on the outside will take as much effort as feeding him or her well on the inside did? Actually, because the basic composition of breast milk isn't directly dependent on what you eat, breastfeeding makes minimal demands on your diet. Quantity isn't affected, either, unless a mom's diet and nutritional reserves are severely deficient (as they might be if she were living under famine conditions). That's because Mother Nature puts a breastfeeding baby's needs first. Skimp on the calories, fall short on the protein, or come up behind on minerals, and your body will tap into its own stores of nutrients to make milk—at least until reserves run out. In other words, your milk isn't likely to become deficient in nutrients, but you could. Eating a well-balanced and well-varied diet will help keep you healthy while your milk helps keep your baby healthy. And because there are fewer restrictions on your diet postpartum, eating well won't be nearly as challenging as when you were pregnant (though finding the time to eat at all, that's a different story).

There's yet another reason to eat a variety of healthy foods when you're breastfeeding—and believe it or not, it's got nothing to do with nutrition. Because what you eat affects the taste and smell of your breast milk, your breastfed baby is exposed to different flavors before he or she is ready for that first bite of solids. In fact, studies have shown that babies fed breast milk are more accepting of new foods when they start on solids than babies who are formula-fed—probably because they've already gotten a taste for them. Enjoy a lot of highly flavored foods while breastfeeding, and your baby's more likely to grow into an adventurous eater. (Forget the chicken fingers, Mom—pass the pad thai!) Eat your vegetables now, and your baby may be more likely to eat his or her vegetables later.

You already know the Daily Dozen drill: lean meat and poultry, low-mercury fish (experts recommend 8 to 12 ounces of fish per week when you're breastfeeding to ensure enough omega-3s in your system and in your breast milk), plenty of fruits and vegetables, whole grains and legumes, and iron-rich foods. Just adjust your servings for breastfeeding. To find out what's back on the menu now that you're no longer pregnant, see the box on page 167. To find out what's off-limits or still restricted, see page 173.

What about lactation foods and supplements you've heard increase your milk supply? Should you be dunking lactation cookies in coconut water, or chasing a bowl of oatmeal down with blue Gatorade? Taking mother's milk tea for two, along with fenugreek capsules and a big spoonful of brewer's yeast? Here's a breakdown of some of the foods, drinks, and supplements that are touted as milk-making miracles but don't necessarily stand up to the science.

■ Fenugreek (and other herbs). The most popular ingredient in the vast

Color Your (Breast Milk) World

You don't have to be Irish to celebrate St. Patrick's Day with green breast milk—all you have to do is eat a plateful of asparagus. What you eat can change the color of your milk (though it doesn't always, and you may not notice the change unless you're pumping), and from there, even the color of your baby's pee. And it's easier being green than you might think. Kelp, green Gatorade or Jell-O, seaweed (in tablet form), and some other natural supplements can be linked with green breast milk. Green not your color? Going carrot crazy can lend a slight orange hue. Eat beets (or red Jell-O), and you may see pink, or slightly red. Unless a color change comes with tummy troubles for your baby, there's no need to worry, or to take a pass on asparagus.

Keep in mind that breast milk naturally comes in slightly different colors. Foremilk (the milk at the beginning of a feed) usually runs a little blue, or somewhat watery looking. Hindmilk (the milk your breasts release later in a feed) is creamier looking, white or yellowish. Blood (usually from cracked nipples) can turn breast milk pink or rusty red—even brown if the blood is residual. Medications you take can also change the color of your breast milk (make sure that any medication or supplement you're taking is cleared by baby's doctor). If there's a mystery in your milk or your baby's pee color that can't be easily solved, or if an unusual color continues, check in with the doctor. Check in with the pediatrician right away if baby's pee is darker and more concentrated than usual or if it is scant, since this can be a sign of dehydration.

CHEW ON THIS. Old wives are fond of passing down this less-than-wise tale: Eating onions and garlic will help with weaning. Obviously, this tale is rooted in another tale—that babies don't like the taste of garlic, onions, or other strong flavors in their breast milk. But studies have shown that this is likely to be the case only when mom's been a bland eater throughout her pregnant and lactating days. In fact, lots of babies especially enjoy breast milk when it's spiked with spices like garlic—possibly because they picked up a taste for garlic-infused amniotic fluid while dining at Café Uterus. If you're a fan of Eggplant with Garlic Sauce, it's likely your baby will be, too.

majority of lactation products, fenugreek also comes alone in capsule, powder, tincture, or tea form (alone or in mother's milk tea blends). Fenugreek has been recommended for centuries by midwives, and more recently by some lactation consultants and mommy bloggers, as a milk-supply booster. While fenugreek is considered safe for most breastfeeding moms when used in moderation (it's smart to check with your doctor first), studies of its effectiveness have been mixed at best. So have real-life results as reported by moms. Some moms challenged by milk-supply issues find it works for them, increasing supply within a day to weeks of starting fenugreek, but others find that it doesn't help a bit. Coming to a scientific conclusion on fenugreek's effectiveness (or lack of it) is complicated by the fact that most women trying fenugreek (and other purported milk makers) are trying something else to boost their supply at the same time—say,

pumping more often or nursing more frequently. Was it the pumping, or the extra feeds, or the fenugreek that did the trick—or was it actually a psychological benefit (placebo effect)? That's hard to identify. Plus there are side effects to fenugreek and products containing it. Some side effects are more or less harmless (like your pee, sweat, and milk—and possibly baby's—smelling like maple syrup). Other side effects are more uncomfortable (for mom these can include loose stool, tummy troubles, and nausea, for baby green, watery stools, and fussiness). And still others are potentially dangerous (severe allergies, hypoglycemia, or worsening asthma symptoms).

What about other herbs, herbal tea blends (including mother's milk tea, which blends fenugreek, fennel, anise, coriander, blessed thistle, and more), other herb-containing lactation products (like chews and bars), and supplements (like garlic and basil)? There are many on the market targeting moms looking to boost their milk supply (or their let-down), but there's little scientific evidence that they actually get the job done. Some carry a risk of side effects in high doses. Another case for: Ask your practitioner or pediatrician before brewing or dropping them into your diet.

■ Oats. Can a bowl full of oatmeal help you make 2 breasts full of milk? Maybe. Certainly, traditional wisdom passed down from mom to mom (and lactation specialist to lactation specialist) indicates that eating oats can boost milk supply. How, exactly? There are several theories. One: by pumping up iron levels—after all, oatmeal is a good source of iron, and low iron levels have been linked to lower supply. Two: with its cholesterol-reducing

Pass the Broccoli ... and the Gas?

Of course you know that gas can't really be passed through breast milk. It's produced in the intestines, and babies normally produce a whole lot of it, due to their age-appropriately immature digestive systems. Still, it's easy to blame baby's tummy troubles, fussiness, or even colic on something you've eaten. Many moms claim that eating gas-producing foods (like cabbage, onions, broccoli, brussels sprouts, or beans) produces gas attacks in their babies. Or that downing dairy causes colic. Or that coffee triggers the fussies (in baby, not mom).

It's just not usually the case. Passing gas and crying are two things that babies do a lot of, usually unrelated to what mom had for breakfast (if she ever got around to eating it) or dinner (ditto). Some babies seem to excel in producing gas, or spitting up, or crying—but every baby does some of all three. And some days will be gassier or fussier than others (and that goes for breastfed and formula-fed babies). The reality is that few babies are actually sensitive to something in their mom's diet, and that gas (or crying bouts, or both) is usually just newborn-baby business as usual. At least that's what the research shows, for the most part.

Still, scientific studies don't amount to a hill of beans when it's your baby who's gassy and uncomfortable after you've wolfed down a burrito. Or is crying overtime after that extra-large latte. And once in a while, a breastfed baby does show sensitivity and a consistent reaction (that gas, that fussiness, that crying) to something in a mom's diet. A super-sensitive baby might even have an allergic reaction (such as a rash, hives, wheezing, diarrhea, or even bloody stool) to something in a mom's diet, but that's even less common.

Thinking that something you're regularly eating or drinking is rubbing your baby the wrong way, or worse? Check with your baby's pediatrician—especially if you think your baby might be allergic to something in your diet. You'll be able to screen for a sensitivity (or allergy) simply by eliminating suspect foods (whether it's those vegetables or that dairy) from your diet one at a time (in the case of dairy, it would mean eliminating the entire dairy category). Eliminate more than one at a time and you'll never know what, if anything, was causing the reaction. If baby's symptoms improve dramatically after 2 to 3 weeks of eliminating that food (though in most babies the symptoms will begin to improve within a week), chances are you've found your culprit. Give that food or drink a break, and then consider reintroducing it at a later date, or just wait until after you wean.

effects, which may (in theory) nudge up milk supply. Three: by offering a nourishing, sustaining dose of comfort food—comfort that can make a mom feel (potentially) more relaxed, which can, in turn, make her produce more milk and let it down more effectively. Plus, oatmeal is a good source of B vitamins, often touted for breast milk boosting (and energy boosting). There's no scientific proof that oat-eating moms produce more milk, but many moms claim success. And with only nutritional upside, there's no reason not to start your day (or your night shift with baby) with a bowl of oats. You can also shake them into a smoothie.

Nursing Twins (or More)

Double (or triple) the mouths to feed? If you're nursing twins or triplets, you'll need extra rest and, yes, extra food—more calories, in fact, than when you were pregnant. Be sure to follow the Postpartum Diet for breastfeeding—increasing your calorie requirement by 500 to 600 calories and adding an extra serving of calcium and protein for each additional baby.

- Lactation cookies, bars, and shakes. You can buy them, you can make them at home, and there's no harm in eating (or drinking) them, as long as they don't include herbs you haven't cleared with your practitioner or baby's pediatrician. But do lactation cookies, bars, and shakes work? Not surprisingly, there's only anecdotal evidence that they do—and there's a chance that much of the reported success may, in fact, be caused by a placebo effect (a mom believes that eating lactation cookies helps her make milk, she relaxes while eating them . . . and the milk magic happens). Most contain oats, often as the first ingredient. Other healthy (if not proven milk-producing) ingredients in many of these lactation treats include flaxseed, peanut butter, nuts, and seeds. Most also contain brewer's yeast (another purported milk booster that isn't evidence backed but can lend a bitter taste to some recipes). And some contain significant amounts of sugar (that's the cookie talking), which brings up the only real downside to eating lots of them: They can add up in the calorie department.

- Electrolyte drinks. From Gatorade (some would specify blue) and other sports drinks to coconut juice blends, you'll find plenty of moms who credit an "electrolyte" beverage for boosting milk supply. But do they work? There's no scientific reason why they would, unless a mom were seriously dehydrated (say, from an extreme workout). Maybe it's the placebo effect at work again, but most experts feel confident that it's not the electrolytes (or the dye that turns Gatorade—and often breast milk— the requisite blue . . . or green). The downside, again, would be the sugar and empty calories in most drinks, along with any artificial flavors and colors. Coconut water is refreshing (look for one that doesn't include added sugar), even if it's not all it's cracked up to be in the milk production department.

- Beer. You've waited 9 months to have one, so go ahead—make your night. But don't count on beer (and make sure you do keep count; see the next page) to boost your milk supply. Again, mom tales (these from way back) may claim otherwise, but there's no evidence that the beer makes milk, as happy as it may make you. In fact, alcohol of any kind is known to decrease supply. The theory is probably rooted in the barley many (but far from all) beers are made from. Some say that barley can increase levels of prolactin (that's the breastfeeding hormone), which in turn bumps up milk supply. Without a doubt, barley's a good whole grain to add to your diet—it's packed with fiber and B vitamins every new mom needs— but it definitely doesn't have to come in the form of a beer, and if it does, it should come only occasionally, in limited amounts.

▪ Chicken soup, papaya, dates, root vegetables—you name it. There are plenty of other foods said (but not conclusively proven) to help with milk production and let-down.

So should you give these foods, drinks, and supplements a try? You could—and when it comes to healthy foods, like oatmeal and root vegetables, you definitely should. But consider, before you spring for big-ticket lactation products or commit to gagging down something you can't stand, that most women who think they have supply issues actually don't. And if you do, the best step you can take (besides taking the many milk-supply-boosting steps listed in *What to Expect the First Year*) is to see a lactation professional who can diagnose the problem and help you find a remedy that's really tried and true, as well as medically sound.

What Not to Eat (or to Limit)

Maybe you barely noticed pregnancy's diet limitations—you weren't a raw fish fan to begin with, you didn't have a soft spot for soft cheese or deli meats, you always took a pass on cocktails. Or maybe aversions or morning sickness had you turned off to all—or some—of the above, making giving them up a piece of cake (especially because you could still have cake). Still, chances are you're looking forward to putting at least one of pregnancy's off-the-menu items back on the table. And for the most part, you can, even while you're breastfeeding. You can tap into beer and pop that champagne. Eat your cold cuts cold, and your oysters raw, and your salmon barely seared. Order your hamburger rare and your steak practically mooing. Embrace the brie and blue cheese, without giving a thought to whether it's pasteurized. And pour the coffee you crave (though you could have poured it while you were expecting, too—at least, in moderate amounts).

But a few restrictions are still standing—some items to keep avoiding, others that can be added back in, but in moderation, and others (like that coffee) that you'll still be limited on. Here's a list of foods and drinks you'll have to watch out for when breastfeeding:

Too much alcohol. The bar has reopened now that you've delivered—just in time to celebrate your baby's arrival. But remember to keep the bar low: no more than 1 drink at a time and preferably no more than 2 servings per week. Have a beer or a glass of wine, but to avoid sharing the alcohol with your baby (it will end up in your breast milk), drink it right after a feeding or pumping. Wait a few hours (2 to 3 is usually enough) before you feed or pump again, since that will allow enough time for the alcohol to be metabolized. Pumping and dumping won't help speed up that process. Not sure whether you've exceeded your alcohol limit or if your body has finished metabolizing it? Put it to the

---

CHEW ON THIS. Here's one more for the old wives' hall of fiction: According to folklore, if you get frightened, your breast milk will go sour. While it's true that stress hormones (produced when you're scared, for instance) may temporarily suppress the let-down reflex, your milk won't taste any different to baby. So go ahead and push "play" on that horror flick. Then take a deep breath, relax, and don't get yourself worked up over sour milk.

Losing the Baby Weight

Here's something you might not have expected when you were expecting: still looking pregnant months after you've delivered. While you'll lose far more weight the day you give birth than you could ever hope to lose in many weeks of dieting (about 12 pounds, give or take), you'll likely have plenty of pounds to shed before you return to your prepregnancy weight. Some will be lost quickly after delivery, thanks to fluid loss. Most will linger a lot longer—and that's what you should expect. Remember, the body lays down extra pounds, beyond what it needs for baby building, to fuel breastfeeding after baby arrives—and that's a good thing.

Yet, if you're eager to wear pants that zip again, it can also be a frustrating thing. Try not to sweat the pounds (you'll be doing plenty of sweating anyway postpartum, nature's way of draining some of those accumulated fluids). Instead, remember that you've earned those inches in the service of a healthy pregnancy—and if you're breastfeeding, in the service of feeding your baby. Wear them with honor for now while looking ahead to reaching a healthy weight sensibly, keeping these tips in mind.

If you're not breastfeeding:

- Take a break. Sure, you're in a hurry to see your waist again. But it's not smart to embark on a weight-loss program until your body has a chance to recuperate from childbirth. So wait until at least 6 weeks postpartum (3 months is considered more reasonable) before starting any weight loss campaign.

- Give yourself time. You didn't put on those pounds overnight, so you can't expect to lose them that quickly either. For most women, it takes 6 months to a year for pregnancy weight to come off.

- Add in exercise. The best way to lose weight postpartum is by combining exercise and diet. Once your practitioner has given the green light, resume or begin an exercise program (preferably one that includes cardio and strength training) to help you shed the pounds.

If you are breastfeeding:

In addition to the tips for nonbreastfeeding new moms above, also:

- Take a longer break. If you're breastfeeding, you should wait at least 3 months before starting any weight-loss effort. Check with your practitioner for specific guidelines for you.

- Go slow. Much of the weight you put on during pregnancy was set aside as fat stores earmarked for lactation. Lose those fat stores too quickly and your milk supply could suffer. Slow and steady will win this race (though it's definitely not a race): Once you start on your weight-loss program, aim to lose no more than half a pound a week (approximately 1 to 2 pounds per month).

- Don't depend on breastfeeding. Although breastfeeding burns about 500 calories a day (the same as a daily 5-mile run, and all without even breaking a sweat), nursing alone won't guarantee weight loss. Though plenty of moms find the pounds melt away when they're breastfeeding, others have trouble losing weight, and some can't manage to lose an ounce until after baby is weaned. As long as the healthy foods in your diet outweigh the unhealthy and you've incorporated a consistent exercise routine into your day, it'll come off eventually.

test with Milkscreen, test strips that detect the volume of alcohol in your breast milk to find out if the level is safe before latching on baby or pumping to feed baby. If the alcohol levels in your breast milk are too high and it's time for a feeding, feed baby from your stash of pre-pumped and stored breast milk instead. If you need to relieve engorgement, you can pump a little, but you'll have to dump it.

Avoid heavy drinking when you're breastfeeding. Not only can large doses of alcohol make baby sleepy, sluggish, unresponsive, and unable to suck well, but too many drinks can also impair your own functioning (whether you're nursing or not), making you more susceptible to depression, fatigue, and lapses in judgment. And even moderate amounts of alcohol can reduce your milk supply.

Too much caffeine. During those early, sleep-deprived postpartum weeks, a little jolt from your local coffee bar may be just the pick-me-up you need. So go ahead and give it a shot—just not too many shots at a time. Sticking to the same 200 mg of coffee (or the equivalent in other caffeinated foods and drinks) per day as you did while you were expecting won't affect your baby, and may actually allow you to stay vertical when you'd really rather be horizontal. But exceeding that limit can make junior jittery and keep you both from getting any sleep—and no amount of caffeine is going to help you then.

Questionable herbs. Watch out for herbs, even some seemingly innocuous herbal teas. Stick to regular (black) tea that comes flavored, or choose other teas that are considered safe during lactation, including white tea, chamomile, and rosehip (you can ask your doctor for a list of safe teas). Read labels carefully

---

Eating Well for the Next Baby

Is there a baby in your near future? If you're planning an encore, there's a lot more to the preparations than figuring out where yet another new nursery will go. You'll also have to prepare your next baby's very first source of bed and board: you. And one of the best ways to get yourself into tip-top baby-making shape during the preconception months is by getting your diet into shape (or getting it back into shape). Even before you start eating for two, you can start eating well for your future baby's health. For all the information you'll need on eating well before you're expecting, see *What to Expect Before You're Expecting*.

---

to make sure other herbs haven't been added to the brew, and drink them only in moderation.

Some herbal preparations touted for their milk-producing properties can have unpleasant side effects, including nausea, and other herbs like chasteberry, jasmine, and sage can actually reduce milk supply. In general, because the FDA doesn't regulate herbs and little is known about how herbs affect a nursing baby, play it safe and consult your doctor before taking any herbal remedy.

Certain sugar substitutes. Most sweeteners are considered safe during lactation in sensible moderation. The one sweetener that's not sweet when you're breastfeeding: Sweet'N Low (aka saccharine). And of course, avoid aspartame entirely if you have PKU or your baby does.

Fish high in mercury. Though it's safe to reel in the sushi again, continue to avoid high-mercury fish, such as shark, swordfish, tilefish from the Gulf of Mexico, king mackerel, bigeye tuna steaks, marlin, and orange roughy, and to limit those that may contain moderate amounts of that heavy metal. But because guidelines recommend that breastfeeding moms eat 8 to 12 ounces per week of low-mercury fish, be sure to cast your net widely to benefit from the brain-boosting nutrients found in safe fish (see page 72 for a list).

CHAPTER 11

Safe Cooking and Prepping When You're Expecting

M aybe you're already hyper when it comes to hygiene around your house, especially in your kitchen. Maybe you're a little laxer about kitchen conditions. Maybe bacteria is always on your mind when you're prepping, cooking, storing, and serving food—or maybe it's on the back burner (literally, because you haven't cleaned the back burner since that soup you were simmering boiled over 4 days ago). Maybe you regularly take your food's temperature before you eat it, check use-by dates religiously, and toss questionable foods without question. Or maybe you've been known to eat straight out of the takeout container that sat out for 3 hours last night before you remembered to stick it in the fridge. Wherever your sanitary standards stand—whether you're sure you'd ace an inspection from your local health department or pretty certain you'd fail—everyone has something to learn about food safety, especially when they're trying to eat safely for two. That's because pregnant women, in general, are more susceptible to food-borne illness—and more likely to get sicker from it.

Consider this chapter your Food Safety 101—the bacteria basics. A little on the boring side, yes. A lot of extra precautions, true. But following at least some of the advice here, at least some of the time, can sure beat getting hit with a bad bug (especially when you're already bugged by pregnancy symptoms). For information on foods you should avoid entirely because of the risk of bacterial infection they may carry, see Chapter 5.

Keeping Your Kitchen Safe

Think that you have months before you'll have to worry about making your kitchen safe for baby? While it's true that you can hold off on installing childproof latches on the cabinets and knob covers on the stovetop, there are many other precautions you should be taking around your kitchen right now to protect your growing baby—not from pinched fingers or accidental burns, but from foodborne bacteria that can make both of you sick. So, before stepping up to the kitchen counter:

Wash your hands. Mom (and the CDC) does know best when it comes to this first rule of safe cooking and eating. Washing your hands in hot soapy water before preparing food is your best line of defense against the spread of bacteria

in the kitchen. Break out the soap, too, after you've handled raw meat, poultry, fish, or eggs—all of which can harbor dangerous bacteria. Stating the obvious but not always observed: Also wash your hands after blowing your nose, going to the bathroom, changing a diaper, or attending to another germ-charged activity.

Wash your towels and sponges. That dish towel you just dried your hands with looks pretty clean, doesn't it? Take a closer look (like under a microscope) and you might change your mind—as well as your towel. Do the same with your sponge (a sponge for bacteria) and you'd do the same. Sponges and dish towels provide a perfect breeding ground for bacteria, which thrive in moist environments. To avoid drying your hands, wiping your counter, and cleaning your dishes with a veritable petri dish of microorganisms, wash dishcloths and towels often in hot soapy water or in the washing machine (with a little bleach if possible). Replace sponges at least once a month, and wash them thoroughly with soap and water or in the dishwasher at the end of the day (microwaving them won't kill all the bacteria). To avoid spreading germs around your kitchen, use paper towels for kitchen cleanup.

Wash (and watch) your surfaces. Bacteria multiply far faster than rabbits, especially when left to their own devices on kitchen surfaces. To keep those bugs from breeding in your kitchen, clean countertops and sinks often with soapy water or cleansers. Take precautions in the fridge, too. Don't put a package of raw chicken or meat or fish directly

---

Home Is Where the Health Is ... or Is It?

Myth: Food prepared at home is much safer than restaurant food. Most foodborne illnesses are contracted from food at restaurants.

Fact: Actually, you're more likely to pick up a bug dining at home than at your local diner. That's because most (though certainly not all) professional food handlers have been trained in hygiene and food safety protocol and are more likely to be careful about following those standards. Plus, they know their restaurant can be shut down if those standards aren't met. Think about this, too: Most home kitchens probably wouldn't pass inspection by the health department.

on the shelf for defrosting (even if it's wrapped, it's likely to leak, so put it on a plate). Wash cutting boards in the dishwasher after each use—or if they're too large to fit, with hot, soapy water. When boards get scarred from too much use, discard them. (Bacteria like to hide—and multiply—in pitted surfaces.)

Cut out cross contamination. One knife that gets around—from the raw chicken breasts to the cheese to the tomatoes—can spread a whole lot of bacteria around your kitchen. If you're using one knife for several food-prep steps, wash between uses with hot soapy water. Better still, keep different knives for different purposes (one for raw meat and poultry, another for produce). Something else to keep separate: cutting boards. Ideally use one for produce, another for fish, meat, and poultry.

Keeping Your Foods Safe

You've shopped for the most nutritious ingredients, and you're ready to test your cooking chops (and your dicing, sautéing, and saucing skills). Or maybe your plan is a little less ambitious—you're going to slice a peach and a banana, toss in some yogurt and nuts, and call it dinner . . . and a night. Or dive into that box of leftover pizza with a side salad. Either way, one thing you'll want to incorporate into your dinner (or breakfast, or lunch) plans is safety. So keep these safe-food strategies in mind when storing, preparing, and serving:

- Don't wait to refrigerate. Make sure anything that must be kept refrigerated (that meat, fish, poultry, cut raw or cooked produce, eggs, cheese, yogurt, milk) finds its way into your fridge as soon as possible after purchase, but definitely within 2 hours (less in warm weather). If you can't get to a fridge that quickly, bring along insulated bags and ice packs to store your cold purchases in until you return home. Clearly, if you've ordered those perishables via an app for delivery, make sure you're home to receive them—or that you will be

CHEW ON THIS. Not surprisingly, old wives have spent a lot of time in the kitchen over the ages—and have stirred up more than a few tales there. Among them—you shouldn't put hot food in the refrigerator because it will spoil. In fact, the old wives are way off base on this one. The longer a food (hot or cold) sits out at room temperature, the greater the chances bacteria will multiply—and the faster it will spoil. A good mantra to remember when cooking foods that won't be eaten right away: Cool slightly—then don't hesitate, refrigerate.

soon—so they're not sitting on a hot doorstep (unless they're packaged in an insulated box).

- Give perishables priority placement. Store highly perishable foods (milk, fish) in the back of the refrigerator. The storage areas on the door are fine for condiments, but they don't stay as cold. Make sure your fridge is set to 40°F or below and your freezer at 0°F or below.

The Dating Game

How can you tell if a food you're about to purchase or that's been sitting in your fridge for a while is too old to eat? Play the dating game by checking out the label.

- Products that aren't perishable, like flour and grains, baked goods, chips, cereals, and some canned goods, generally read "Best if used before" or "Best if used by" or "Best before." These foods generally won't be dangerous to dig into after the date given, but they'll probably start to taste stale. Best to toss them.

- Perishable products that require refrigeration and have a shorter shelf life (like cheese, yogurt, or eggs) will have an expiration, use-by, or use-before date. In general, it means the food should no longer be consumed after that date passes.

- Milk comes with a sell-by date—and though the milk should be pulled from the grocer's shelves after that date, it will usually be safe to use for another week if it's refrigerated at home. Ditto for some other dairy products, like parmesan cheese.

- Meat that's bought fresh can be refrigerated and safely used within 3 to 5 days (2 days for ground meat) after that sell-by date. Freeze meat that you won't be using within that time frame. Fresh poultry and seafood should be consumed within 2 days of the sell-by date. How long frozen meat, poultry, and seafood will last in the freezer (whether you've frozen it yourself or bought it frozen) depends on how well it is wrapped and how cold your freezer is.

- Frozen foods (the kind you get from the freezer section of the supermarket, not the leftovers you've frozen) will last for 6 to 12 months in the freezer. The dates on the packages let you know when they won't taste as good as intended. That's because flavor and texture break down over time.

Another trick of the dating game? To bring home foods with the latest dates possible, check the back of the supermarket shelf. It's common grocery store practice to put the older items up front (to get rid of them before they expire).

- Cook or freeze promptly. Didn't have time to cook that salmon or those chicken breasts, as planned? If you haven't gotten around to cooking fresh poultry, fish, or ground meats within 2 days of purchasing it, wrap it up and stick it in the freezer. Don't keep other cuts of meat in the fridge for longer than 3 to 5 days—freeze or cook before they've reached that window.

- Heat it like you mean it. That stew that you turned off after simmering for hours, because your dinner guests were running late? Bring it back up to a rolling boil before you dig in. Ditto gravies and soups. Reheat leftovers thoroughly until hot and steaming.

- Don't let your buffet overstay. Here's a buffet table buzzkill: Food shouldn't be left at room temperature for more than 2 hours (1 hour outside on a hot day or in a hot room—so beware the summer BBQ spread or the Fourth of July picnic). Love lingering with your guests when the party's over? Make sure you refrigerate those leftovers first.

- Refuse to refreeze. Don't refreeze foods that have been thawed at room temperature, or have been brought to room temperature after thawing, or have been kept more than a day or two after thawing, even in the refrigerator.

- Go by "sell by" and "use by" dates (see the box on the facing page). When in doubt, throw it out—even if there are no obvious signs of spoilage. Definitely throw out any food that has an off color or odor.

- Don't double dip (dip a carrot into salsa, take a bite, and then dip the same carrot again) or eat straight from a container unless you're planning to finish off the contents. Bacteria from your mouth (transferred via the spoon, vegetable, cracker, or chip you're snacking from) can contaminate the food—even if it's refrigerated afterward.

- Wash the lids of canned foods before opening to keep dirt and bacteria from getting into the food. Also, clean the blade of the can opener or drop it into the dishwasher after each use.

Safe Produce

Nothing is more wholesome than fresh fruits and vegetables, right? For the most part, yes. That is, unless that fresh peach or carrot or apple you're eyeing is covered in bacteria—courtesy of a picker, a store worker, or even a customer who didn't wash his or her hands before handling the produce you're about to plop into your cart. Or bacteria that comes from the cart itself, or the conveyer belt at checkout, if you haven't bagged your produce in clean reusable or plastic bags.

According to the CDC, nearly half of all foodborne illness has its roots in fruits and vegetables. Luckily, the overall risks are low, and they're lower still if you take steps to make sure the produce that's supposed to keep you healthy won't make you sick:

- Cook your produce. One of the best ways to bid bacteria bye-bye is to cook your fruits and veggies—sauté that kale, steam those carrots, bake that apple (yes, even grill that watermelon, those romaine hearts). But clearly, not every member of the produce family can take the heat (say, cantaloupe)—and just as clearly, there will be many times when you'll want your carrots raw, your salad crisp, and your apple crunchy. So read on for how to safely eat it raw.

- Give all produce that isn't prewashed a good wash. Thoroughly rinse the surfaces of all fruits and vegetables with water (the FDA recommends skipping any cleaners, even produce wash), and then pat them dry with a clean towel or paper towels—not only to keep them fresher and crunchier, but to rub off even more surface germs. Do this just before serving, preparing, or cooking—not when you bring the produce home (unless you're planning to cut up and stash that watermelon for easy munching right from the fridge). If necessary, use a scrub brush or mitt designed for scrubbing produce to remove visible dirt (use a softer brush for mushrooms, a stiffer brush for potatoes), and wash the brush after use with hot soapy water or in the dishwasher. Don't skip that rinse because you're planning to peel before serving anyway—otherwise the knife or peeler you're using can pick up surface germs and transmit them to the part you'll be eating. So rinse that avocado, that lemon, that cantaloupe before slicing into it, that carrot before peeling. Stick to rinsing rules, too, even if you just picked a basket of organic (or locally grown) strawberries at the local farmers market—those berries are just as likely to be sprinkled with bacteria as those from the supermarket, and either can make you sick if you're not careful. Will rinsing remove all bacteria? No, but it's an important precaution to take.

■ Double-check before you don't wash. Most packaged lettuce is already washed—usually triple-washed—but read the fine print before serving. Don't rewash produce that's already been washed unless you're cooking it or eating it right away.

■ Screen precut fruit and veggies. They're the ultimate convenience (those neat cubes of honeydew, those berry medleys just begging to be popped into your mouth, those sliced carrots and cucumbers). But even if you're happy to pay the price of conveniently precut produce, make sure you don't inadvertently pay another price, in the form of a tummy ache or worse. Be sure to check use-by dates and select only ready-to-eat produce that's been kept refrigerated while on display. That goes for half watermelons and coconuts. Refrigerate at 40°F or less as soon as possible after purchase.

■ Buy local, when you can. For one thing, local produce is usually fresher than imports, which means it's likely to retain more nutrients (same goes for seasonal produce). For another, while any produce can wear bacteria home from the market or stand, locally grown may be less likely to be contaminated than imported, since regulations on sanitation are more lax in some foreign countries.

■ Go organic, when you can. Whenever it's available and affordable and looks good, opt for organic. It isn't less likely to contain bacteria, but at least it won't be covered with pesticides. Check out page 66 to see when an upgrade to organic is worth the extra cost and when it probably isnt.

■ Be picky when picking fruits and veggies, even when you're picking them from your fridge. That 2-for-1 deal on raspberries sounded like a great deal—but try to buy only what you can eat before it spoils. Check for soft spots, little bits of fuzzy mold, a funny smell, a damp look, or brown

---

Recall Alert

A great way to stay on top of food safety is by staying on top of food recalls. The FDA and CDC will, from time to time, issue recalls on foods that are found to carry unsafe bacteria, from E. coli in ground beef to salmonella in precut cantaloupe, or that are unsafe for other reasons. For the latest recalls, keep an eye on your newsfeed and visit foodsafety.gov/recalls, where you can also sign up for automatic alerts to let you know when there's a food recall.

edges on all produce before buying, and then again before eating. Bruised isn't a biggie, though.

- Date your produce. Always check expiration dates on bagged or boxed produce when buying and before eating.

- Keep up to date on produce recalls and safety warnings (see the box on the facing page).

Safe Meat, Poultry, and Fish

Building a baby? There's no more efficient source of baby-building protein than lean meat, poultry, and fish. To cash in on the protein without tapping into any bacteria that may have come along for the ride—and might make you sick—try to keep these tips in mind:

- When freezing store-bought meat, poultry, or fish, remove the plastic or paper wrapping it came in and seal in plastic wrap and then heavy-duty aluminum foil or specially designed freezer bags to prevent freezer burn.

Alternatively, using foil or plastic wrap, wrap around the original wrapping. Don't forget to label your packets so you won't be left with unidentified frozen objects—and to date them, so you don't let them overstay their welcome in the freezer.

- Defrost appropriately wrapped meats, poultry, or fish in the refrigerator, in cold water (changing the water every 30 minutes), or in a microwave oven on "defrost," rather than at room temperature. Food defrosted

---

Now You Tell Me (Part Two)?

Already ordered your hamburger rare before finding out you shouldn't have it your way when you're expecting (unless your way is medium-well)? Poked around in the poke department before you discovered that well marinated isn't the same as well cooked when it comes to fish? Didn't know you should be running from runny eggs? Gobbled those strawberries right out of the farmers market basket without washing them first? Not to worry. First, because foodborne illness are relatively uncommon in the United States. And second, because in the case of most of the bacteria (or parasites) that can cause these illnesses, the only risk is getting really sick (and if you didn't get really sick pretty fast, that risk has already passed). The exceptions are Listeria and toxoplasmosis, which can be more dangerous during pregnancy (see page 82 for the lowdown on Listeria).

The bottom line on bacteria when you're expecting: It's best to avoid those that can make you sick. Worrying yourself sick about what you've eaten—or what you might eat inadvertently—isn't best. Take what precautions you can (and know about), and then sit back at the dinner table and relax.

Is It Done Yet?

How do you make sure that your dinner isn't half baked (or half grilled or half roasted)—and still potentially harboring germs that could make you sick? By taking its temperature. Reaching the right temperature means your meat, fish, or poultry won't be serving you a side of bacteria. Don't rely on the pop-up thermometers that come with some poultry—invest in a good-quality instant-read or leave-in meat thermometer, and use it faithfully (wash it after each use with hot soapy water). Of course, you'll also need to know where to stick it—as well as what temperature to look for once you have. Here's a guide:

For roasts, steaks, or chops made from beef, veal, pork, or lamb: Insert the thermometer in the center or the thickest part of the meat, away from any bone, fat, or gristle.

For ground meat or poultry, cutlets, fish, and casseroles: Insert the thermometer in the thickest part of the food. For burgers, insert sideways.

For chicken, turkey, duck, or goose: Insert the thermometer in the inner thigh area, where the leg meets the body of the bird (but be sure the thermometer isn't touching the bone).

The following foods can be considered safely cooked when they reach these temperatures:

- Beef, veal, lamb, pork roasts, chops, or steaks: 145°F

- Ground beef, veal, lamb, pork: 160°F

- Precooked ham: 140°F

- Whole chicken or turkey, ground chicken or turkey: 165°F

- Chicken breasts: 165°F

- Stuffing (cooked in bird or alone): 165°F

- Fish: 145°F

- Egg dishes: 160°F

---

in the microwave should be cooked immediately.

- Marinate meat, poultry, or fish in the refrigerator, not at room temperature. Don't reuse marinade that has touched raw meat or poultry. Set some marinade aside before pouring it all on the raw meat, poultry, or fish if you'd like to use it for basting (change the utensil between bastings so you don't double dip) or for sauce.

- Keep hot meats hot and cold meats cold. If you're bringing chicken salad to a picnic, be sure it's transported and served on ice. Don't let cooked

hot meats stay out at room temperature for more than 2 hours (1 on a hot day or in a very warm room).

- Don't stuff meat or poultry until it is ready to go into the oven. Stuff lightly (about ¾ pound of stuffing per pound of turkey), keep it moist, and cook until the center of the stuffing reaches at least 165°F on a meat thermometer. After cooking, store the stuffing and meat separately. Safer still, don't stuff at all. Bake the stuffing in a separate pan, basting occasionally with broth. A bonus: The stuffing will develop a crusty top. If you prefer soft stuffing, bake it covered with foil.

- Cook meat to medium. Yes, it's true what you've heard (and you may not be pleased about it): Rare meat is off the menu when you're expecting. But when cooking, don't rely on color, which can vary too much. Use a meat thermometer to get a better reading of meat safety (see the box on the facing page for information on what temperature to cook foods to). Order beef, pork, lamb, and other meat "medium" or "well" in restaurants, just to be on the safe side. With a thick fillet, that might mean asking for it to be "butterflied" before cooking.

- Cook chicken and other poultry through. The easiest way to see if poultry is safely cooked is to take its temperature—in the center, not near the bone (see the box on the facing page). Juices should run clear, too. You can't tell bone-in chicken by its color near the bone (traces of pink may remain even after it's well cooked, because of leaching from the bone). Unfortunately for rare-duck-breast lovers (there aren't many rare-chicken lovers), these rules apply to any form of poultry. Order duck "well" in restaurants, too.

- Don't eat it raw. Any raw meat, from tartare to carpaccio (even if it's seared) to traditional raw meats served in certain cuisines, is considered unsafe during pregnancy. Meat can harbor microorganisms when it isn't cooked through—you can't see them, you can't taste them, but they can make you sick. See page 83 for more.

- Don't eat it raw, fish edition. In case you haven't had the pregnancy briefing yet from your doctor or midwife: Raw or rare fish or seafood is also off the menu when you're expecting. Rolls containing only cooked fish or seafood

Mold and Moms-to-Be

You had good intentions of filling your fridge (and your tummy) with nutritious goodies when you bought that extra container of cottage cheese and pint of strawberries. But somehow you never got around to eating them, and when you finally dig them out for a healthy breakfast, blue fuzz has started multiplying across the top of the cottage cheese, and a green one is sprouting on the strawberries. Do you scrape and eat them, or dump them? Here are some guidelines about mold for the mom-to-be:

- If small fruits (grapes, berries, strawberries) become moldy, throw them out. If a few berries at the top of a box are moldy, it's okay to eat the rest as long as you've screened them carefully.

- If a hard fruit or vegetable (apple, potato, broccoli, onion, for instance) or hard cheese has a small area of mold, it's safe to cut the mold away (plus a half-inch margin of safety) and eat the rest. Moldy soft fruits (peaches, plums, melons, tomatoes) should be tossed in their entirety.

- Soft dairy products (cottage cheese, yogurt, sour cream, butter) that are sprouting mold should be discarded—even if the mold is only on top. Ditto moldy meat and leftovers.

- Moldy bread, grains, peanut butter, nuts, sauces, and jams should be thrown away (even if the mold is only visible in a single area).

And always remember—when in doubt, throw it out. Especially when you're expecting.

(not seared) are a safe pick from the sushi bar, while cooked shrimp or crab can be selected from the raw bar (as long as they're handled separately and stored separately from raw options). All fish (including salmon, often prepared "medium rare," because it's inarguably yummy that way) and seafood should be cooked through (see the box on page 184). See page 72 for a list of fish that's safe to eat, and page 81 for information about the safety of smoked seafood.

- Heat ready-to-eat hot dogs, sausages, and deli meat and meat or poultry leftovers until steaming hot all the way through.

For more on meat and poultry safety, call the USDA meat and poultry hotline at (888) 674-6854.

A Meat Myth That's All Wet

Myth: Raw meat, poultry, and fish should always be rinsed before cooking to wash away the bacteria on the surface.

Fact: Cooking meats, poultry, and fish to the right internal temperature (see the box on page 184) will almost always kill all the bacteria lurking on the surface—and inside. Rinsing doesn't wash enough bacteria away—however, it does splash germs and bacteria into the sink (and, if you're not careful, onto countertops). So, both pointless and counterproductive.

Safe Dairy

There's no quicker way to fill your calcium requirement (and to pick up a good bonus of protein) than to stop at your market's dairy case. And most dairy products are as safe as they are nutritious. To ensure safe dairy eating:

- Steer clear of raw (unpasteurized) milk or cheeses. See page 81 for more.

- Store all dairy products in the refrigerator (even pasteurized products can become contaminated), and don't use them after the expiration date (see page 180) or if they smell or look off.

Safe Eggs

Eager to crack open a great source of pregnancy protein (and in the case of certain eggs, of omega-3 fatty acids)? Though the cholesterol in eggs isn't considered a problem in pregnancy, contamination with salmonella could be.

So before cracking open that carton of eggs, consider these rules of egg safety:

- Buy refrigerated eggs. The vast majority of eggs sold in the U.S. are sold refrigerated, making this an easy rule

CHEW ON THIS. Expectant moms in Mexico are often told that eating eggs during pregnancy can make their babies smell bad after birth. Take it from the egg-sperts: All babies smell amazing, no matter how many eggs their moms eat.

to follow. The next rule is also a cinch: Store eggs you've bought refrigerated in the fridge until you use them, and use them by their expiration date. When is it safe to break the refrigerated egg rule? If you're buying (and using) those eggs in a part of the world (like Europe) where eggs are carefully regulated for safety instead of refrigerated for safety. Large egg farmers in the U.S. are required to wash eggs after laying. This process strips the protective cuticle off the outer shell of the egg, making refrigeration necessary afterward. European farmers are prohibited from washing their eggs, keeping that protective cuticle intact and making them safe to store at room temperature. Instead, chickens are vaccinated against salmonella (the dangerous bacteria that sometimes spreads in chicken coops). In fact, health regulations in Europe discourage the refrigeration of eggs in the store or at home, because when chilled eggs are brought back to room temperature, they can "sweat," cracking the door to mildew growth and possible bacterial contamination.

What about those room-temperature eggs you see at the farmers market or at a farm stand? If they're from a small farm and you're certain they've never been washed or refrigerated, they're considered safe to buy and to store on the countertop. No need to wash them when you bring them home, though if there's visible dirt on them,

you can wipe it off. Only rinse with water to remove visible dirt immediately before you use them. Refrigerated eggs will have an expiration date on the carton. Farm-fresh and unrefrigerated eggs will last 2 weeks to a month on the counter (they'll taste best eaten within 2 weeks).

- Refrigerate cooked eggs. Even hard-boiled eggs can become contaminated, so don't leave them at room temperature for longer than 2 hours (and don't eat hard-boiled eggs from an unrefrigerated buffet table or salad bar if you're not sure how long they've been out there). Eat refrigerated unpeeled hard-boiled eggs within a week. Peeled hard-boiled eggs are best eaten right away and not longer than 4 or so days after peeling.

- Don't crack open an egg that's already cracked. Whether it was cracked when you bought it or cracked on the way home, toss it. Disease-causing organisms can get in through cracks too easily.

- Order your eggs pregnancy-style. Unless eggs are pasteurized (a process that kills harmful bacteria), it's safest to cook or order them cooked until whites are set and the yolks have begun to thicken. Scrambles and omelets should be cooked through. Poached or soft-boiled eggs should not be runny. And raw eggs shouldn't be eaten during pregnancy at all (see page 82).

- Go uncaged when you can. The more room chickens have to roam around, the better. That's because cramped coops are breeding grounds for infectious bacteria, like salmonella, which can end up in your eggs. See page 62 for more about what cage-free and pasture-raised means when it comes to eggs.

PART 2

Cooking Well

E ating well for pregnancy isn't all that different from eating well at any other time in your life—and the same goes for cooking well. Most nutrition-forward, health-conscious, lean-leaning, whole food–focused recipes are pregnancy-appropriate, even pregnancy-perfect, sometimes with just a few tweaks for safety's sake (say, cooking the salmon all the way through instead of searing it rare, making sure those goat cheese crumbles are pasteurized before they top your salad) or with a nod to aversions or super-sensitive sniffers or troubled tummies.

So by all means, tap into recipes you've collected that fit the Pregnancy Diet profile (you know, concentrating on those Daily Dozen heavy hitters: veggies, fruits, grains, lean protein and dairy, and healthy fats) and pore over those health-foodie blogs and cooking sites for more. Tweak as needed for safety or your own personal eating quirks, punch up the nutrients when you can (add red pepper to that sauce, carrots to that stew, swap romaine for the iceberg), and enjoy.

But also turn to the pages that follow, where you'll find recipes that are made for the pregnant you in mind. Most of them are quick to prepare, so you'll be eating in a hurry and with a minimum of muss, fuss, and standing on the feet you'd so much rather put

up. Many of them are quease-easing, or may be easily adjusted to steer clear of tastes you're finding offensive. All of them pack plenty of nutrients—and of course, all of them are delicious.

From soothing smoothies to soups that eat like a meal, from breakfast muffins to one-pan dinners, pancakes to pasta, from sweet to spicy to a little bit of both, Asian to Italian to Mexican to all-American, from healthy twists on classic comfort foods (mac and cheese!) to tasty but enlightened takes on guilty pleasures (Alfredo!)—you'll find something to satisfy your every craving and every nutritional requirement, usually in the same bite.

Happy cooking well—and eating well!

Breakfast

....

M om said it first and best (and most often, probably repeating it every time you tried to sneak out to the school bus without your cereal, toast, and OJ): Nothing starts the day off like a good breakfast. And that's especially true now that you're on your way to being a mom yourself (or adding another baby love muffin to your family). A healthy breakfast will provide the fuel both you and baby need to start the day off right. Plus, it can mean the difference between a day filled with nausea, heartburn, and fatigue and a day filled with . . . well, less nausea, heartburn, and fatigue. Still sneaking out the door without breakfast these days? Whether you're breakfast phobic or time challenged, the recipes in this chapter are tempting and quick enough to lure you back to the table (though you can take many of these breakfast champions on the morning commute or to the office, too). From easy Diner Eggs and a sumptuous Tomato and Roasted Red Pepper Frittata to portable Breakfast Burritos and Stuffed French Toast, you'll have no problem braking for breakfast.

Diner Eggs

SERVES 1

H ome fries and eggs rolled into one, minus the greasy-spoon heartburn—plus, you get an added healthy dose of vitamin A from the red bell pepper.

1½ teaspoons olive oil
2 small red potatoes with their skins on, cooked and diced (about ¼ cup)

½ small onion, chopped
¼ teaspoon dried oregano or thyme
Salt and black pepper
2 large eggs
½ medium-size red bell pepper, diced
¼ cup finely shredded cheddar or
    Monterey Jack cheese

From the Test Kitchen

Looking to score another yellow vegetable serving with your Diner Eggs? Substitute sweet potatoes for the red potatoes. Want something more adventurous to toss into your morning skillet? Try any of the following (depending, of course, on your tastes and your morning nausea status): diced apple, chopped avocado, diced tomatoes, steamed broccoli florets, sliced mushrooms, or jalapeño peppers.

1. Heat the olive oil in an 8-inch non-stick skillet over medium heat. Add the potatoes, onion, and herbs and cook until browned, about 4 minutes, stirring occasionally. Season with salt and pepper to taste.

2. Meanwhile, place the eggs in a small bowl and whisk. When the potatoes and onion are browned, add the bell pepper and cook until it is slightly softened, about 1 minute. Pour the eggs into the skillet but do not stir them. Lower the heat to low and cook until the eggs are cooked through, about 3 minutes, lifting the edge to let the uncooked egg run underneath.

3. Sprinkle the cheese over the eggs and serve.

NUTRITION INFO: 1 portion provides:

Protein: 1 serving

Calcium: 1 serving

Vitamin C: 2½ servings

Vitamin A: 1 serving

Other fruits and vegetables: ½ serving

Fat: ½ serving

Omegas: some, if using omega-3 eggs

It's No Yolk

Cholesterol's not a worry for most pregnant women. But if you're in the market for a particularly low-calorie omelet, or you're feeding someone who's watching his or her cholesterol, just leave out the yolks. To make a basic egg white omelet, whisk 4 egg whites with 2 teaspoons water. Cook them as you would a regular omelet and add your choice of fillings. You can also find compromise in a 1 whole egg, 2 egg white omelet.

Mushroom and Spinach Omelet

SERVES 1

This veggie-stuffed omelet makes for one easy, hearty breakfast, or a filling brunch or dinner when paired with a simple side salad.

1½ teaspoon olive oil
¼ cup minced shallots (optional)
1 clove garlic, minced
¼ cup sliced white button mushrooms
1 sprig fresh thyme (¼ teaspoon dried)
3 ounces fresh baby spinach
    (about 4 cups, packed)
Pinch of salt
Pinch of pepper
2 large eggs
2 teaspoons butter
2 slices provolone cheese
    (about 1½ ounces total)

1. Heat the olive oil in an 8-inch non-stick skillet over medium heat. Add the oil. Add the shallots, if using, garlic, mushrooms, and thyme and sauté for 7 minutes, or until the mushrooms are browned. Add the spinach and sauté for 4 minutes, or until the liquid has almost completely evaporated. Remove the vegetable mixture from the pan; discard the thyme sprig. Wipe the pan clean.

2. Place the salt, pepper, and eggs in a small bowl and whisk to mix.

3. Melt the butter in the skillet over medium heat. Pour the egg mixture into the pan and cook for 1 minute, until the eggs start to set on the bottom. Lift the edge of the omelet with a rubber spatula to let the uncooked egg run underneath. Cook for 1 minute more, or until the center of the omelet just begins to set. Place the provolone on top and spoon the vegetable mixture over the cheese. Run the spatula around the edge and under the omelet to loosen it from the pan, fold it in half, and slide it onto a plate. Serve.

NUTRITION INFO: 1 portion provides:

Protein: 1 serving

Calcium: 1½ servings

Vitamin C: 4 servings

Vitamin A: 4 servings

Other fruits and vegetables: 2 servings

Iron: some

Fat: 1 serving

Omegas: some, if using omega-3 eggs

Egg Bites

SERVES 4

Order up an easy breakfast or snack with these tasty egg bites—easier still if you've made them ahead for speedy reheating. Add a salad and a whole grain roll for a light lunch or dinner.

Cooking oil spray

1 tablespoon olive oil or butter

3 cups broccoli florets, chopped into small pieces

2 teaspoons chopped fresh thyme

¾ cups shredded sharp white cheddar cheese (about 3 ounces)

½ cup whole milk

4 large eggs

1 teaspoon salt

¼ teaspoon pepper

1 tablespoon chopped fresh chives, for serving (optional)

From the Test Kitchen

Fill these bites with whatever you like. change up the cheese (Swiss, provolone, Jack). Or swap any of the following for the broccoli, or do a mix and match depending on what you're hungry for and what you have on hand.

- Sauteed baby spinach
- Sauteed mushrooms
- Cooked turkey sausage, crumbled or diced

---

1. Preheat the oven to 375°F. Spray 8 cups of a 12-muffin pan with cooking oil spray.

2. Heat the oil or melt the butter in a large nonstick skillet over medium heat. Add broccoli, and cook, stirring occasionally, until softened but not browned, about 6 minutes. Add the thyme, and cook until fragrant and broccoli is tender, about 1 minute more. Remove from heat. Let cool slightly, then distribute the broccoli evenly among the prepared muffin cups.

3. Whisk together the cheese, milk, eggs, salt, and pepper in a medium bowl. Pour about ¼ cup of the egg mixture over the broccoli in each muffin cup. Bake at 375°F until set and a knife inserted into the center comes out clean, about 13 minutes.

4. Let cool for 3 minutes before removing from the muffin tins. To remove, run a knife around the edges, and then gently lift each quiche out of the muffin tin. Sprinkle with chives and serve immediately.

The egg bites can be stored in the refrigerator in an airtight container for up to 3 days. To reheat, wrap in aluminum foil and heat in a preheated 375°F oven until warmed through, 8 to 10 minutes. If using a microwave, loosely wrap in paper towels and cook on high for 1 to 2 minutes.

NUTRITION INFO: 1 portion (2 bites) provides:

Protein: ½ serving

Calcium: 1 serving

Vitamin C: 1 serving

Vitamin A: 1 serving

Tomato and Roasted Red Pepper Frittata

SERVES 2

A brunch-worthy dish that cooks up in minutes—especially if you use leftover or store-bought roasted red peppers. Add a salad and some whole-grain bread, and call it dinner, too.

4 large eggs

4 teaspoons milk

½ cup grated Parmesan or sharp provolone cheese

1 clove garlic, minced

Salt and black pepper

2 small tomatoes, seeded and chopped

1 tablespoon chopped fresh basil or 1 teaspoon dried basil

1 tablespoon olive oil

½ cup coarsely chopped roasted red bell pepper (about 1 large pepper; leftover or from a jar)

1 tablespoon chopped fresh flat-leaf (Italian) parsley or 1 teaspoon dried parsley (optional)

1. Place the eggs, milk, cheese, and garlic in a medium-size bowl. Add a pinch each of salt and black pepper and whisk to mix. Add the tomatoes and basil and stir gently to combine.

2. Heat the olive oil in a medium-size skillet over medium-low heat. Pour the egg mixture into the skillet and cook until nearly set, 5 to 8 minutes, lifting the edge to let the uncooked egg run underneath.

From the Test Kitchen

Have some leftover steamed broccoli from last night's dinner? Toss it in the skillet along with the eggs and buy yourself an extra serving of green leafies and vitamin C.

3. Sprinkle the roasted red pepper on top of the frittata and cook until completely set, 1 to 2 minutes longer.

4. Slide the frittata onto a plate and sprinkle the parsley on top, if desired, before serving.

NUTRITION INFO: 1 portion provides:

Protein: 1 serving

Calcium: 1 serving

Vitamin C: 2½ servings

Vitamin A: 1½ servings

Fat: ½ serving

Omegas: some, if using omega-3 eggs

Breakfast Burritos

SERVES 1

The ultimate in portable breakfasts, a Breakfast Burrito brimming with avocado, tomato, black beans, eggs, and salsa can find its way to your mouth almost as quickly as the fast-food variety (more quickly if there's a wait at the drive-thru) but contains much less fat and is much more nutritious.

Olive oil cooking spray
¼ cup drained canned black beans, rinsed and drained
2 tablespoons store-bought tomato-based salsa
1 scallion (white and light green parts), trimmed and thinly sliced
1 tablespoon chopped fresh cilantro
2 large eggs, lightly beaten
1 whole-wheat tortilla or wrap (12-inch diameter)
¼ medium-size avocado (preferably Hass), chopped (optional)
½ roma tomato, seeded and chopped
¼ cup shredded cheddar, Monterey Jack, or Colby cheese

1. Coat a medium-size skillet with olive oil cooking spray and heat over medium heat. Add the black beans, salsa, scallion, and cilantro and cook until heated through, about 2 minutes. Add the eggs and cook, stirring gently, until completely set, about 3 minutes. Remove from the heat.

2. Place the tortilla on a microwave-safe plate or paper towel and heat for 15 seconds in the microwave.

3. Place the tortilla on a work surface or on a plate. Spoon the egg and black bean mixture in the center. Sprinkle the avocado, if using, tomato, and cheese on top.

From the Test Kitchen

Beans aren't exactly what the doctor (or the guy who sits next to you at work) ordered? If tummy troubles have you avoiding gas makers, skip the beans and toss in a cup of cooked edamame (soybeans); you'll be getting some additional protein in the bargain. For that matter, you can roll up just about any steamed or sautéed veggie (think last night's leftovers) in a Breakfast Burrito.

4. Fold the top and bottom of the tortilla into the center. Starting at one side, roll up the tortilla to enclose the filling.

NUTRITION INFO: 1 portion provides:

Protein: 1 serving

Calcium: 1 serving

Vitamin C: 1 serving

Other fruits and vegetables: 1 serving

Whole grains and legumes: 2½ servings

Iron: some

Omegas: some, if using omega-3 eggs

Baby's Big Bite

SERVES 1

Egg on a muffin without the McFat, but with plenty of grains and calcium. Pack one of these quick and convenient babies to go tomorrow morning.

1 whole-grain English muffin, split, or
  2 slices whole-grain bread
1 tomato, sliced
1 slice Swiss or cheddar cheese
1 large egg
1 tablespoon milk
1½ teaspoons oil or butter

1. Toast the English muffin.

2. Place the muffin halves split side up on a microwave-safe plate and arrange half of the tomato slices on each. Top each half with a slice of cheese. Microwave on high power until the cheese is slightly melted, about 30 seconds.

3. Place the egg and milk in a small bowl and whisk until well combined. Heat the olive oil in a small skillet over medium-high heat. Add the egg mixture and cook, stirring gently, until completely set, about 1 minute.

4. Spoon the scrambled egg on a muffin half and top with the other half.

From the Test Kitchen

Extra hungry this morning? Heat diced turkey breast or cooked crumbled turkey, chicken, or vegetarian sausage, then add them to the egg while it cooks.

NUTRITION INFO: 1 portion provides:

Protein: 1 serving

Calcium: 1 serving

Vitamin C: ½ serving

Whole grains and legumes: 2 servings

Fat: ½ serving

Omegas: some, if using omega-3 eggs

Stuffed French Toast

SERVES 1

Want a sandwich that eats like breakfast—only neater? Slices of whole-grain bread stuffed with fresh peaches or banana and fruit preserves hit the spot when you're craving something sweet.

1 tablespoon peanut or almond butter

2 slices whole-grain bread

2 teaspoons all-fruit preserves
   (any flavor)

½ fresh or frozen peach or banana,
   very thinly sliced

1 large egg

¼ cup milk

½ teaspoon vanilla extract

½ teaspoon ground cinnamon

1½ teaspoons canola oil or butter

1. Spread 1½ teaspoons of the almond butter on one side of each slice of bread. Spread the preserves over one coated slice of bread. Arrange the peach slices over the preserves, then top with the other slice of bread to make a sandwich.

2. Place the egg, milk, vanilla, and cinnamon in a shallow bowl and whisk to mix.

3. Place the sandwich in the egg mixture and let it soak for 1 minute on each side.

4. Heat the oil in a small skillet over medium-high heat. Cook the sandwich until browned, 2 to 3 minutes per side.

5. Cut the sandwich in half and serve warm.

From the Test Kitchen

Not in the mood for sweet? Make a savory Stuffed French Toast instead: Substitute cooked turkey sausage (protein) and Swiss cheese (calcium), or Swiss and thinly sliced tomato, for the almond butter and fruit.

NUTRITION INFO: 1 portion provides:

Protein: ½ serving

Vitamin A: ½ serving if made with peach

Other fruits and vegetables: ½ serving if made with banana

Whole grains and legumes: 2 servings

Fat: 1½ servings

Any Day Breakfast Parfait

SERVES 1

Getting your Daily Dozen doesn't get any easier than this. Or any cooler. This parfait teams fresh fruit, yogurt, and granola for a refreshing breakfast at home or on the go.

**1 ripe yellow peach or nectarine or
½ mango, coarsely chopped
1 cup fat-free vanilla Greek yogurt
½ cup granola
½ cup blueberries or sliced strawberries
Mint sprig (optional)**

Arrange the chopped peach, yogurt, granola, and berries in alternating layers in a bowl or glass. Top with a mint sprig, if desired. Want to take the parfait with you? Layer the ingredients in a plastic container or cup, or a medium-size mason jar.

NUTRITION INFO: 1 portion provides:

Protein: ½ serving

Calcium: 1½ servings

Vitamin C: 1 serving if made with strawberries; 2 if made with strawberries and mango

Vitamin A: 1 serving

Other fruits and vegetables: 1 serving if made with blueberries

Whole grains and legumes: 1 serving

From the Test Kitchen

Any fruit that suits your fancy—or fills your fridge—can be layered into a yogurt parfait. Try raspberries, blackberries, plums, cherries, pineapple, or bananas, too. If winter leaves you with slim pickings in the produce department, opt for frozen fruit, but thaw and drain it first. And there's always room for some dried or crunchy freeze-dried fruit. Toasted nuts make a great topping, too.

Whole-Wheat Buttermilk Pancakes

MAKES ABOUT 12 PANCAKES

Pancakes made with only white flour just can't stack up to these. Plus, you won't have to give up fluffiness for nutrition—these pancakes have plenty of both.

1¼ cups whole-wheat flour
½ cup all-purpose white flour
3 tablespoons ground flaxseed, oat bran, or wheat germ
1 teaspoon baking powder
1 teaspoon baking soda
1 teaspoon ground cinnamon
Pinch of ground nutmeg
Pinch of salt
1¾ cups buttermilk
¼ cup milk
1 teaspoon sugar
2 large eggs
1 teaspoon vanilla extract
2 tablespoons plus 2 teaspoons canola oil

1. Place the whole-wheat and white flours, flaxseed, baking powder, baking soda, cinnamon, nutmeg, and salt in a medium-size bowl and stir to combine.

2. Place the buttermilk, milk, honey, eggs, vanilla, and 2 tablespoons of the oil in another bowl and whisk to mix. Pour the buttermilk mixture into the flour mixture and beat just until smooth. If possible, let the batter rest for up to 30 minutes at room temperature before cooking the pancakes.

3. Heat the remaining 2 teaspoons oil in a 9-inch skillet over medium-high heat. Cook the pancakes two at a time, using ¼ cup batter per pancake, until the batter bubbles on top and the pancakes are firm on the bottom, about 3 minutes. Turn the pancakes over and continue cooking until the second side is brown, about 3 minutes. Repeat with the remaining batter.

4. Serve the pancakes warm. They can be frozen for up to 2 weeks: Let them cool completely, then wrap them in a single layer or individually in aluminum foil. To reheat, unwrap a pancake and microwave it on high power for 2 minutes, or heat it in a 350°F oven for 10 minutes.

NUTRITION INFO: 1 portion (about 4 pancakes) provides:

Protein: ½ serving

Calcium: ½ serving

Whole grains and legumes: 2 servings

Iron: some

Fat: 1 serving

Pancake Add-Ins

Make basic whole-wheat pancakes anything but basic by tossing in:

- Finely chopped apple or pear
- Chopped banana
- Blueberries—fresh, thawed frozen, dried, or freeze-dried
- Dried cranberries or cherries
- Raisins
- Chopped dried apricots
- Chopped pineapple, peaches, cherries, or mango
- Chopped pecans, almonds, or walnuts

Ginger-Blueberry Whole-Wheat Pancakes

MAKES 10 TO 12 PANCAKES

Feeling a little green this morning? Try some blues. These pancakes, infused with ginger and packed with blueberries and whole wheat, make a soothing and nutritious morning meal. What's better still is that these pancakes are surprisingly light—even with the whole-wheat flour.

1½ cups whole-wheat flour
1 teaspoon ground ginger
1 teaspoon ground cinnamon
Pinch of ground allspice
1 teaspoon baking soda
1 cup milk
1 tablespoon butter, melted
2 medium-size eggs
2 teaspoons granulated sugar
1½ cups fresh or unthawed frozen
    blueberries or 1 cup freeze-dried
2 teaspoons canola oil

1. Place the whole-wheat flour, ginger, cinnamon, allspice, and baking soda in a large bowl and stir to combine. Set aside.

2. Place the milk, butter, eggs, and sugar in a medium-size bowl, and whisk to blend. Add the milk mixture to the flour mixture and whisk until blended. Add the blueberries and stir gently to combine.

3. Heat the canola oil in a 9-inch skillet over medium-high heat. Cook the pancakes two at a time, using about ¼ cup batter per pancake, until they are golden brown on the bottom, 2 to 3 minutes. Turn the pancakes over and continue cooking until the second side is golden brown, about 2 minutes. Repeat with remaining batter.

4. Serve the pancakes warm with maple syrup or a Quick Fruit Syrup (see below). The pancakes can be frozen for up to 2 weeks: Let them cool completely, then wrap them in a single layer or individually in aluminum foil. To reheat, unwrap a pancake and microwave it on high power for 2 minutes or heat it in a 350°F oven for 10 minutes.

NUTRITION INFO: 1 portion
(about 4 pancakes) provides:

Other fruits and vegetables: ½ serving

Whole grains and legumes: 2 servings

Quick Fruit Syrups

Feeling fruity? Warm some all-fruit preserves in the microwave on medium-high power, then serve them syrup style over pancakes. If you like your syrup thinner, add some water after heating the preserves.

Power Breakfast Bars

MAKES ABOUT 20 BARS

These pack a lot more nutrition than the bars you buy. Pack them to go—with a side of yogurt or cheese, they make the perfect take-along breakfast, mini meal, or snack.

¼ cup packed dark brown sugar
¼ cup maple syrup or honey
¼ cup creamy peanut butter
2 large eggs
4 tablespoons canola oil
2 tablespoons butter, melted
1 teaspoon vanilla extract
2½ cups old-fashioned rolled oats
1 cup whole-wheat flour
½ teaspoon baking soda
1 teaspoon ground cinnamon
2 tablespoons oat bran or ground flaxseed
1 cup chopped walnuts or almonds
1 cup chopped raisins or mixed dried fruit such as chopped apricots, blueberries, cranberries, and/or cherries

1. Preheat the oven to 375°F.

2. Place the sugar, maple syrup, peanut butter, eggs, oil, butter, and vanilla in a mixing bowl and beat until well mixed.

3. Place the oats, whole-wheat flour, baking soda, cinnamon, oat bran, walnuts, and raisins in another mixing bowl and stir to mix. Add the oat mixture to the sugar and oil mixture and stir until thoroughly combined.

4. Line a baking sheet with parchment paper. Shape heaping tablespoons of the batter into bars about 2 x 4 inches, arranging them about 1 inch apart. Bake the bars until the bottoms are brown and the tops are golden brown, about 15 minutes. For crisper bars, reduce the oven temperature to 200°F and bake for 10 minutes longer.

5. Let the bars cool completely before sliding them off the baking sheet. Wrap individually in foil or plastic wrap if you plan to transport them. The bars can be stored in an airtight container for 3 days at room temperature or frozen for up to 1 month.

NUTRITION INFO: 1 portion (2 bars) provides:

Protein: ½ serving

Vitamin C: ½ serving

Vitamin A: ½ serving if made with apricots

Other fruits and vegetables: ½ serving

Whole grains and legumes: 1½ servings

Iron: some

Fat: 1 serving

Omegas: some

No-Bake Energy Bites

MAKES ABOUT 18 BALLS

These easy-to-make energy bites can pull triple duty as breakfast, snack, or wholesome dessert. Store them in an airtight container in the fridge.

1 cup old-fashioned rolled oats
½ cup creamy peanut butter
¼ cup ground flaxseed
½ cup mini dark chocolate chips
¼ cup honey
⅓ cup raisins or dried chopped cherries
1 teaspoon vanilla extract
½ teaspoon salt

1. Stir the oats, peanut butter, flaxseed, chocolate chips, honey, raisins or cherries, vanilla, and salt together in a medium bowl until thoroughly mixed. Cover and chill in the refrigerator for about 30 minutes.

2. Lay out a sheet of waxed paper on a work surface. For each bite, scoop out a heaping tablespoon of the mixture, roll into a 1-inch ball, and set it on the waxed paper. Store in the refrigerator in an airtight container, with the layers separated with waxed paper, for up to 1 week.

NUTRITION INFO: 1 portion (2–3 balls) provides:

Whole grains and legumes: 1 serving

Iron: some

Omegas: some

Muffins

....

Mad about muffins but wondering whether there's a place for these sweet breakfast treats now that you're trying to eat healthier? Good news! While many store-bought or bakery muffins may be lightweights when it comes to nutrition (and heavyweights when it comes to calories), the sugar-free muffins in this chapter are tasty and nutritious. Start a queasy morning with a Ginger and Carrot Muffin. Spice up a snack with a Pumpkin Pie Muffin or linger over brunch with a Triple Blueberry Muffin. Whatever flavor you're craving, there's a muffin here for you.

So many muffin cravings, but so little time? Bake a few batches at once, and freeze the extras for munching later on. And don't stop with breakfast. A wholesome muffin (especially when teamed with a piece of cheese) makes the perfect pick-me-up when your blood sugar starts to take a midmorning or midafternoon dive. And, with a glass of milk, there's no better bedtime snack.

Triple Blueberry Muffins

MAKES 12 MUFFINS

Triple the blueberries—preserves, frozen, and dried—means triple the taste in these yummy muffins. The addition of old-fashioned rolled oats lends a chewier texture and nuttier taste, plus nets extra fiber.

¾ cup whole-wheat flour

¼ cup ground flaxseed

2 teaspoons baking powder

1 teaspoon baking soda

1½ cups old-fashioned rolled oats

1 cup honey or maple syrup

½ cup all-fruit blueberry preserves

2 large eggs, lightly beaten

3 tablespoons canola oil

2 teaspoons vanilla extract

¾ cup frozen blueberries

½ cup dried or freeze-dried blueberries

1. Preheat oven to 375°F. Line a standard-size 12-cup muffin tin with paper liners.

2. Place the flour, flaxseed, baking powder, and baking soda in a large bowl and stir to mix. Add the oats and stir until well combined. Place the honey, preserves, eggs, oil, and vanilla in a medium-size bowl and stir to mix well. Add the blueberry mixture to the flour mixture and stir gently just until thoroughly blended; be careful not to overmix. Gently fold in the frozen and dried blueberries.

3. Spoon the batter into the prepared muffin tin, dividing it evenly among the muffin cups. Bake until a toothpick inserted into the center of a muffin comes out clean, 18 to 20 minutes.

4. Transfer the muffins to a wire rack and cool completely. The muffins can be stored in an airtight container for up to 3 days or individually wrapped in plastic wrap and frozen for up to 3 months.

NUTRITION INFO: 1 portion (1 muffin) provides:

Vitamin C: ½ serving

Whole grains and legumes: 1 serving

Iron: some

Going Fruity? Getting Nutty?

Add an additional ¼ cup of all-fruit preserves (any flavor) to any muffin batter, or better still, cut baked muffins in half and slather them with the preserves. Are you tired of raisins? Explore other dried fruit options, and chop them as needed—from apricots to mangos, apples to pears, cherries to blueberries. And don't forget to go nutty—add ½ cup of whatever coarsely chopped nuts you like (almonds, hazelnuts, pecans, walnuts, to name a few) to the muffin batter. Toast them first for even more flavor (see page 217 for toasting tips). Or toss in ½ cup of unsweetened coconut flakes.

Gluten-Free Carrot and Almond Muffins

MAKES 8 TO 10 MUFFINS

Ditch the gluten and the dairy without losing the nutrients or the flavor with these moist muffins. The coconut oil supplies a subtle tropical note, but if it's not a shelf staple in your kitchen, canola oil will work just as well.

2 cups finely ground almond flour
½ teaspoon salt
½ teaspoon baking soda
1 teaspoon ground cinnamon
½ teaspoon ground nutmeg
3 large eggs, at room temperature
¼ cup coconut oil, melted and cooled
¼ cup maple syrup
1 cup finely shredded peeled carrots

1. Preheat oven to 350°F. Line 8 to 10 cups of a standard-size muffin tin with paper liners.

2. In a large bowl, whisk the almond flour, salt, baking soda, cinnamon, and nutmeg to combine. In a medium-size bowl, whisk the eggs, oil, and maple syrup. Add the egg mixture to the almond flour mixture and stir until mixed. Stir in the carrots.

3. Spoon about ¼ cup of the batter into each muffin cup. Bake until a toothpick inserted into the center of a muffin comes out clean, about 20 minutes.

4. Transfer the muffins to a wire rack and cool before serving. Store in an airtight container in the refrigerator for up to 3 days or wrap individually in plastic wrap and store in the freezer for up to 3 months.

NUTRITION INFO: 1 portion (1 muffin) provides:

Protein: 1 serving

Vitamin A: ½ serving

Omegas: some

Flour Power

Any muffin batter can benefit from the addition of omega-3-rich (and constipation-combating) ground flaxseed. Substitute ¼ cup of flaxseed for ¼ cup of flour. If it's fiber you're looking for, substitute ¼ cup of wheat bran for ¼ cup of flour (although flax will give you the same results, more nutritiously). Want a nuttier flavor, protein boost, and some healthy fatty acids? You can use ¼ cup of ground nuts to take the place of ¼ cup of flour. For extra nutrients substitute ¼ cup of wheat germ or oat bran for ¼ cup of flour. For more protein use soy flour in place of up to a third of the flour in your recipe. Want to lighten things up? Substitute ½ cup of unbleached white flour for ¼ cup of whole-wheat flour.

Savory Spinach Cheddar Muffins

MAKES 12 MUFFINS

Looking for a savory spin on a breakfast or snack muffin, or for the perfect sidekick for your lunchtime soup that also kicks up nutrition? Look no further.

2 cups white whole-wheat flour
¼ cup oat bran
1 tablespoon baking powder
½ teaspoon salt
2 large eggs
1 cup milk
½ cup canola oil
1 cup coarsely chopped fresh spinach,
    tough stems removed
¾ cup shredded cheddar cheese
    (about 3 ounces)
1 tablespoon minced fresh chives

1. Preheat oven to 400°F. Line a standard-size 12-cup muffin tin with paper liners.

2. In a large bowl, mix together the flour, oat bran, baking powder, and salt. In a medium-size bowl, whisk together the eggs, milk, and oil. Add the egg mixture to the flour mixture and stir just until blended. Gently stir in the spinach, cheddar cheese, and chives; be careful not to overmix.

3. Spoon the batter into the prepared muffin tin, dividing it evenly among the muffin cups. Bake until a toothpick inserted in the middle comes out clean, 15 to 18 minutes.

4. Transfer the muffins to a wire rack and cool before serving. Store in an airtight container for up to 5 days or wrap individually in plastic wrap and store in the freezer for up to 3 months.

NUTRITION INFO: 1 portion (1 muffin) provides:

Protein: ½ serving

Vitamin A: ½ serving

Whole grains and legumes: 1 serving

Iron: some

Fat: ½ serving

Muffins Now, Muffins Later

Are 12 muffins 11 muffins too many? Fortunately, the muffins you bake today can be enjoyed tomorrow and next week—and even for months to come. To store muffins at room temperature, place them in an airtight container or ziplock bag; they'll keep for up to 3 days. Still haven't polished them off? Wrap each muffin individually in plastic wrap or aluminum foil and freeze them for up to 3 months. To thaw, simply take a muffin out of the freezer and allow it to come to room temperature. Prefer a muffin that tastes fresh out of the oven? Wrap the thawed muffin loosely in foil and place it in a preheated 350°F oven for 7 to 10 minutes until it's warmed through.

Raisin Bran Muffins

MAKES 12 TO 18 MUFFINS

Sure, all that bran will get things going—but these muffins are so delicious, you'll want to eat them on a regular basis even when you're regular.

1½ cups oat bran
1 cup whole-wheat flour
1 cup old-fashioned rolled oats
2 teaspoons ground cinnamon
½ cup chopped toasted nuts, such as
    walnuts, pecans, or almonds
    (see page 217)
2 teaspoons baking soda
1 teaspoon baking powder
1 cup honey or maple syrup
1¼ cups buttermilk
2 large eggs, lightly beaten
3 tablespoons canola oil
2 teaspoons vanilla extract
1 cup raisins

1. Preheat the oven to 400°F. Line a standard-size 12-cup muffin tin with paper liners.

2. Place the oat bran, flour, oats, cinnamon, nuts, baking soda, and baking powder in a large bowl and stir to mix. Place the honey, buttermilk, eggs, oil, and vanilla in a medium-size bowl and mix well. Add the honey mixture to the bran mixture and stir gently just until thoroughly blended; be careful not to overmix. Gently fold in the raisins.

3. Spoon the batter into the prepared muffin cups, dividing it evenly. (You may have extra batter. If so, just bake a few more muffins.)

4. Bake until a toothpick inserted into the center of a muffin comes out clean, 15 to 18 minutes.

5. Transfer the muffins to a wire rack and cool completely before serving. The muffins can be stored in an airtight container for up to 3 days or individually wrapped and frozen for up to 3 months.

NUTRITION INFO: 1 portion (1 muffin) provides:

Protein: ½ serving

Vitamin C: 1 serving

Whole grains and legumes: ½ serving

Iron: some

Omegas: some

Pumpkin Pie Muffins

MAKES 12 MUFFINS

Do you wish every morning were Thanksgiving morning? Here's the spicy, sweet taste of your favorite holiday pie in a wholesome everyday muffin.

1 cup whole-wheat flour
¼ cup oat bran
¼ cup ground flaxseed
2 teaspoons baking powder
1½ teaspoons baking soda
2 teaspoons ground cinnamon
¼ teaspoon ground ginger
¼ teaspoon ground cloves
¼ teaspoon ground nutmeg
¾ cup solid-pack pumpkin puree
2 large eggs, lightly beaten
3 tablespoons canola oil
1 cup maple syrup
2 teaspoons vanilla extract
½ cup chopped toasted walnuts
    (see page 217; optional)

1. Preheat the oven to 400°F. Line a standard-size 12-cup muffin tin with paper liners.

2. Place the flour, oat bran, flaxseed, baking powder, baking soda, cinnamon, ginger, cloves, and nutmeg in a large bowl and stir to mix. Place the pumpkin, eggs, oil, maple syrup, and vanilla in medium-size bowl and mix well. Add the pumpkin mixture to the flour mixture and stir gently just until blended; be careful not to overmix. Gently fold in the walnuts, if using.

3. Spoon the batter into the prepared muffin tin, dividing it evenly among the muffin cups. Bake until a toothpick inserted into the center of a muffin comes out clean, 15 to 18 minutes.

4. Transfer the muffins to a wire rack and cool completely. The muffins can be stored in an airtight container for up to 3 days or individually wrapped and frozen for up to 3 months.

NUTRITION INFO: 1 portion (1 muffin) provides:

Vitamin C: ½ serving

Vitamin A: ½ serving

Whole grains and legumes: 1 serving

Iron: some

Omegas: some

Sandwiches

....

Lunchtime boredom sending you out for fast food? Stop filling your brown bag with the same old sandwiches. There's a lot more you can put between two slices of bread than turkey and cheese—in fact, sandwiches become even more interesting if you skip traditional bread altogether. So wrap your mouth around a tasty wrap (the perfect take-along lunch, since they're so neat to eat), stuff a pita or tortilla, layer a bagel, or fill a roll—and meet a surprising number of Daily Dozen requirements while you're at it. It's food to go that's good for you.

A Better BLT

MAKES 1 SANDWICH

Here's a great way to get your BLT without the F (fat). A white bean spread stands in for mayo, adding a tasty fourth dimension. It's a BLT that's built for baby-building—and mom satisfaction.

2 slices whole-grain toast
2 tablespoons White Bean Spread
    (recipe follows)
½ cup sliced red leaf lettuce
¼ cup shredded carrot
4 slices vegetarian bacon or turkey bacon
    (about 4 ounces), cooked
½ medium-size avocado (preferably
    Hass), sliced
1 roma tomato, sliced

Spread both slices of toast with the bean spread. Layer the lettuce, carrot, bacon, avocado, and tomato on one slice, then top with the other slice.

NUTRITION INFO: 1 portion provides:

Protein: ½ serving

Vitamin C: 1 serving

Vitamin A: 1½ servings

Other fruits and vegetables: 1 serving

Whole grains and legumes: 2 servings

White Bean Spread

MAKES ABOUT 1 CUP

Hold the mayo, and use this creamy spread on your sandwiches instead. Makes a great dip for crudités and pita strips, too.

2 tablespoons olive oil

1 large clove garlic, peeled and crushed (optional; if raw garlic bothers you, see the box on page 262)

1 can (about 15 ounces) cannellini or Great Northern beans, drained and rinsed

2 tablespoons coarsely chopped fresh cilantro or flat-leaf (Italian) parsley

Juice of 1 large lemon

1 teaspoon tahini (optional)

Salt and black pepper

Place the olive oil, garlic, beans, cilantro, lemon juice, and tahini, if using, in a food processor and process until a smooth puree forms. Season with salt and pepper to taste. Serve at room temperature, or warm in the microwave or on top of the stove. The bean spread can be refrigerated, covered, for up to 5 days.

From the Test Kitchen

For a spicier spread, substitute chickpeas (garbanzo beans) in the White Bean Spread, and add 1 teaspoon ground toasted cumin seeds and a pinch of hot paprika and/or cayenne pepper (add both if you you really want to turn up the heat). You can kick it up with more garlic, too.

Prefer a BLT that's tidier to eat? Layer the filling inside a whole-grain roll, pita, or wrap.

NUTRITION INFO: 1 portion (¼ cup) provides:

Whole grains and legumes: ½ serving

Iron: some

Fat: ½ serving

What a Spread: Not Honey Mustard

Craving a sweet spread on your sandwich? Try this Not Honey Mustard spread. It's sweet like honey mustard, but has a more complex flavor. Yummy on chicken, turkey, or meat sandwiches—or anywhere else where you'd enjoy honey mustard. Mix together ¼ cup each Dijon mustard and all-fruit apricot preserves. Enjoy!

Chicken Burgers with Mango Relish

MAKES 4 BURGERS

These chicken burgers are cheese-burgers with a twist. Topping the burgers with mango relish as they grill adds an unexpectedly exotic taste. And traditional burgers can't beat this: Each chicken burger contains a hefty serving of vitamin A, compliments of the mango.

**4 frozen chicken burger patties,
    3 to 4 ounces each**
**½ cup shredded cheddar, Monterey Jack,
    or Colby cheese**
Mango Relish (recipe follows)
4 whole-grain rolls

1. Prepare the chicken patties according to package instructions.

2. Preheat the broiler to high. Sprinkle the cheese evenly over the cooked burgers and broil until browned, 1 to 3 minutes.

3. Spread a spoonful of the mango relish over each burger. Serve the burgers on whole-grain rolls with extra mango relish, if desired.

NUTRITION INFO: 1 portion (1 burger without Mango Relish) provides:

Protein: 1 serving

Calcium: ½ serving

Whole grains and legumes: 2 servings

Mango Relish

MAKES 1½ CUPS

Scoop up this sweet and spicy salsa with whole grain tortilla chips, but don't stop there. It'll add a kick to grilled chicken, fish, or pork, sass to sandwiches and wraps, and plenty of vitamins A and C to anything you top with it or spread it on. Too much of a kick? Turn the heat down by cutting the amount of jalapeno you add (or cutting it out altogether).

**2 ripe medium-size mangos, peeled,
    pitted, and cut into ½-inch pieces**
¼ cup (packed) chopped fresh cilantro
**2 tablespoons chopped shallot or
    scallions**
2 tablespoons fresh lime juice
**1 tablespoon white wine vinegar
    (or extra lime)**
**1½ tablespoons seeded and chopped
    jalapeno pepper (about 2 peppers), or
    to taste**
½ teaspoon kosher salt

Place the mangos, cilantro, shallot, lime juice, vinegar, jalapeno, and salt in a small bowl and stir to mix. Or for a finer mixture, pulse everything in a food processor until finely chopped, about 5 times. Leftovers will last 2 days refrigerated in an airtight container.

NUTRITION INFO: 1 portion (3 tablespoons) provides:

Vitamin C: 1 serving

Vitamin A: 1 serving

Fill 'er Up

Tired of the same old sandwich? Add a few of these into your brown-bag rotation. Don't be afraid to mix and match proteins or leave out any ingredient you're not currently feeling or don't have handy. And, of course, add pickles and pepperoncini (or anything you're craving). No need to explain—you're pregnant.

- Sliced beef, whole-grain mustard, spinach, fresh basil leaves, and tomato slices, on a whole-grain roll

- Sliced beef, Pesto with Sunflower Seeds (page 245), fresh basil leaves, roasted red pepper, and roasted red onion, wrapped in a whole-wheat tortilla

- Grilled chicken breast, Not Honey Mustard (page 211), Swiss cheese, romaine lettuce, and thinly sliced mango, in a pita

- Sliced chicken, Pesto with Sunflower Seeds (page 245) or whole-grain mustard, shaved Parmesan cheese, fresh basil leaves, and roasted red pepper, in a whole-grain wrap

- Sliced turkey breast, sharp cheddar cheese, arugula, and cranberry sauce or relish, on a whole-grain roll

- Sliced hard-boiled egg, shaved Parmesan cheese, baby spinach leaves, and tomato slices, on a whole-wheat English muffin

- Egg salad, whole-grain mustard, shaved Parmesan cheese, romaine or arugula, and tomato slices, on a whole-wheat bagel

- Cheddar cheese, Not Honey Mustard (page 211), thinly sliced apple or ripe pear, and arugula, on whole-grain bread

- Provolone cheese, Creamy Kale Pesto (page 216), tomato slices, fresh basil leaves, and arugula, in a whole-grain pita

- Sliced pasteurized mozzarella cheese, Creamy Kale Pesto (page 216), tomato slices, roasted red pepper, and a roasted portobello mushroom, on a whole-grain roll or in a whole-grain wrap

- Grilled eggplant, shredded romaine, hummus, and shredded Swiss cheese, in a whole-wheat pita

- Smashed ripe avocado on multigrain toast with a squeeze of lime juice (add a layer of sliced hard-boiled egg for a protein boost, hot sauce for a kick)

- Cheddar cheese and mango chutney, on whole-grain toast

- Any cheese and any jam on whole-grain toast

- Hummus, sliced avocado and tomato, and flaky salt, open-faced on whole-wheat toast

- Faux tuna salad: a cup of chickpeas mashed with a fork and mixed with a little mayo, mustard, and chopped celery

- Peanut butter and banana on whole-wheat bread; dark chocolate chips

- Peanut butter, sriracha, and thinly sliced cucumbers on whole-grain toast with a squeeze of lime

- Cottage cheese, sliced avocado, chopped tomato, chopped cucumber, minced chives optional, on whole-grain bread

Chicken Caesar Wrap

MAKES 1 SANDWICH

Next time you have a craving for chicken Caesar salad, leave the fork behind. Romaine, cheese, roasted red bell pepper, and chicken team up with a creamy dressing to create a salad that's high in flavor but low in fat. And it gets better—rolled up, the tasty salad becomes a super sandwich to go, so you can satisfy those cravings on the road. If you're leaning more plant-based, you can replace the chicken with an equal amount of thinly sliced firm or extra-firm tofu. Smoked tofu, if you can find it, would be particularly tasty here.

1 cup shredded romaine lettuce

¼ cup shredded provolone cheese

2 tablespoons grated Parmesan cheese

1 tablespoon Simple Caesar Dressing
   (page 263), plus more to taste

3 ounces cooked chicken or turkey,
   sliced thinly

4 strips roasted red bell pepper
   (left over or from a jar)

1 whole-grain tortilla or wrap (12-inch
   diameter), or whole-grain pita

1. Place the romaine, provolone and Parmesan cheeses, and Caesar dressing in a bowl and toss to mix. Add more dressing, if desired.

2. Layer the chicken and roasted pepper strips on the tortilla and top with the romaine salad. If you're using a pita, trim ½ inch off an edge of the pita and stuff it into the bottom of the pita. Fill the pita with the chicken and roasted pepper strips, then add the romaine salad.

3. Fold the sides of the tortilla or wrap over the filling.

NUTRITION INFO: 1 portion (without dressing) provides:

Protein: 1 serving

Calcium: 1 serving

Vitamin C: 2 servings

Vitamin A: 2 servings

Whole grains and legumes: 2 servings

Omegas: some

All Washed Up

Many of these recipes call for greens such as arugula, watercress, and romaine lettuce, and herbs including cilantro, parsley, dill, and basil. As with all fruits and vegetables, you'll need to thoroughly rinse the greens and herbs and pat them dry before adding them to sandwiches.

If your produce is "prewashed," don't wash it again. According to food safety experts, you could actually up your odds of introducing bacteria by washing it again at home. See page 181 for more tips on washing produce.

Curried Chicken Pita

MAKES 1 SANDWICH

A departure from the deli, this low-fat, creamy, Indian-inspired chicken salad sandwich really hits the spot when you're looking for something out of the ordinary. A cool combination of tomato, cucumber, and greens is tossed with diced chicken spiced up with curry and cilantro, stuffed into a pita, and topped with a sprinkling of raisins and sunflower seeds.

¾ cup diced cooked chicken or turkey (about 4 ounces)

3 tablespoons plain Greek yogurt (use 2% or whole-milk yogurt for a creamier dressing)

2 teaspoons mayonnaise

¼ cup diced peeled hothouse (seedless English) cucumber

1 roma tomato, diced

1 teaspoon chopped fresh cilantro, or more, to taste

½ teaspoon curry powder

Pinch of ground cumin

Hot red pepper sauce, such as Tabasco (optional)

Salt and black pepper

1 whole-wheat pita

½ cup shredded butter lettuce or romaine

1 tablespoon raisins, optional

1 tablespoon toasted sunflower seeds, optional (see page 217)

1. Place the chicken, yogurt, mayonnaise, cucumber, tomato, cilantro, curry powder, and cumin in a mixing bowl and stir to mix. Season with hot sauce, if desired, and salt and pepper to taste.

2. Trim ½ inch off an edge of the pita and stuff it into the bottom of the pita. Fill the pita with the lettuce, then add the chicken salad. Top with the raisins and sunflower seeds, if using.

Nutrition Info: 1 portion provides:

Protein: 1 serving

Vitamin C: 1 serving

Vitamin A: ½ serving

Other fruits and vegetables: ½ serving

Whole grains and legumes: 2 servings

Fat: ½ serving

Chicken for Days

Prepare and freeze a big batch of chicken breasts so you can put together sandwiches in a flash.

Place chicken in a single layer in a baking dish. Salt and pepper generously. Bake in a 375°F oven until the chicken's internal temperature reads 165°F (about 25–30 minutes). If you're eating it immediately, cover the chicken with foil and let it rest for 15 minutes before slicing. If you're going to freeze the chicken, the let the breasts cool completely before wrapping them tightly in foil and placing them in a large freezer bag. Leftover chicken can be stored in an airtight container in the refrigerator for up to 3 days or frozen for up to 2 months.

Salmon Pocket

MAKES 1 SANDWICH

Looking for a home for leftover cooked or canned salmon? How about this tasty Salmon Pocket? It combines greens, tomato, avocado, and pesto with salmon for a lunch or dinner that packs in not only protein but also those baby-friendly omega-3 fatty acids.

1 whole-wheat pita, or 2 slices
    whole-grain bread
½ cup flaked cooked salmon
    (fresh or canned)
2 tablespoons Pesto with Sunflower
    Seeds (page 245) or Creamy Kale
    Pesto (recipe follows)
1 small plum tomato, thinly sliced
¼ medium-size avocado
    (preferably Hass), thinly sliced
½ cup arugula, or other tender greens

Trim ½ inch off an edge of the pita and stuff it into the bottom of the pita. Fill the pita with the salmon, then spoon the pesto over it. Top with the tomato, avocado, and arugula.

NUTRITION INFO: 1 portion (without pesto) provides:

Protein: 1 serving

Calcium: 1 serving if made with canned salmon with bones

Vitamin C: 1 serving

Vitamin A: ½ serving

Other fruits and vegetables: ½ serving

Whole grains and legumes: 2 servings

Omegas: some

Creamy Kale Pesto

MAKES ABOUT 1 CUP

The kale in this peppy pesto kicks up flavor and nutrition, while the yogurt slims down the fat content of this Mediterranean classic. It's creamy enough to use as a dip for veggies or a spread for sandwiches, but don't forget to use it the traditional way—tossed with pasta and cheese, and maybe some chicken or shrimp. Any kale will work, but if kale doesn't work for you at all (or you can't find it), you can switch it out for extra spinach. Hungry for even more flavor? Toast the walnuts before adding them (see the box on the facing page).

2 cups torn kale leaves, rinsed,
    patted dry, ribs removed
2 cups baby spinach
½ cup grated Parmesan cheese
¼ cup walnuts
2 cloves garlic, minced
    (optional; If raw garlic bothers you,
    see the box on page 262)
2 tablespoons plain Greek yogurt,
    plus more as needed
1 tablespoon fresh lemon juice,
    plus more as needed
2 tablespoons olive oil, plus more
    as needed
Salt and cracked black pepper

Place the kale, spinach, Parmesan, walnuts, and garlic in a food processor and process until finely minced. Add the yogurt, lemon juice, and olive oil and process until well blended. Too thick?

A Toast to Toasted Nuts

Tempted to skip the toasting when a recipe calls for toasted nuts or seeds? You'll be skipping more than you think. Toasting brings out the true nutty flavor, adding a memorably rich dimension to any salad, sandwich, pasta, poultry—you name it. There are several ways to toast nuts or seeds.

On the stovetop: Sprinkle ½ cup nuts or seeds in an ungreased heavy skillet (don't use a nonstick one). Cook over medium heat, stirring frequently, until the nuts begin to brown, 5 to 7 minutes.

In the oven: Spread ½ cup nuts or seeds in an ungreased shallow pan. Bake uncovered in a 350°F oven, stirring frequently, until the nuts are light brown, about 10 minutes.

In the microwave: Spread ½ cup nuts or seeds evenly in a flat microwave-safe dish. Cook on high power until they are lightly browned, 2 to 3 minutes, stirring halfway through.

Toasted nuts will continue to darken after you remove them from the heat. A good test for doneness, along with color, is when you can smell a toasted (not burnt—that's overdone) aroma.

When toasting small seeds in a skillet, use a splatter screen, if possible. The seeds tend to pop around.

For ground nuts or seeds, you can grind toasted nuts or seeds in a food processor or mini grinder. Just be careful not to overprocess them, or you'll end up with nut or seed butter.

Add a little more yogurt, olive oil, and/or lemon juice. Season with salt and pepper to taste. The pesto can be refrigerated, covered tightly, for up to 5 days.

NUTRITION INFO: 1 portion (¼ cup) provides:

Vitamin C: 1 serving

Vitamin A: 1 serving

Iron: some

Fat: ½ serving

Omegas: some

From the Test Kitchen

For a more traditional pesto, substitute 1 cup basil leaves for 1 cup of the kale. For a zippier pesto, substitute arugula for the spinach. For a creamier sandwich spread, add a tablespoon or two of mayonnaise to the pesto along with the yogurt.

Black Bean Quesadilla

MAKES 1 QUESADILLA

Quesadillas—Mexican-style grilled cheese sandwiches—are quick to make and easy to customize. Packed with authentic flavor and an impressive array of nutrients, this Black Bean Quesadilla features Monterey Jack cheese, tangy black bean salsa, avocado, and tomato. Off to work? Take it cold, then heat it in the office microwave.

1 whole-grain tortilla or wrap
   (12-inch diameter)
½ cup shredded Monterey Jack or
   cheddar cheese
⅓ to ½ cup Black Beans in Lime and
   Cumin Vinaigrette (recipe follows)
¼ medium-size avocado
   (preferably Hass), sliced
½ medium-size tomato, chopped
½ medium-size red bell pepper, chopped
2 tablespoons chopped fresh cilantro,
   or to taste (optional)
Lime wedge for serving

1. Line a microwave-safe plate with a paper towel and place the tortilla on top. Sprinkle half of the cheese over half of the tortilla. Top the cheese with the Black Beans in Lime and Cumin Vinaigrette (page 219), avocado, tomato, and bell pepper. Sprinkle the remaining cheese on top.

2. Fold the bare half of the tortilla over the filling, covering it. Microwave on high power until the cheese melts, 1 to 2 minutes.

3. Remove and discard the paper towel, then cut the quesadilla into wedges. Sprinkle the cilantro over it and add a squeeze of lime, if desired, before serving.

From the Test Kitchen

There's more than one way to fill a tortilla—dozens, in fact. Here's one more: Spread 3 to 4 tablespoons fat-free refried beans over a tortilla. Top with 3 tablespoons of your favorite salsa. Sprinkle ¼ cup of your choice of shredded cheese over the salsa and microwave the tortilla on high power until the cheese melts, 1 to 2 minutes. Roll the tortilla and enjoy it immediately, or wrap it to go. Have leftover chicken, pork, steak, fish, or shrimp? Layer it on the tortilla, too. And that's a wrap!

NUTRITION INFO: 1 portion (without beans) provides:

Protein: 1 serving

Calcium: 2 servings

Vitamin C: 2½ servings

Vitamin A: 1 serving

Other fruits and vegetables: ½ serving

Whole grains and legumes: 2 servings

Black Beans in Lime and Cumin Vinaigrette

SERVES 4

These marinated black beans show off bold Southwestern flavors. Try using them in your next burrito, or on the side of grilled meat, chicken, or seafood.

1 can (about 15 ounces) black beans, drained and rinsed
1 medium-size red bell pepper, finely chopped
1 medium-size tomato, finely chopped
4 scallions (white and light green parts), trimmed and sliced
2 tablespoons chopped fresh cilantro
1 tablespoon chopped fresh flat-leaf (Italian) parsley
2 tablespoons fresh lime juice
1 tablespoon olive oil
½ teaspoon ground cumin, plus more to taste
Salt and black pepper

Place the black beans, bell pepper, tomato, and scallions in a salad bowl and stir to mix. Add the cilantro, parsley, lime juice, olive oil, and cumin and toss to mix. Taste for seasoning, adding salt and pepper and more cumin if necessary. The beans can be refrigerated, covered, for up to 2 days.

From the Test Kitchen

B eans are a great source of protein—but they can also be a great source of gas. Keep the protein and skip the gas by substituting cooked edamame.

NUTRITION INFO: 1 portion provides:

Protein: ½ serving

Calcium: ½ serving

Vitamin C: 1½ servings

Vitamin A: ½ serving plus

Whole grains and legumes: 1 serving

Iron: some

Fruity Turkey Salad

SERVES 2

A chewy (and vitamin-packed) surprise—dried apricots—makes this salad a treat for the taste buds. Nuts add crunch and important omegas. Serve the turkey salad with red leaf lettuce in a pita or on bread. And chicken can sub for the turkey.

1¼ cups chopped cooked turkey or chicken breast (about 7 ounces)

1 medium-size rib celery, thinly sliced

6 dried apricot halves, coarsely chopped

2 tablespoons coarsely chopped toasted walnuts (see page 217)

2 tablespoons chopped red onion or scallion (white and light green parts)

3 tablespoons plain Greek yogurt (whole-milk yogurt makes a creamier dressing)

1 tablespoon mayonnaise

1 tablespoon whole-grain mustard

1 tablespoon all-fruit apricot preserves (finely chop any pieces of fruit)

1 tablespoon fresh lemon juice, plus more to taste

1 tablespoon chopped fresh flat-leaf (Italian) parsley

Salt and black pepper

1. Place the turkey, celery, apricots, nuts, and onion in a bowl and stir to mix.

2. Place the yogurt, mayonnaise, mustard, apricot preserves, lemon juice, and parsley in a small bowl and stir to mix. Taste for seasoning, adding more lemon juice as necessary, and salt and pepper to taste.

3. Add the yogurt mixture to the turkey mixture, and stir to coat well.

NUTRITION INFO: 1 portion provides:

Protein: 1 serving

Vitamin A: ½ serving

Other fruits and vegetables: 1 serving

Fat: ½ serving

Iron: some

Omegas: some

Greek Salad Sandwich

SERVES 1

Can't decide between a salad and a sandwich? Here's a Greek salad that eats like a sandwich, neatly tucked into a pita. It's flexible, too. Keep it veggie or add the protein of your choice.

1 plum tomato, ripe but firm, seeded and diced

½ Persian or Kirby cucumber, seeded and diced

1 (¼-inch-thick) slice red onion, cut in half, rings separated, rinsed and drained

2 tablespoons crumbled pasteurized feta cheese

4 pitted kalamata olives, chopped

1 or 2 pepperoncini, drained and diced

1 teaspoon red wine vinegar

2 teaspoons extra-virgin olive oil

Salt and black pepper

1 small or ½ large whole-wheat pita,
   lightly toasted

1½ teaspoons mayonnaise

2 large-size leaves of romaine lettuce

1. In a medium bowl, combine half the tomato, the cucumber, onion, feta, olives, and pepperoncini. Add more tomato if desired. Toss with the vinegar and olive oil. Sprinkle with salt and pepper to taste.

2. Cut the pita in half and gently open. Spread mayonnaise on the inside bottom of each half, tuck in a lettuce leaf, and scoop the salad mixture evenly into each pita half. Serve immediately.

NUTRITION INFO: 1 portion (1 pita) provides:

Calcium: ½ serving

Vitamin C: 2 servings

Other fruits and vegetables: 1 serving

Whole grains and legumes: 2 servings

Fat: 2 servings

Spicy Egg Salad

SERVES 2

This kicked-up classic is perfect on its own or served on toast with lettuce leaves. Other add-ins could be fresh herbs, chopped dill pickle, or walnut pieces.

From the Test Kitchen

- Use omega-3 eggs for even more baby brain-boosting power. For an Asian twist, swap the Tabasco sauce with 1 teaspoon of sriracha and add a squeeze of lemon.

- Fortify your sandwich and score a protein serving by adding diced cooked chicken or chopped cooked shrimp.

4 hard-cooked eggs, peeled and
   coarsely chopped

2 tablespoons mayonnaise

1 tablespoon finely chopped celery

2 teaspoons Dijon mustard

2 teaspoons hot red pepper sauce,
   such as Tabasco

Salt and black pepper

Place the eggs, mayonnaise, celery, mustard, and hot sauce in a medium bowl. Stir gently to combine. Season to taste with salt and pepper.

NUTRITION INFO: 1 portion provides:

Protein: ½ serving

Fat: 1½ servings

Omegas: some

Soups

....

"S oup's on" can mean lots of things. For a cool, elegant start to a summer brunch, think Tomato Soup with Avocado. For a hearty, soul-warming meal in a bowl on a winter's evening, there's Broccoli and Cheese Soup or Turkey Chili. And for a nourishing pick-me-up in the middle of a long afternoon, pick Vegetable and Edamame Soup or Red Lentil and Tomato Soup. But there's one thing that all these soups and chilies serve up: plenty of delicious nutrients in a soothing form, a definite plus if you're finding sipping easier than chewing on queasy days.

Butternut Squash and Pear Soup

SERVES 4

Creamy and fragrant, this bisque only looks like it took a lot of effort. It's easier and faster to cook than you'd think, and you'll rack up powerful nutritional rewards. The sweet and subtly spiced combination of squash and pears will reward your taste buds, too.

1½ pounds precut diced butternut
   squash
3 cups low-sodium vegetable broth or
   chicken broth
Salt
1 tablespoon butter or canola oil
1 small onion, very thinly sliced
2 red pears, peeled, cored, and coarsely
   chopped

2 teaspoons curry powder
½ teaspoon ground ginger (optional)
⅓ cup plain whole-milk Greek yogurt
White pepper
½ cup finely shredded cheddar cheese,
   for serving

1. Place the squash, 2½ cups of the broth, and a pinch of salt in a large saucepan over medium-high heat and let it come to a boil. Reduce the heat and let it simmer until the squash softens, about 35 minutes. Set the squash aside with its cooking liquid.

2. While the squash is cooking, melt the butter or heat the oil in a large skillet

over medium heat. Add the onion and cook, stirring frequently, until softened, about 5 minutes. Add the pears and cook, stirring frequently, until softened, about 5 minutes. Add the curry powder, turmeric, and ginger, if using, and the remaining ½ cup broth and let it come to a simmer. Cover the skillet and let the mixture cook until the flavors blend, about 10 minutes.

3. Add the onion and pear mixture to the cooked squash. Let the mixture cool slightly, then working in batches if necessary, transfer it to a blender or food processor and puree until smooth.

4. Return the soup to the saucepan, add the yogurt, and season with salt and pepper to taste. Place the saucepan over low heat and let the soup heat through, stirring frequently, 2 to 3 minutes. Do not let it boil. Pour the soup into serving bowls and top each with 2 tablespoons cheddar cheese.

From the Test Kitchen

Only serving two (and a half) for dinner tonight? Make the Butternut Squash and Pear Soup through Step 3, then divide it in half. Continue with Step 4, using 3 tablespoons yogurt and ¼ cup cheddar cheese. The rest of the soup can be refrigerated, covered, for up to 2 days. Reheat it before continuing with Step 4. Want to double up on calcium? Double the cheese you sprinkle.

NUTRITION INFO: 1 portion (1 bowl) provides:

Calcium: ½ serving

Vitamin A: 2 servings

Other fruits and vegetables: 1 serving

The Cream of the Crop

Love cream soups but don't love all the calories that come with them? Get creamy the low-fat way.

Say potato: Adding a diced Yukon Gold potato to a soup before cooking it will result in a very creamy texture for a pureed soup that's creamless.

Milk it. Evaporated skim milk and evaporated low-fat milk are more concentrated than regular milk and will make soup creamier. Buttermilk also adds more creaminess than regular milk, along with a tangier taste. Add evaporated milk or buttermilk just before you are ready to serve; gently bring the soup back to a simmer over very low heat, whisking as it warms.

Go yogurt. Adding yogurt will make soup creamier and thicker. For a richer flavor, use whole-milk yogurt, which while higher in fat still has far less than cream. All with a calcium bonus. Whisk yogurt into the hot soup, then serve it immediately.

Try tofu. Adding 4 ounces well-drained, pureed soft tofu to a warm pureed soup will lend creaminess without the cream, and with no noticeable taste.

Ginger and Carrot Soup

SERVES 4

Ginger and carrot soup makes a soothing way to take your vitamins, especially when morning sickness outlasts the morning.

2 teaspoons olive oil or butter
1 medium-size sweet onion, chopped
1 clove garlic, minced (optional)
1 package (16 ounces) baby carrots
    (about 3 cups)
2-inch piece fresh ginger, peeled and
    thinly sliced
4 cups low-sodium chicken broth or
    vegetable broth
Fresh lemon juice
Salt and black pepper
Plain low-fat Greek yogurt, for serving

1. Heat the olive oil in a large saucepan over medium heat. Add the onion and garlic, if using, and cook until softened, about 5 minutes. Add the carrots and ginger and cook until the ginger is fragrant, about 2 minutes, stirring frequently.

2. Add the broth, raise the heat to medium-high, and let the soup come to a boil. Cover the saucepan, reduce the heat, and let the soup simmer until the carrots are very soft, about 15 minutes.

3. Let the soup cool slightly, then working in batches if necessary, transfer it to a blender or food processor and puree it until velvety smooth.

4. Return the soup to the saucepan and season it with lemon juice, salt, and pepper to taste. Let the soup come to a simmer over medium-low heat and cook

From the Test Kitchen

Don't have the time—or the stomach—to sauté the onions and carrots for Ginger and Carrot Soup? Place the carrots, onion (you don't even have to chop it, quartering will do, and you can leave out the garlic), and ginger in a pot with the broth. Bring it to a boil and let simmer until the carrots are soft, then puree it. Add a little lemon juice and some salt and pepper and you've got a lighter soup without that lingering onion odor in your kitchen.

until heated through. Pour the soup into serving bowls and top each with a large spoonful of yogurt. The soup can be refrigerated, covered, for 2 days.

NUTRITION INFO: 1 portion (1 bowl) provides:

Vitamin C: ½ serving

Vitamin A: 3 servings

Other fruits and vegetables: ½ serving

Sweet Potato Vichyssoise

SERVES 4

With more flavor and nutrition than traditional vichyssoise, making the soup with sweet potatoes is an elegant way to serve up your yellow vegetables.

1 tablespoon butter or olive oil

2 large leeks (white and light green parts), trimmed, rinsed well and thinly sliced

2 medium-size sweet potatoes, peeled and chopped

3 cups low-sodium chicken broth or vegetable broth

¼ cup chopped fresh flat-leaf (Italian) parsley

Salt and black pepper

1. Melt the butter or heat the olive oil in a saucepan over medium-high heat. Add the leeks and cook until they soften, about 3 minutes. Add the sweet potatoes and cook until they begin to soften, about 5 minutes. Add the broth and parsley and let the soup come to a boil. Reduce the heat and let it simmer until the sweet potatoes are completely soft, about 10 minutes.

Make Soup a Meal

Topped with shredded cheese and served with a salad and some whole-grain bread, most soups make an easy but sustaining meal at the end of a long day. Or pack a thermos of soup, with cheese already melted on top, to take to work with you.

From the Test Kitchen

If you'd like this soup a little more sippable, add some milk or buttermilk after it cools. You'll get a creamier taste and a calcium bonus.

2. Let the soup cool slightly, then working in batches if necessary, transfer it to a blender or food processor and puree it until smooth. Season the soup with salt and pepper to taste. The soup can be served either hot or cold. Reheat it over low heat after pureeing, if desired. The soup can be refrigerated, covered, for up to 4 days.

NUTRITION INFO: 1 portion (1 bowl) provides:

Vitamin C: ½ serving

Vitamin A: 1 serving

Other fruits and vegetables: ½ serving

Spiced-Up Gazpacho

SERVES 6

Like a salad you can sip, this soup is especially easy going down. Easy prepping, too. No cooking means no cooking smell or mess, plus once you make it, you can enjoy it for several days as a starter or a snack. Adding olive oil will make a richer gazpacho, but the soup is refreshing without it.

6 large plum tomatoes or 3 medium-size
    tomatoes, coarsely chopped
1 medium-size hothouse
    (seedless English) cucumber,
    peeled and coarsely chopped
1½ large red bell peppers, chopped
1 small red onion, chopped
1 clove garlic, minced (optional; if raw
    garlic bothers you, see the box on
    page 262)
3 tablespoons chopped fresh flat-leaf
    (Italian) parsley
2 tablespoons chopped fresh basil
4 cups tomato juice or vegetable juice,
    such as V8
3 tablespoons red wine vinegar
3 tablespoons olive oil (optional)
1 tablespoon fresh lemon juice,
    plus more to taste
Salt and black pepper
Tabasco sauce

1. Place the tomatoes, cucumber, bell peppers, onion, garlic, if using, parsley, basil, tomato juice, vinegar, olive oil, if using, and lemon juice in a food processor and pulse until the vegetables are finely chopped but not pureed.

2. Transfer the gazpacho to a large bowl and season it with salt, black pepper, and Tabasco sauce to taste. Add more lemon juice, if desired. Refrigerate the soup, covered, until chilled through, at least 2 hours or up to 3 days. Serve in

From the Test Kitchen

There are any number of possible variations on this gazpacho. Here are just a few:

- For a chunkier gazpacho, don't run the vegetables through the food processor. Or process only half the veggies.

- For a little taste of Mexico, substitute 2 tablespoons chopped fresh cilantro for the basil and fresh lime juice for the lemon juice; garnish the soup with chopped avocado.

- Chop two hard-cooked eggs and add them just before serving.

- For a more substantial soup, cut chilled cooked shrimp or scallops in half lengthwise and float them on top. Feeling really flush? Add chunks of chilled cooked crab or lobster.

- For a more sippable soup, use a whole 46-ounce bottle of juice.

soup bowls or in glasses. The soup can be refrigerated, covered, for up to 4 days.

NUTRITION INFO: 1 portion (1 bowl) provides:

Vitamin C: 3 servings; 3½ if made with vegetable juice

Vitamin A: 2½ servings; 3 if made with vegetable juice

Other fruits and vegetables: 1 serving

Fat: ½ serving if made using olive oil

Tomato Soup with Avocado

SERVES 4

This versatile and vitamin-packed soup is yummy hot and refreshing chilled.

2 teaspoons olive oil

3 scallions (white and light green parts), trimmed and thinly sliced

½ teaspoon coarsely chopped garlic (from 1 clove)

1½ cups canned crushed tomatoes, with their juices

4 cups tomato juice or vegetable juice, such as V8

¼ cup loosely packed fresh basil leaves, thinly sliced

Salt and black pepper

Diced avocado, for serving

½ red bell pepper, finely chopped, for serving

4 lime wedges, for serving

1. Heat the olive oil in a saucepan over medium heat. Add the scallions and garlic and cook until softened, about 2 minutes.

2. Add the tomatoes, tomato juice, and basil, raise the heat to medium-high, and let the soup come to a boil. Reduce the heat and let it simmer until the flavors are well blended, about 15 minutes. Season with salt and pepper to taste.

From the Test Kitchen

Substitute chopped cilantro for the basil, add some hot sauce, and your soup becomes a *sopa*.

3. Pour the soup into serving bowls, sprinkle avocado and bell pepper on top, and serve the lime wedges alongside. The soup can also be served chilled. It can be refrigerated, covered, for up to 2 days.

NUTRITION INFO:

Vitamin C: 2½ servings if made with tomato juice; 3 if made with vegetable juice

Vitamin A: 1½ servings if made with vegetable juice

Red Lentil and Tomato Soup

SERVES 2

Besides being prettier to look at than green or brown lentils, red lentils have a creamier texture and a milder taste. Teamed with chunky tomatoes, carrot, and celery, they make a rich-tasting, nutritious, and sustaining soup that's gentle on the stomach.

1 tablespoon olive oil

1 medium-size onion, chopped

½ teaspoon ground cumin

½ teaspoon ground turmeric

½ teaspoon ground allspice

½ tablespoon fresh ginger, peeled and
minced

2½ cups low-sodium vegetable broth or
chicken broth

½ cup red lentils

1 large rib celery, chopped

1 medium-size carrot, peeled and
chopped

4 roma tomatoes, coarsely chopped
(set aside 1 chopped tomato)

Salt and black pepper

1. Heat the olive oil in a large saucepan over medium heat. Add the onion and cook until softened, about 5 minutes.

2. Add the cumin, turmeric, allspice, and ginger and cook, stirring frequently, until fragrant, about 1 minute.

3. Add the broth, lentils, celery, carrot, and 3 of the chopped tomatoes, raise the heat to medium-high, and let the soup come to a boil. Reduce the heat and let it simmer until the lentils are tender, about 30 minutes.

From the Test Kitchen

Substitute any lentil for the red (they come in green, black, and basic brown)—though simmer time may need to be adjusted. Don't have all those spices on your shelf or fresh ginger handy? Just substitute 1 teaspoon of any of these: cumin, paprika, curry powder, or chili powder.

4. Add remaining tomato and season with salt and pepper to taste. Let the soup simmer until heated through, about 3 minutes. The soup can be refrigerated, covered, for up to 2 days.

NOTE: If you are serving only half of the soup now, add half of 1 chopped roma tomato at this stage. Add the second half after the rest of the soup has been reheated.

NUTRITION INFO: 1 portion (1 bowl) provides:

Protein: ½ serving

Vitamin C: 1 serving

Vitamin A: 2 servings

Other fruits and vegetables: ½ serving

Whole grains and legumes: 1½ servings

Iron: some

Fat: ½ serving

Roasted Vegetable Soup

SERVES 4

Thick and rich-tasting, but without a drop of cream, this soup is super satisfying. Add a handful of shredded cheese and some crusty whole-grain bread and your soup becomes supper. Just plan ahead for roasting time.

Cooking oil spray

2 medium-size carrots, cut into 1-inch chunks (about 1½ cups)

2 medium-size parsnips, cut into 1-inch chunks (about 1 cup)

1 cup 1-inch chunks peeled broccoli stems

1 small red onion, quartered, each quarter cut in half

1 tablespoon olive oil

Salt and black pepper

4 teaspoons fresh thyme leaves

3 to 4 cups low-sodium chicken broth

Toasted pumpkin seeds (see page 217), for serving

Chopped fresh flat-leaf (Italian) parsley, for serving

1. Preheat the oven to 400°F. Spray a large rimmed baking sheet with cooking oil spray, or just line an unsprayed sheet with parchment paper.

2. Place the carrots, parsnips, broccoli, and onion in a large bowl, add the olive oil, and toss to coat evenly. Spoon the vegetable mixture in an even layer onto the prepared baking sheet. Sprinkle some salt and pepper and 3 teaspoons of the thyme leaves on top.

3. Roast the vegetables until tender, about 45 minutes, stirring occasionally.

4. Transfer the roasted vegetables to a large saucepan and add 3 cups of the broth and the remaining 1 teaspoon thyme leaves. Let the soup come to a boil over high heat, then reduce the heat and let it simmer until the vegetables are very tender, about 15 minutes.

5. Let the soup cool slightly, then working in batches if necessary, transfer it to a blender or food processor and puree it until slightly chunky or smooth, as you prefer. If the soup is too thick, add more broth to thin it. Taste for seasoning, adding more salt and/or pepper as necessary.

6. If the soup has cooled down too much, return it to the saucepan and gently reheat it over low heat. Sprinkle pumpkin seeds and parsley on top just before serving. The soup can be refrigerated, covered, for up to 2 days.

NUTRITION INFO: 1 portion (1 bowl) provides:

Vitamin A: 1½ servings

Other fruits and vegetables: 1 serving

Iron: some

Vegetable and Edamame Soup

SERVES 4

This hearty but quick-cooking vegetable soup combines the best in beans—in this case white beans and protein-packed edamame (soybeans). The soup is half pureed, half chunky, so you get an interesting mix of textures, too. Provolone or cheddar cheese—your choice—adds even more flavor and a serving of calcium, too.

1 tablespoon olive oil
1 small onion, chopped
1 clove garlic, minced (optional)
4 plum tomatoes, coarsely chopped
2 medium-size carrots, coarsely chopped
3 to 4 cups low-sodium vegetable broth or
    chicken broth
2 teaspoons fresh thyme leaves
¼ cup chopped fresh flat-leaf (Italian)
    parsley
1 cup shelled cooked edamame
1 can (about 15 ounces) Great Northern
    beans, drained and rinsed
Salt and black pepper
1 cup shredded provolone or cheddar
    cheese, for serving

1. Heat the olive oil in a large saucepan over medium heat. Add the onion and garlic, if using, and cook until softened, about 5 minutes. Add the tomatoes and carrots and cook, stirring often, until the carrots are softened, about 10 minutes. Set aside 1 cup of the cooked vegetables.

2. Add 3 cups of the broth, the thyme, and the parsley to the saucepan. Raise the heat to medium-high and let the soup come to a boil, then cover the saucepan and reduce the heat to low. Let the soup simmer until the vegetables are very tender, about 15 minutes.

3. Let the soup cool slightly, then transfer it to a blender or food processor, working in batches if necessary, and puree the soup.

4. Return the soup to the saucepan and add the reserved cooked vegetables, edamame, and beans. If the soup is too thick, add more broth to thin it. Bring the soup to a simmer over medium heat and cook until the beans are heated through, about 5 minutes. Season the soup with salt and pepper to taste. Sprinkle the cheese over the soup before serving. The soup can be refrigerated, covered, for up to 2 days.

NUTRITION INFO: 1 portion (1 bowl) provides:

Protein: ½ serving

Calcium: 1 serving

Vitamin C: 1 serving

Vitamin A: 1 serving

Whole grains and legumes: 1 serving

Iron: some

Broccoli and Cheese Soup

SERVES 2

Broccoli, cheese, and potatoes are friends from way back. This velvety-smooth and vitamin-rich soup brings them together for a delicious reunion. You'll never miss the cream—or the calories it would add. Save time by using a package of precut broccoli florets.

1 tablespoon butter or olive oil
½ medium-size yellow onion, chopped
1 clove garlic, minced (optional)
2 cups broccoli florets
1 medium-size Yukon Gold potato, diced
2½ cups low-sodium chicken broth or vegetable broth
½ cup finely shredded cheddar cheese
¼ cup buttermilk, or more to taste
Salt and black pepper

1. Melt the butter or heat the oil in a large saucepan over medium heat. Add the onion and garlic, if using, and cook until softened, about 5 minutes.

2. Add the broccoli, potato, and broth, raise the heat to high, and let it come to a boil. Reduce the heat, cover the saucepan, and let the soup simmer until the broccoli and potato are softened, about 7 minutes.

3. Let the broccoli mixture cool slightly, then transfer it to a blender or food processor, and working in batches if necessary, puree it until satiny smooth.

4. Return the soup to the saucepan, add ¼ cup of the cheese and the buttermilk. Cook the soup over low heat until the cheese melts (do not let it come to a boil), about 3 minutes. Season with salt and pepper to taste. Pour the soup into serving bowls and top each with 2 tablespoons of the remaining cheese.

NUTRITION INFO: 1 portion provides:

Protein: ½ serving

Calcium: almost 2 servings

Vitamin C: 2 servings

Vitamin A: 2 servings

Other fruits and vegetables: ½ serving

Fat: ½ serving

Burn, Baby, Burn?

If pregnancy indigestion has you feeling the burn, try omitting garlic and/or onion from your soups, or subbing a sprinkle of garlic or onion powder.

Turkey Chili

SERVES 6

Leaner than your average chili, but no less flavorful. You can adjust the amount of chili powder to sound as many—or as few—alarms as you and your heartburn can handle. Substitute lean ground beef for the turkey if you'd like to up your iron. Want to steer clear of tummy troubles? Use edamame instead of the black beans.

1 tablespoon olive oil
1 medium-size onion, chopped
2 cloves garlic, minced (optional)
1½ pounds ground turkey breast
1 medium-size red bell pepper, chopped
1 medium-size yellow bell pepper, chopped
1 small jalapeno pepper, seeded and
    diced (optional)
2 tablespoons chili powder, or more or
    less to taste
1 tablespoon ground cumin
1 tablespoon tomato paste
1 can (about 15 ounces) red kidney beans,
    drained and rinsed
1 can (14½ ounces) diced tomatoes,
    with their juices (try fire-roasted
    tomatoes)
1½ cups shredded cheddar cheese,
    for serving
2 tablespoons chopped fresh cilantro,
    for serving

1. Heat the olive oil in a large saucepan over medium heat. Add the onion and garlic, if using, and cook until they begin to soften, about 2 minutes. Add the turkey, red and green bell peppers, and jalapeño, if using, and cook, stirring occasionally to break up the turkey, until the peppers begin to soften, about 3 minutes. Stir in the chili powder, cumin, and tomato paste and cook until fragrant, about 2 minutes.

2. Add the beans and tomatoes and let the chili come to a simmer. Reduce the heat and let it simmer until the flavors are blended, about 10 minutes.

3. Spoon the chili into serving bowls and top with the cheese and cilantro. (Garnish just before serving.) The chili can be refrigerated, covered, for up to 3 days.

NUTRITION INFO: 1 portion (1 bowl) provides:

Protein: 1 serving plus

Calcium: 1 serving

Vitamin C: 2 servings

Vitamin A: 1 serving

Whole grains and legumes: ½ serving

Iron: some

Wrap It Up,
I'll Eat It Here

Wrap leftover turkey or vegetarian chili, along with a little chopped tomato, avocado, cheese, and maybe a spoonful of salsa or low-fat sour cream, in a warm whole-wheat tortilla for a quick but satisfying lunch or dinner.

Mexican Tortilla Soup

SERVES 4

This authentically flavored meal in a bowl will take you south of the border in 25 minutes or less. Leaving the garlic unpeeled produces a heady flavor without the burn—plus it saves chopping time.

4 whole-grain corn tortillas
    (each 6 inches in diameter)
1 large head garlic
2 tablespoons olive oil
2 medium-size onions, finely chopped
1 pound skinless, boneless chicken
    breasts, cut into 1-inch strips
2 medium-size carrots, peeled and
    finely chopped
2 bay leaves
1 teaspoon ground cumin
4 cups low-sodium chicken broth
1 can (14½ ounces) diced tomatoes
¼ cup chopped fresh cilantro
4 lime wedges, for serving

1. Preheat the oven to 300°F.

2. Cut the tortillas into ½-inch-wide strips and place them flat on a large rimmed baking sheet. Bake the tortillas until crisp, about 20 minutes. (The baked tortilla strips can be stored in an airtight container at room temperature for up to 1 week.)

3. Meanwhile, remove and discard the loose papery skin on the outside of the head of garlic. Place the head of garlic on its side on a work surface and, holding it steady, use a sharp knife to cut it in half crosswise. Set the garlic aside.

4. Heat the olive oil in a large saucepan over medium heat. Add the onions and cook until they begin to soften, about 2 minutes. Add the chicken, carrots, bay leaves, cumin, and the two half-heads

From the Test Kitchen

Add even more flavor, texture, and nutrition to the tortilla soup with any of the following:

- Diced avocado
- Diced red bell pepper
- Minced pickled jalapeno peppers
- Shredded Monterey Jack cheese

garlic and cook until the chicken browns and the carrots begin to soften, about 3 minutes.

5. Add the broth and tomatoes, raise the heat to medium-high, and let the soup come to a boil. Reduce the heat and let it simmer until the flavors are well blended, about 10 minutes.

6. Remove and discard the garlic and bay leaves. If you will be serving only half of the soup, set aside the rest. (It can be refrigerated, covered, for up to 3 days.) Pour the hot soup into bowls, sprinkle each with cilantro and a squeeze of lime. Scatter tortilla strips on top and serve.

NUTRITION INFO: 1 portion (1 bowl) provides:

Protein: 1 serving

Vitamin C: ½ serving

Vitamin A: 1½ servings

Other fruits and vegetables: 1 serving

Whole grains and legumes: 1 serving

Fat: ½ serving

Hearty Fish and Potato Chowder

SERVES 2

Go ahead—chow down on this creamy-but-creamless chowder. Add a green salad and dinner's a done deal.

1 tablespoon olive oil
1 medium-size onion, chopped
1 rib celery, chopped
1 medium-size carrot, chopped
1½ cups low-sodium chicken broth or
    vegetable broth
1 cup whole milk
4 small red potatoes, scrubbed and
    quartered
Salt and black pepper
½ pound skinless salmon, tilapia,
    or red snapper fillets, cut into
    1-inch cubes
1 tablespoon chopped fresh dill, or
    1 teaspoon dried dill
½ medium-size red bell pepper
    (optional), finely diced

1. Heat the olive oil in a large saucepan over medium heat. Add the onion, celery, and carrot and cook until the vegetables are softened, about 5 minutes.

2. Reduce the heat to low, add the broth and milk, and let the soup come to a simmer.

3. Add the potatoes, let the soup return to a simmer, and cook until the potatoes are tender, about 10 minutes. Season the soup with salt and black pepper to taste. The soup can be prepared up to this point and refrigerated, covered, for 1 day. Reheat the soup gently over low heat before proceeding with Step 4.

From the Test Kitchen

Like to cover even more Daily Dozen bases in your bowl of fish chowder? Substitute cubes of sweet potato for the red ones and score an extra Vitamin A serving. Prefer a seafood chowder? Sub peeled, deveined shrimp for the fish.

4. Add the fish and dill and let the soup simmer until the fish is just cooked through (don't overcook it). Pour the soup into serving bowls and top with a sprinkling of bell pepper, if desired.

NUTRITION INFO: 1 portion (1 bowl) provides:

Protein: 1 serving

Calcium: ½ serving

Vitamin C: 1½ servings

Vitamin A: 1½ servings

Other fruits and vegetables: 1 serving

Fat: ½ serving

Omegas: some, if using salmon

Pasta

....

Nothing satisfies a carb craving or comforts a tumultuous tummy like a plateful of pasta. And there's good news for pregnant pasta lovers: Though pasta of the past was almost always made with refined wheat, you can now find an impressive selection of whole-grain, high-protein, and legume-based pasta alongside that white stuff. Not only are these pasta options more nutritious, with more fiber, more trace minerals, and more naturally occurring vitamins, their chewier bite and nutty taste bring a new dimension to standard pasta recipes.

You can toss virtually anything—seafood, poultry, vegetables, cheese—with pasta and call it a meal. From Linguine with Shrimp and Red Pepper to Chickpea Pasta with Chicken, Tiny Tomatoes, and Spinach, you're bound to find the one-bowl dinner of your dreams in the recipes that follow.

Pasta Presto

Looking for a way to shave time off your pasta prep? Try this trick: Add the contents of an entire box of pasta to a pot of boiling salted water and cook it for 5 minutes. Remove half the pasta (or as much as you want to save for later) from the pot and drain it. Toss this pasta with about 2 tablespoons olive oil (just enough to coat it lightly) and ¼ cup chopped fresh flat-leaf parsley. Let the pasta cool to room temperature, then refrigerate it in an airtight container until you're ready for another pasta fest—up to 1 week, if you can wait that long. Continue cooking the remaining pasta until it's done and use it for tonight's dinner. When you're next in the mood for pasta, simply heat a sauce or broth in a saucepan and add the partially cooked pasta. Let the pasta simmer until it has finished cooking, then serve.

Fettuccine with Turkey and Wild Mushrooms

SERVES 2

Take a walk on the wild side and explore the intriguing texture wild mushrooms add to fettuccine. Yogurt makes the sauce Alfredo-like, without Alfredo's fat. Not feeling wild? Use white button or brown (cremini) mushrooms or portobellos instead.

¼ pound whole-grain fettuccine
1 tablespoon olive oil
½ pound raw turkey breast, thinly sliced
    across the grain
3 cups sliced wild mushrooms
    (such as shiitakes; about ½ pound)
2 shallots, minced
1 teaspoon fresh thyme leaves
⅓ cup plain Greek yogurt (whole-milk
    yogurt makes a creamier sauce)
3 tablespoons minced fresh flat-leaf
    (Italian) parsley
½ cup grated Parmesan cheese
Salt and black pepper
2 tablespoons toasted pine nuts or
    walnuts (see page 217; optional)

1. Bring a large pot of water to a boil over medium-high heat. Add the fettuccine and cook it according to the directions on the package.

2. Meanwhile, heat the olive oil in a large nonstick skillet over medium heat. Add the turkey and cook, stirring occasionally, until almost cooked through, about 3 minutes. Add the mushrooms, shallots, and thyme and cook until the mushrooms soften, 3 to 4 minutes. Add the yogurt and parsley and toss to mix. Set the turkey and mushroom mixture aside until the fettuccine is ready, covering it to keep warm.

From the Test Kitchen

Sliced carrots, steamed or microwaved until just tender, would add extra Vitamin A, a bit of crunch, and a little color to the Fettuccine with Turkey and Wild Mushrooms. Toss them in after the mushrooms have cooked for about 2 minutes.

---

3. Drain the fettuccine, shaking off any excess water. Reserve ½ cup pasta water. Toss the fettuccine with the turkey and mushroom mixture and the Parmesan cheese. Add pasta water 2 tablespoons at a time until a sauce forms, then season with salt and pepper to taste. Sprinkle the nuts over the fettuccine, if desired.

NUTRITION INFO: 1 portion provides:

Protein: 1½ servings

Calcium: 1 serving plus

Vitamin C: ½ serving

Vitamin A: ½ serving

Other fruits and vegetables: 3 servings

Whole grains and legumes: 2 servings

Fat: ½ serving

Omegas: some

Chickpea Pasta with Chicken, Tiny Tomatoes, and Spinach

SERVES 2

Chicken, cherry tomatoes, and spinach make a colorful and nutritious combo for a light yet zesty sauce that's a flash in the pan to prepare.

¼ pound chickpea spirals or rotini, such as Banza
1 tablespoon olive oil
½ pound skinless, boneless chicken breasts or turkey cutlets, thinly sliced
2 shallots, thinly sliced
1 clove garlic, thinly sliced (optional)
1 cup cherry or grape tomatoes
1 bag (about 6 ounces) baby spinach
2 tablespoons sliced fresh basil leaves (optional)
½ cup shredded mozzarella cheese
¼ cup grated Parmesan cheese
Cracked black pepper
Grated zest of 1 medium-size lemon

1. Bring a large pot of water to a boil over medium-high heat. Add the pasta and cook it according to the directions on the package.

2. Meanwhile, heat the olive oil in a large skillet over medium-high heat. Add the chicken and cook, stirring occasionally, until it registers 165°F at its thickest part, 3 to 5 minutes. Remove the chicken from the skillet and set aside.

3. Add the shallots and garlic, if using, to the skillet and cook over medium heat until softened, about 3 minutes. Add the tomatoes and cook until they soften, about 3 minutes. Return the chicken to the skillet, then add the spinach and basil, if using. Cover the skillet and cook until the spinach wilts, about 1 minute. Set the chicken mixture aside until the pasta is ready, covering it to keep warm.

4. Drain the pasta, shaking off any excess water. Toss the pasta with the mozzarella, Parmesan cheese, and cracked black pepper. Divide the pasta between 2 serving bowls. Spoon the chicken mixture over it, then sprinkle the lemon zest on top.

NUTRITION INFO: 1 portion provides:

Protein: 2 servings

Calcium: 1½ servings

Vitamin C: 2 servings

Vitamin A: 3 servings

Whole grains and legumes: 2 servings

Iron: some

Fat: ½ serving

Omegas: some

Alotta Broccoli with Chicken and Penne

SERVES 2

A plateful of broccoli never tasted so good. Not surprising, considering the tasty company it keeps: chicken, cheese, and crunchy walnuts. The result is a lightly sauced but flavor-filled pasta dish.

Chickened Out?

You can substitute turkey cutlets or tenderloins, sliced lean beef, scallops, or peeled and deveined shrimp in almost any pasta recipe that calls for chicken. Shrimp and scallops won't need to cook as long; simmer or sauté them only until they're firm and opaque—don't let them overcook.

For a vegetarian alternative, use vegetable broth and swap chunks of well-drained extra-firm tofu for the chicken. Add the tofu after the other ingredients have cooked through. If you have the time, it will pick up more flavor if you let it cook briefly. Or just get your protein fix by using bean or legume pasta.

For extra spice, add ½ teaspoon (or more) crushed red pepper flakes to any pasta dish.

¼ pound whole-grain or legume penne
2 cups broccoli florets
1 tablespoon olive oil
1 small onion, chopped
1 clove garlic, minced (optional)
½ pound skinless, boneless chicken breast, cut into ½-inch strips
¼ cup low-sodium chicken broth, plus more if necessary
½ teaspoon dried oregano
½ cup grated cheddar cheese
½ cup grated Parmesan cheese
1 tablespoon chopped fresh flat-leaf (Italian) parsley
2 tablespoons coarsely chopped toasted walnuts (see page 217)
Cracked black pepper

1. Bring a large pot of water to a boil over medium-high heat. Add the penne and cook according to the directions on the package.

2. Meanwhile, steam the broccoli following the instructions on page 315 until crisp-tender, about 5 minutes.

3. Heat the olive oil in a large nonstick skillet over medium-low heat. Add the onion and garlic, if using, and cook, stirring, until they begin to soften, about 3 minutes. Add the chicken and cook, stirring occasionally, until it registers 165°F at its thickest part, about 4 minutes. Add the broth and oregano and cook until heated through, about 1 minute.

4. Remove the broccoli from the steamer and add it to the chicken. Reduce the heat to low and cook, stirring frequently, until the flavors blend, about 2 minutes. Set the chicken and broccoli mixture aside until the penne is ready, covering it to keep warm.

5. Drain the penne, shaking off any excess water. Add the penne, cheddar, ¼ cup of the Parmesan, and the parsley to the chicken and broccoli mixture and toss to mix. If the penne seems too dry, add more broth.

6. Divide the penne among four serving bowls. Top it with the remaining ¼ cup Parmesan and the walnuts. Sprinkle cracked black pepper over the penne and serve at once.

NUTRITION INFO: 1 portion provides:

Protein: 1½ servings; 2 if made with legume pasta

Calcium: 1½ servings

Vitamin C: 2 servings

Vitamin A: 2 servings

Other fruits and vegetables: 1 serving

Whole grains and legumes: 2 servings

Fat: ½ serving

Omegas: some

Pasta Primer

Don't know fusilli from fettuccine? Not to worry. Most recipes will work no matter what pasta you pick. Still, some pasta shapes are better suited to certain types of dishes than others. Here's a handy guide:

- Regular spaghetti is typically served with light tomato-based sauces.

- The skinniest pastas, such as angel hair and vermicelli, work best in broths and with thinner sauces.

- Long, flat pastas, like fettuccine and linguine, stand up to thicker, creamier sauces.

- Specialty pasta shapes, such as bow ties, shells, corkscrews, rotelle, radiatori (radiators), cavatappi, and so on, can trap chunkier sauce and hold it as it travels from plate to mouth (so you won't end up with quite so many stains on your belly). Most are also sturdy enough to use in pasta salads and baked casseroles.

- Tubular pasta, like penne or ziti, is the pasta of choice for salads, thick sauces, and casseroles. Tubes with grooves on the exterior, like fusilli, penne rigate, and rigatoni, do a better job of securing sauces.

Penne with Chicken and Cheesy Skillet Tomato Sauce

SERVES 2

Why settle for pasta with tomato sauce from a jar when you can make a healthier and tastier version in just a few minutes? Want an extra serving each of Vitamin A and Vitamin C? Add a cup of steamed broccoli florets.

¼ pound whole-grain or legume penne
1 tablespoon olive oil
½ pound skinless, boneless chicken breast, thinly sliced
1 clove garlic, thinly sliced (optional)
½ small onion, finely chopped
1 medium-size red bell pepper, chopped
2 cups chopped canned tomatoes
1½ teaspoons chopped fresh oregano, or ½ teaspoon dried oregano
1 tablespoon chopped fresh basil, or ½ teaspoon dried basil (optional)
½ cup grated Pecorino Romano cheese
½ cup grated Parmesan cheese
2 tablespoons chopped fresh flat-leaf (Italian) parsley

1. Bring a large pot of water to a boil over medium-high heat. Add the penne and cook according to the directions on the package.

2. Meanwhile, heat the olive oil in a large nonstick skillet over medium heat. Add the chicken and cook, stirring, until it registers 165°F at its thickest part, about 4 minutes. Add the garlic, if using, and cook until the flavor releases, about 1 minute. Add the onion and bell pepper and cook until they begin to soften, about 3 minutes. Add the tomatoes, oregano, and basil, if using, and let

> ## From the Test Kitchen
>
> Don't have both kinds of cheese on hand? Just substitute a cup of either Parmesan or Pecorino Romano.

the sauce simmer until the flavors are well blended, about 4 minutes. Set the chicken sauce aside until the penne are ready, covering it to keep warm.

3. Drain the penne, shaking off any excess water. Toss the penne with the Pecorino Romano, ¼ cup of the Parmesan, and the parsley. Divide the penne between two serving bowls and top it with the chicken sauce and the remaining ¼ cup Parmesan.

NUTRITION INFO: 1 portion provides:

Protein: 1½ servings; 2 if using legume pasta

Calcium: 2 servings

Vitamin C: 3 servings

Vitamin A: 2 servings

Whole grains and legumes: 2 servings

Fat: ½ serving

Omegas: some

Alfredo Light

SERVES 2

Craving a creamy Alfredo, but wish you could dig in without spooning up all that fat? This enlightened alternative to the uber-caloric classic may be your pasta dream come true. Add in steamed sugar snap peas, asparagus tips, peas, or any of your favorite greens for a veggie-forward meal, sautéed chicken strips or shrimp for a protein boost. Use chickpea pasta for protein plus-plus.

¼ pound whole-grain or chickpea
    cavatappi (such as Banza)
1 tablespoon olive oil
1 clove garlic, minced
    (about 1 teaspoon, optional)
1¼ cups 2% milk
1 teaspoon all-purpose flour
6 tablespoons cream cheese
1 teaspoon kosher salt
½ teaspoon black pepper
½ cup grated Pecorino Romano cheese

1. Bring a large pot of water to a boil over high heat. Add the cavatappi and cook according to the directions on the package.

2. Meanwhile, heat the oil in a large skillet over medium heat. Add the garlic, if using, and cook, stirring constantly, until fragrant, about 1 minute. Whisk together the milk and flour in a small bowl. Pour the milk mixture into the skillet; bring to a boil, and cook, stirring occasionally, until slightly thickened, about 1 minute. Whisk in the cream cheese, salt, and pepper, stirring until the cream cheese melts. Reduce the heat to low and stir in the Pecorino.

3. Drain the cavatappi, shaking off any excess water. Stir into the sauce until well coated. Serve immediately.

NUTRITION INFO: 1 portion provides:

Protein: ½ serving

Calcium: 1 serving

Whole grains and legumes: 2 servings

Fat: 1 serving

Red Pepper and Edamame Peanut Noodles

SERVES 2

A super nutritious twist on an Asian favorite that satisfies many of pregnancy's most common cravings, all in one dish: sweet, salty, spicy, crunchy . . . and peanut butter. Double the recipe to double the pleasure later in the week— no heating means speedy, easy eating.

¼ pound uncooked whole-wheat linguini
    or buckwheat soba noodles
1 cup frozen shelled edamame, thawed
¼ cup low-sodium soy sauce
¼ cup creamy peanut butter
2 tablespoons packed brown sugar
1 tablespoon canola oil
1 tablespoon minced peeled fresh ginger
1 teaspoon sesame oil (optional)
1 clove garlic, minced (if raw garlic
    bothers you, see the box on page 262)
1 teaspoon sriracha sauce or ½ teaspoon
    hot red pepper sauce, such as
    Tabasco
1½ cups packaged coleslaw mix
1 medium-size red bell pepper,
    thinly sliced
2 teaspoon sesame seeds, toasted
    (optional, see page 217)

1. Bring a large pot of water to a boil over medium-high heat. Add the linguine and cook it according to the directions on the package. Drain the linguine in a colander.

From the Test Kitchen

For extra protein, toss in or top with cooked chicken or shrimp.

2. Meanwhile, bring another pot of water to a boil and cook the edamame according to the package directions. Drain with the linguine.

3. Whisk together the soy sauce, peanut butter, brown sugar, canola oil, ginger, sesame oil, if using, garlic, sriracha, and sesame seeds (if using) in a small bowl.

4. Combine the coleslaw mix, bell pepper, linguine, and edamame in a large bowl. Add the dressing and toss to coat. Serve at room temperature or chilled. Store leftovers in the refrigerator, covered, for up to 3 days.

NUTRITION INFO: 1 portion provides:

Protein: 1 serving

Vitamin C: 2 servings

Vitamin A: 2 servings

Whole grains and legumes: 2 servings

Fat: 1½ serving

Macaroni and Cheese, Outside the Box

SERVES 4

Comfort food at its most nutritious, this macaroni and cheese is definitely different from the orange stuff you get in a box. It's a whole lot tastier, too. Four cheeses add flavor and calcium, and kale adds vitamins. Plus you'll love the leftovers—they reheat in the microwave in minutes.

½ pound whole-grain or legume elbow
    macaroni or shells
2 tablespoons butter
1½ tablespoons whole-wheat flour
1 cup milk
½ cup grated Gouda cheese
½ cup shredded mild cheddar cheese
1 cup shredded pasteurized part-skim
    mozzarella cheese
Hot red pepper sauce, such as Tabasco
    (optional)
Salt and black pepper
1 cup chopped cooked kale
2 tablespoons grated Parmesan cheese
1½ tablespoons whole-wheat bread
    crumbs

1. Preheat the oven to 350°F.

2. Bring a large pot of water to a boil over medium-high heat. Add the pasta and cook it according to the directions on the package.

3. Meanwhile, melt the butter in a nonstick saucepan over medium heat. Add the flour and cook, stirring, until a paste forms, 1 to 2 minutes. Add the milk and let it come to a boil, stirring constantly. When the sauce thickens slightly, remove it from the heat and add the Gouda, cheddar, and mozzarella. Stir until the cheeses melt. Season the cheese sauce with a dash of hot sauce, if desired, and salt and pepper to taste, then set it aside.

From the Test Kitchen

For a bigger protein punch, toss diced tofu, cooked chicken, or edamame with the macaroni and cheese. You can also add another vegetable—or more than one. Try 1 cup chopped roasted red bell peppers, cooked broccoli florets, yellow corn kernels, green peas, or chopped cooked spinach. To go white-on-white, use 1 cup chopped cooked cauliflower instead of the kale. You won't even notice that you're eating your vegetables.

4. Drain the pasta, shaking off any excess water, and return it to the pot. Add the cheese sauce and stir to coat evenly. Add the kale and stir to combine. Place the pasta mixture in a 9 x 13-inch baking dish.

5. Place the Parmesan and bread crumbs in a small bowl and stir to mix, then sprinkle over the pasta.

6. Bake the pasta and cheese until hot and bubbly, about 10 minutes.

NUTRITION INFO: 1 portion provides:

Protein: 2 servings

Calcium: 2½ servings

Vitamin C: ½ serving

Vitamin A: 1 serving

Whole grains and legumes: 2 servings

Fat: ½ serving

Creamy Linguine with Shrimp and Red Pepper

SERVES 2

No need to skimp on this scampi, lightened up with chicken broth but rich in flavor. It's easy and cheesy, packing protein not only from the shrimp but the chickpea pasta. Red peppers and parsley add a pop of color and a side of baby-friendly nutrients.

¼ pound chickpea or other legume
    linguine
1 tablespoon olive oil
1 teaspoon chopped garlic or 2 cloves
    garlic, thinly sliced (optional)
1 medium-size red bell pepper,
    thinly sliced
½ pound shelled and deveined large
    shrimp
2 cups low-sodium chicken broth,
    fish broth, or shellfish broth
½ cup grated provolone cheese
¼ cup grated Parmesan cheese
5 ounces zucchini noodles
    (about 4 cups)
2 tablespoons chopped fresh flat-leaf
    (Italian) parsley
Cracked black pepper
¼ teaspoon crushed red pepper flakes,
    or to taste (optional)

1. Bring a large pot of water to a boil over medium-high heat. Add the linguine and cook according to the directions on the package.

2. Meanwhile, heat the olive oil in a skillet over medium heat. Add the garlic, if using, and cook until just golden, 2 minutes. Add the bell pepper and cook until slightly softened, about 2 minutes. Add the shrimp and cook until cooked through and opaque, about 4 minutes. Remove the bell pepper and shrimp from the skillet and set aside, covered, to keep warm.

3. Add the broth to the skillet and let come to a simmer. Add the provolone and Parmesan, zucchini noodles, parsley, and pepper to taste. Stir to combine.

4. Drain the linguine, shaking off any excess water. Divide the linguine between two serving bowls. Spoon the broth and zucchini over it and top with the shrimp and bell peppers. If you like a little spice, sprinkle red pepper flakes on top.

NUTRITION INFO: 1 portion provides:

Protein: 1½ servings

Calcium: 1½ servings

Vitamin C: 1 serving

Vitamin A: 1 serving

Other fruits and vegetables: 2 servings

Whole grains and legumes: 2 servings

Iron: some

Fat: ½ serving

Omegas: some

Extra (Pasta) Sauce

At a loss for pasta sauce? You won't be if you make extra-large batches of these sauces. Toss with pasta and whatever veggies and protein you like, and you'll have a meal in minutes!

Pesto with Sunflower Seeds

MAKES ABOUT 2 CUPS

Instead of the traditional pine nuts, this pesto gets its rich flavor—and healthy fatty acids—from sunflower seeds (or, if you prefer, pumpkin seeds). Spoon this zesty pesto on pasta, into sandwiches, on poultry, or on anything else that could use a pick-me-up.

2 cups (firmly packed) fresh basil leaves
½ cup shelled lightly toasted sunflower or pumpkin seeds
1½ teaspoons chopped garlic (if raw garlic bothers you, see the box on page 262), optional
2 tablespoons olive oil, plus more for storing
Juice of 1 medium-size lemon
½ cup grated Parmesan cheese
Salt and black pepper

1. Place the basil, sunflower seeds, and garlic in a food processor and process until finely chopped.

2. With the motor running, add the olive oil and lemon juice in a steady stream through the feed tube.

From the Test Kitchen

Really want to up the omega-3 ante? Substitute toasted walnuts for the seeds.

3. Transfer the pesto to a small bowl. Fold in the Parmesan cheese, and salt and pepper to taste. To use, toss 2-ounce servings of hot pasta with several tablespoons of pesto. To store, place the pesto in a small airtight container and float a thin layer of olive oil over the top to keep the basil from turning brown. The pesto can be refrigerated for 2 weeks.

NUTRITION INFO: 1 portion (½ cup) provides:

Calcium: ½ serving

Vitamin C: 1 serving

Vitamin A: 1 serving

Fat: ½ serving

Omegas: some

Turkey Bolognese Sauce

MAKES ABOUT 6 CUPS

Have a beef with greasy meat sauce? This Bolognese swaps out the beef with turkey, for a leaner profile and a light taste. Miss the beef but not the grease? Use extra-lean ground beef.

1 tablespoon olive oil
1 medium-size onion, chopped
3 medium-size carrots, peeled and
    chopped
2 ribs celery, chopped
2 cloves garlic, peeled and crushed, or
    1 teaspoon chopped garlic (optional)
1½ pounds ground turkey
1 can (28 ounces) diced tomatoes,
    with their juices
1 can (about 28 ounces) tomato puree
1½ teaspoons dried oregano
2 bay leaves
¼ cup chopped fresh flat-leaf (Italian)
    parsley
Salt and black pepper

1. Heat the olive oil in a saucepan over medium heat. Add the onion and cook until slightly softened, about 1 minute. Add the carrots, celery, and garlic, if using, and cook until the carrots and celery start to soften, about 2 minutes.

2. Add the turkey and cook, chopping up the pieces with a wooden spoon, until the turkey is cooked through, about 10 minutes.

3. Add the diced tomatoes, tomato puree, oregano, bay leaves, and parsley. Let the sauce come to a simmer and cook it until the flavors blend, about 15 minutes. Let it cool to room temperature, add salt and pepper to taste, then remove and discard the bay leaves. Spoon the sauce into three 1-pint containers. The sauce can be refrigerated for 3 days or frozen for up to 2 months. Let it thaw in the refrigerator overnight before reheating.

NUTRITION INFO: 1 portion (1 cup) provides:

Protein: 1 serving

Vitamin C: 2 servings

Vitamin A: 2 servings

Saucy Secrets

Feel like you can't look at another carrot or red bell pepper or another piece of broccoli or cauliflower? Don't look at them—hide them in tomato sauce. Tomato sauces, or tomato-and-meat sauces, can camouflage just about any vegetable, which is why you'll want to keep this trick up your sleeve when you start feeding a picky toddler. And what you can't see or smell won't be off-putting to you. If you're making sauce from scratch, add the finely chopped vegetable or vegetables when you sauté the onion and garlic. If you're opening up a jar, just simmer the vegetables in the sauce until they're tender enough to be inconspicuous. If you're adding ground meat to store-bought sauce, add the veggies when you brown the meat.

Salads

....

S ure, you can fill a bowl with lettuce and tomato, douse it with bottled dressing, and call it a salad. But why settle for that when there are so many exciting salad combinations just waiting to be tossed your way? Whether a salad's a side dish or the main event, all the varieties you'll find here deserve a starring role on the table. There's a salad in here for everybody (and any of the salads that serve two can easily be doubled).

Side Salads

W ant a little salad with your dinner? Try one of these tasty side salads. Each crunchy serving will satisfy your taste buds and your nutritional requirements. Don't have room on the side, or don't want to overload your tummy with too much at a time? Serve your salad first. Starting with a salad can also help you pace yourself, so you don't get too full too fast (slow and steady always wins the pregnancy eating race).

Enough Is Like a Feast

S alad eaters come in all kinds of packages, including the kind who can eat their way through a whole bag of salad—and the kind who can barely make it through leaf one. The salad servings in this section are geared to that salad eater in the middle: the one who can happily manage about 2 cups of greens (which, when dressed, wilt down to considerably less). If the recipe makes too much salad for you, cut the servings by half. If the recipe doesn't make enough salad, double the recipe—and double the nutrients you'll be able to score.

Spicy Watermelon, Cucumber, and Feta Salad

SERVES 2

Watermelon makes your mouth water? Wait until your mouth gets a load of a mom-to-be's favorite melon tossed with salty feta, zesty lime, and a kick of mint. Add grilled shrimp or scallops, and it's dinner. Ot top with cottage cheese for a yummy meatless meal.

¼ cup freshly squeezed lime juice
    (about 3 limes)
2 teaspoons honey
¼ teaspoon kosher salt
¼ teaspoon crushed red pepper
    flakes
2 tablespoons extra-virgin olive oil
5 cups cubed seedless watermelon
    (¾-inch pieces)
2 cups chopped hothouse
    (seedless English) cucumber
½ cup crumbled pasteurized feta cheese
¼ cup thinly sliced red onion (optional)
2 tablespoons chopped fresh mint leaves

1. Whisk together the lime juice, honey, salt, and pepper flakes in a small bowl. Gradually whisk in the oil until completely incorporated.

2. Stir together the watermelon, cucumber, feta, and onion in a large bowl to combine. Gently stir in 2 tablespoons of the dressing. Chill at least 20 minutes or up to 2 hours.

3. Just before serving, gently stir in the mint. Whisk the dressing to recombine it and drizzle over the salad.

NUTRITION INFO: 1 portion provides:

Calcium: 1 serving

Vitamin C: 2 servings

Other fruits and vegetables: 2 servings

Fat: 1 serving

Ginger Melon Salad

SERVES 2

Always save your fruit salad for dessert? This melon mix makes a refreshing first course or side for grilled chicken or fish. Best of all, it's a comforting way to tuck away vitamins—without vegetables.

1 tablespoon honey
½ tablespoon minced peeled fresh
    ginger
½ tablespoon chopped fresh mint
½ teaspoon grated lime zest
2 tablespoons fresh lime juice
1 cup 1-inch watermelon cubes
1 cup 1-inch cantaloupe cubes

**From the
Test Kitchen**

For a calcium bonus and a salty contrast to the sweet melon, toss in or top the salad with ½ cup pasteurized feta or goat cheese.

1. Place the honey, ginger, mint, lime zest, and lime juice in a small bowl and stir to mix.

2. Place the watermelon and cantaloupe cubes in a large salad bowl, pour the lime and ginger mixture over them, and toss to coat evenly. Cover the salad and refrigerate for at least 1 hour before serving.

NUTRITION INFO: 1 portion provides:

Vitamin C: 1½ servings

Vitamin A: 1 serving

Other fruits and vegetables: 1 serving

Mucho Mango Salad

SERVES 2

Few fruits—or even vegetables— bring as many vitamins to the table as the sweet mango. This salad doubles the mango, and the nutrients, by using it in the dressing, too.

1½ large ripe mangoes, cubed
2 tablespoons plain whole-milk yogurt
1½ tablespoons fresh lime juice
1½ tablespoons fresh orange juice
2 teaspoons grated peeled fresh ginger
½ teaspoon ground coriander (optional)
Salt and black pepper
½ cup cubed peeled kiwi
½ cup fresh blueberries
2 cups mild baby greens
2 tablespoons chopped macadamia nuts
Lime wedges, for serving

1. Place about one third of the mango cubes, the yogurt, lime juice, orange juice, ginger, and coriander, if using, in a food processor and process until smooth. Season the dressing with salt and pepper to taste.

2. Place the remaining mango cubes, kiwi, and blueberries in a large salad bowl, pour the dressing on top, and toss to coat evenly. Divide the greens between two salad plates, top each with half of the mango salad, then sprinkle the nuts on top. Serve with lime wedges.

NUTRITION INFO: 1 portion provides:

Vitamin C: 3½ servings

Vitamin A: 2 servings

Mango and Orange Salad

SERVES 2

Mango, orange, and mint mingle with a red wine vinegar dressing in a refreshing salad that's just about bursting with flavor.

1 ripe mango, peeled and pitted
1 medium-size seedless orange, peeled
    and white pith removed
1 tablespoon red wine vinegar
1 teaspoon chopped fresh mint leaves
Coarse salt, to taste (optional)

Cut the mango into thin slices and place in a bowl. Segment the orange and add to the bowl. Add the vinegar and mint and toss to mix. Sprinkle with salt if desired.

NUTRITION INFO: 1 portion provides:

Vitamin C: 2 servings

Vitamin A: 1 serving

Crunchy Pear Salad

SERVES 2

Pick a pear that's ripe enough to be fragrant, yet firm enough to lend crunch to this lovely fall salad.

1 ripe pear, halved, cored, peeled, and
    thinly sliced
4 cups (packed) baby spinach or arugula
2 tablespoons balsamic vinegar
2 tablespoons olive oil
1 teaspoon Dijon mustard
1 teaspoon minced shallot, optional
Salt and black pepper
½ cup Parmesan cheese shavings
    (about 2 ounces; see page 251)
¼ cup toasted walnut pieces
    (see page 217)

1. Place the pear and spinach in a salad bowl and stir to mix.

2. Place the balsamic vinegar, olive oil, mustard, and shallot in a small bowl and whisk to mix, then season with salt and pepper to taste. Toss the salad with enough dressing to coat it evenly. Divide the salad between two smaller salad bowls and top with the Parmesan shavings and walnut pieces.

NUTRITION INFO: 1 portion provides:

Protein: ½ serving

Calcium: 1 serving

Vitamin C: 1 serving if made with spinach; ½ serving if made with arugula

Vitamin A: 2 servings

Other fruits and vegetables: ½ serving

Iron: some

Fat: 1 serving

Omegas: some

Pomegranate Salad

SERVES 2

In this sassy spin on a standard salad, pomegranate seeds add crunch and a tangy sweetness to the greens, while pomegranate juice lends a rich flavor to the dressing. Both are great sources of vitamins and antioxidants. Parmesan cheese adds a salty component.

½ cup pomegranate juice
1 tablespoon balsamic vinegar
1 tablespoon olive oil
1 teaspoon whole-grain mustard
1 shallot, minced, optional
Fresh lemon juice
Salt and black pepper
4 cups (packed) baby greens, such as
    baby spinach or spring mix
Seeds from ½ pomegranate,
    about ½ cup (see Note)
½ cup Parmesan cheese shavings,
    about 2 ounces (see A Quick Shave)

1. Place the pomegranate juice in a small saucepan and bring to a boil over medium heat. Reduce the heat and let the juice simmer until it is reduced to about 2 tablespoons, about 10 minutes. Remove from the heat and let cool.

A Quick Shave

Those fancy curls of Parmesan cheese only look like they take forever—and a culinary degree—to create. They're actually as easy as this: Let a chunk of Parmesan soften slightly at room temperature, then use a potato peeler to peel off thin shavings. That's all there is to it!

From the Test Kitchen

Turn Pomegranate Salad into a main dish by doubling the recipe and topping it with grilled shrimp or chicken.

2. Add the balsamic vinegar, olive oil, mustard, and shallot, if using, to the reduced juice and whisk to mix. Season with lemon juice, salt, and pepper to taste.

3. Place the greens and pomegranate seeds in a large salad bowl. Toss with enough dressing to coat evenly. Divide the salad between two smaller salad bowls, sprinkle the Parmesan shavings on top, and serve immediately.

NOTE: Some stores carry packaged pomegranate seeds in the refrigerated aisle of the produce department.

NUTRITION INFO: 1 portion provides:

Calcium: 1 serving

Vitamin C: 1 serving

Vitamin A: 2 servings

Other fruits and vegetables: 1 serving

Iron: some

Fat: ½ serving

Fig and Arugula Salad with Parmesan Shavings

SERVES 2

Fresh figs make this a very sexy salad. Can't get fresh (figs, that is)? Use sliced dried figs instead.

1 teaspoon minced shallot, minced
2 tablespoons balsamic vinegar
2 tablespoons extra-virgin olive oil
1 teaspoon whole-grain mustard
Salt
8 fresh figs, cut in half vertically
4 cups (packed) arugula
Black pepper
½ cup Parmesan cheese shavings
    (about 2 ounces; see the box on
    page 251)

1. Place the shallot, balsamic vinegar, olive oil, mustard, and a pinch of salt in a large salad bowl and whisk to mix. Add the figs, toss to coat them evenly, and let them stand, covered with plastic wrap, for 20 minutes.

2. Add the arugula to the figs and toss to mix. Season with salt and pepper to taste, then toss well. Divide the fig salad between 2 smaller salad bowls and top with the Parmesan shavings.

NUTRITION INFO: 1 portion provides:

Calcium: 1 serving

Vitamin C: 1 serving

Vitamin A: 2 servings

Fat: 1 serving

Omegas: some

Move Over, Croutons

Crave a crunch on your salad? Think outside the crouton box to these tasty toppings:

Parmesan Crisps: Preheat the oven to 325°F. Coat a baking sheet with olive oil cooking spray. Mound heaping tablespoons of freshly grated Parmesan cheese on the baking sheet. Using the back of a spoon, pat each mound into a 3-inch circle. Bake until the cheese is bubbling, 6 to 8 minutes. Let the crisps cool slightly, then use a spatula to transfer them to paper towels to finish cooling and crisping. Serve on top of any cheese-friendly salad. They also make a super soup-topper. Or just snack on them.

Crunchy Chickpeas: Preheat the oven to 375°F. Drain a can of chickpeas (garbanzo beans) and pat them dry thoroughly with paper towels. Spread the chickpeas out on a rimmed baking sheet, spray them with olive oil cooking spray, and sprinkle them with grated Parmesan cheese. Bake the chickpeas until crunchy, about 30 minutes. Use the chickpeas to top salads or soups or just enjoy them by the handful. Experiment with other yummy flavor combos: parmesan and garlic powder, paprika and cumin, lime juice and chili powder, even cinnamon and a sprinkle of sugar.

Arugula, Shaved Fennel, and Roasted Pepper Salad

SERVES 2

Serve this classic Italian salad along-side or as a tasty bed for grilled or broiled meat, chicken, salmon, or shrimp—or as a first stop on the way to a pasta dinner. For a milder salad, substitute baby spinach or mixed baby greens for the arugula. Or kick it up a notch with baby kale.

4 cups (packed) arugula
2 tablespoons chopped fresh flat-leaf (Italian) parsley
1 small fennel bulb, trimmed, halved, and very thinly sliced crosswise
2 to 4 tablespoons Lemon Vinaigrette (recipe follows)
1 roasted red bell pepper (leftover or from a jar), sliced into strips
½ cup Parmesan cheese shavings (about 2 ounces; see the box on page 251)

1. Place the arugula, parsley, and fennel in a salad bowl and toss to mix. Toss with enough Lemon Vinaigrette to coat the salad evenly.

2. Divide the salad between 2 salad plates, then top it with the roasted peppers and Parmesan shavings.

From the Test Kitchen

Cheese up the Lemon Vinaigrette by adding ¼ cup of grated Parmesan cheese. Add extra Italian flavor with a sprinkling of dried oregano.

NUTRITION INFO: 1 portion (without dressing) provides:

Protein: 1 serving

Calcium: 1 serving

Vitamin C: 2½ servings

Vitamin A: 3 servings

Lemon Vinaigrette

MAKES ABOUT ½ CUP

This simple dressing can zest up almost any salad green. It's also delicious on grilled veggies.

4 tablespoons fresh lemon juice
4 tablespoons olive oil
Grated zest of 1 lemon
1 clove garlic, minced (if raw garlic bothers you, see the box on page 262), optional
Salt and black pepper

Combine the lemon juice, olive oil, lemon zest, and garlic in a small bowl and whisk to mix. Season the vinaigrette with salt and pepper to taste. The dressing can be stored in an airtight container or jar for up to 1 week. Whisk or shake to recombine before using.

NUTRITION INFO: 1 portion (2 tablespoons) provides:

Vitamin C: ½ serving

Fat: 1 serving

Omegas: some

It's Mediterranean to Me Salad

SERVES 2

This salad combines the best of Greece and Italy for a delicious Mediterranean hybrid.

2 cups chopped romaine lettuce
½ small red bell pepper, diced
½ medium-size avocado
　(preferably Hass), diced
¼ hothouse (seedless English)
　cucumber, peeled and diced
¼ medium-size red onion, chopped
　(optional)
2 roma tomatoes, seeded and diced
½ cup cubed sharp provolone cheese or
　other sharp Italian cheese
⅓ cup drained canned chickpeas
　(garbanzo beans), rinsed
1 tablespoon chopped fresh flat-leaf
　(Italian) parsley
1 teaspoon chopped fresh oregano
　leaves or ¼ teaspoon dried oregano
1 teaspoon chopped fresh mint leaves or
　¼ teaspoon dried mint (optional)
¼ cup sliced pitted kalamata olives
2 tablespoons balsamic vinegar
2 tablespoons olive oil
1½ teaspoons fresh lemon juice, plus
　more to taste
1 small clove garlic, minced
　(optional; if raw garlic bothers you,
　see the box on page 262)
Salt and black pepper

1. Place the romaine, bell pepper, avocado, cucumber, onion if using, tomatoes, cheese, chickpeas, parsley, oregano, mint, if using, and olives, if using, in a large salad bowl and stir to mix.

From the Test Kitchen

Here's a time-saving hint: Chop everything except the avocado early in the day and store the ingredients separately in the fridge. Toss the salad right before serving. Make it a meal by adding cubes of cooked chicken or turkey, chilled grilled shrimp, chunks of cold leftover salmon, or even canned tuna or salmon.

2. Place the balsamic vinegar, olive oil, lemon juice, and garlic, if using, in a small bowl and whisk to mix. Season with salt and black pepper to taste. Toss the salad with enough dressing to coat evenly. Taste for seasoning, adding more lemon juice, salt, and/or black pepper if desired. Divide the salad between 2 smaller salad bowls and serve.

NUTRITION INFO: 1 portion provides:

Calcium: 1 serving

Vitamin C: 1½ servings

Vitamin A: 1½ servings

Other fruits and vegetables: 1 serving

Iron: some

Fat: 1 serving

Broccoli, Tomato, and Mozzarella Salad

SERVES 2

Sure, tomato and mozzarella are made for each other—especially when fresh basil joins the party. But did you ever think of adding crunchy broccoli to the mix? You should—your taste buds will thank you.

1½ cups small broccoli florets
2 ripe roma tomatoes, seeded and
   coarsely chopped
½ cup cubed pasteurized part-skim
   mozzarella (about 2 ounces)
3 tablespoons sliced fresh basil leaves
2 tablespoons balsamic vinegar
1 to 2 tablespoons olive oil
Fresh lemon juice
Salt and black pepper
2 tablespoons toasted pine nuts
   (see page 217)

1. Steam the broccoli following the instructions on page 315 until crisp-tender, 3 to 5 minutes. Set the broccoli aside in a large salad bowl and let it cool completely. Add the tomatoes, mozzarella, and basil, and toss to mix.

2. Place the balsamic vinegar and olive oil in a small bowl and whisk to mix.

From the Test Kitchen

Not feeling the love for broccoli? Leave it out and substitute 2 sliced medium-size tomatoes.

Pour the dressing over the salad and toss well to coat evenly. Squeeze a little lemon juice on top, season with salt and pepper to taste, and toss again. Divide the salad between two smaller salad bowls, then sprinkle the pine nuts on top.

NUTRITION INFO: 1 portion provides:

Calcium: 1 serving

Vitamin C: 2 servings

Vitamin A: 1½ servings

Fat: ½ serving if made with 1 tablespoon oil; 1 serving if made with 2

Spicy Greens with Ginger Dressing

SERVES 2

The greens may be wilted, but the flavor will be lively. Add a dash of crushed red pepper flakes if you'd like it livelier still.

3 tablespoons seasoned rice vinegar
1 tablespoon low-sodium soy sauce
1 tablespoon sesame oil
2 teaspoons minced peeled fresh ginger
2 tablespoons chopped fresh cilantro
 (optional)
3 scallions (white and light green parts),
 trimmed and sliced
1 package (5 ounces) Asian salad mix
 (see Note) or baby spinach
1 tablespoon toasted sesame seeds
 (see page 217)

1. Place the rice vinegar, soy sauce, sesame oil, and ginger in a small saucepan over low heat and cook, stirring, until hot but not boiling, about 3 minutes. Stir in the cilantro, if using.

2. Place the scallions and salad mix in a heatproof bowl and toss to mix. Pour the hot dressing over the greens, sprinkle the sesame seeds on top, and toss well. Serve immediately.

NOTE: Asian salad mix is a spicy combination of greens such as spinach, mizuna, chard, and red mustard. Packages are available in supermarket produce sections.

NUTRITION INFO: 1 portion provides:

Vitamin C: 1 serving

Vitamin A: 3 servings

Iron: some

Fat: ½ serving

Ginger Cucumber Salad

SERVES 2

This crunchy salad pulls double duty as either a snack or a side dish. Pair it with your favorite Asian-style chicken, fish, or pork main.

3 cups thinly sliced hothouse
 (seedless English) cucumber,
 peeling optional
½ cup thinly sliced red onion (optional)
1½ teaspoons grated peeled fresh ginger
¼ cup coarsely chopped fresh cilantro
 leaves (or mint)
3 tablespoons unseasoned rice vinegar
2 teaspoons low-sodium soy sauce
1 tablespoon sesame oil
Thinly sliced scallions (optional)

Place the cucumbers, onion, ginger, cilantro, vinegar, soy sauce, and sesame oil in a medium bowl. Toss to combine. Let stand for 5 minutes. Sprinkle with scallions, if desired, and serve.

NUTRITION INFO: 1 portion provides:

Other fruits and vegetables: 2 servings

Fat: ½ serving

Asian Slaw

SERVES 2

Move over, bland deli coleslaw. Rice vinegar, sesame oil, ginger, and cilantro give this tangy slaw an Asian kick. Packaged coleslaw mix saves time.

1 cup coleslaw mix
½ medium-size red bell pepper,
   thinly sliced
1 cup shredded carrots
3 tablespoons seasoned rice vinegar
1 tablespoon fresh lime juice
1 tablespoon sesame oil
1 tablespoon olive oil (optional)
1 tablespoon grated peeled fresh ginger
1 tablespoon honey, or to taste
Pinch of crushed red pepper flakes
3 tablespoons chopped fresh cilantro
1 tablespoon toasted sesame seeds
   (see page 217)

1. Place the coleslaw mix, bell pepper, and carrots in a large salad bowl and toss to mix.

2. Place the rice vinegar, lime juice, sesame oil, olive oil, if using, ginger, honey, pepper flakes, and cilantro in a small bowl and whisk to mix.

From the Test Kitchen

For a crunchy and extra-nutritious slaw, substitute 1 cup broccoli slaw (available prepacked at the supermarket) for the coleslaw mix.

3. Just before serving, pour the dressing over the slaw mixture and toss to coat evenly. Sprinkle with sesame seeds and serve.

NUTRITION INFO: 1 portion provides:

Vitamin C: 2 servings

Vitamin A: 3½ servings

Fat: ½ serving without olive oil; 1 serving with it

Curtido

SERVES 4

This Mexican-style slaw takes only moments to prep, but it's a dish that keeps on giving—unlike most slaws, it actually tastes even better the day after. Top tacos with curtido or serve it alongside sandwiches.

2 cups packaged green cabbage
    angel hair slaw (or very thinly sliced
    green cabbage)
½ cup very thinly sliced red onion
½ cup shredded peeled carrots
1 small jalapeno pepper, seeded and
    minced (optional)
¼ cup apple cider vinegar
2 teaspoons sugar
1 teaspoon kosher salt

Place the cabbage, onion, carrot, and jalapeno, if using, in a large bowl and stir to mix. Place the vinegar, sugar, and salt in a small saucepan and cook over medium heat, stirring, until the salt and sugar are dissolved. Pour the dressing over the vegetables and stir to mix. Cover and refrigerate for at least 1 hour before serving.

From the Test Kitchen

Not only does curtido have staying power (you can store it in the fridge in an airtight container for about a week), but the flavor actually improves with age.

NUTRITION INFO: 1 portion (scant 1 cup) provides:

Vitamin C: ½ serving

Vitamin A: 1 serving

Carrots Only

Can't stomach cabbage? Try a vitamin-packed all-carrot slaw instead: Drain 1 cup canned crushed pineapple (packed in juice) and mix it with 2 cups shredded carrots, ½ cup raisins, and ½ cup plain whole milk Greek yogurt. Add 2 teaspoons fresh lemon juice, honey to taste, a pinch of ground cinnamon, and 1 teaspoon grated peeled fresh ginger or ¼ teaspoon ground ginger. Chill the slaw. Just before serving, stir in 2 tablespoons chopped toasted walnuts (see page 217). The slaw can be refrigerated for up to 3 days.

Dinner Salads

Looking for a light and easy way to end a long day? Turn off the oven and chill out with a dinner salad. Pretty much any salad (from Caesar to Greek) can be turned into a meal when you top it with your choice of protein (fish, seafood, beef, poultry, eggs, or cheese). To keep things really cool, use last night's leftovers for your salad topper—you'll save yourself time and effort. Serve dinner salads with crusty whole-grain bread or rolls. And, of course, don't forget to take them to lunch, too.

Curried Chicken Salad

SERVES 4

Have some leftovers from last night's chicken dinner? Chop them up to make this yummy salad. Or simply simmer a couple of chicken breasts in broth until cooked through, let them cool, and you're ready to start. Serve the salad on top of greens or in a cantaloupe half (don't forget to count them in your Daily Dozen). Any chicken salad you have left over will make a great sandwich for tomorrow—and the day after. Just pile into a pita and you're good to go.

½ cup plain low-fat Greek yogurt
2 tablespoons mayonnaise
2 to 3 teaspoons curry powder
1 tablespoon fresh lime juice
2 teaspoons grated peeled fresh ginger
Salt and black pepper
1 pound cooked skinless, boneless
    chicken breasts or turkey breast, cut
    into ½-inch pieces (about 3 cups)
4 scallions (white and light green parts),
    trimmed and sliced

1 firm but ripe mango, chopped
½ cup chopped Granny Smith apple
½ red bell pepper, minced
⅓ cup toasted cashews (see page 217),
    coarsely chopped

Place the yogurt, mayonnaise, curry powder, lime juice, and ginger in a large salad bowl and stir to mix. Season with salt and pepper to taste. Add the chicken, scallions, mango, apple, bell pepper, and cashews and toss gently to combine. The salad can be refrigerated, covered, for up to 3 days.

NUTRITION INFO: 1 portion provides:

Protein: 1 serving

Vitamin C: 1 serving

Vitamin A: ½ serving

Fat: ½ serving

Omegas: some

Taco Salad

SERVES 2

Unlike most taco salads, which tend to be off the charts in fat and calories, this one's extra lean. Luckily, it's also extra tasty.

1 tablespoon olive oil

2 cloves garlic, minced

1 medium-size red bell pepper, chopped

½ medium-size yellow bell pepper, chopped

½ small onion, chopped

8 ounces lean ground beef or ground buffalo

2 teaspoons chili powder

1 teaspoon ground cumin

½ cup drained canned pinto or kidney beans, rinsed

1½ cups store-bought tomato-based salsa

2 tablespoons chopped fresh cilantro (optional)

Hot red pepper sauce, such as Tabasco (optional)

4 cups shredded romaine lettuce

2 large roma tomatoes, seeded and chopped

½ cup shredded cheddar or Monterey Jack cheese

½ cup slightly crumbled whole-grain or bean tortilla chips

1. Heat the olive oil in a large skillet over medium heat. Add the garlic, bell peppers, and onion, and cook until softened, about 5 minutes.

From the Test Kitchen

Add a dollop of 2% Greek yogurt and maybe a squeeze of lime for a little tang.

2. Add the beef, chili powder, and cumin and cook, stirring frequently, until the meat is crumbly and cooked through, 3 to 4 minutes. Add the beans and salsa, bring to a boil, reduce the heat, and let simmer until the beans are heated through and the flavors are blended, about 2 minutes. Add the cilantro and Tabasco to taste, if using.

3. Divide the lettuce between two large plates or bowls, then top each with half of the meat mixture. Scatter half of the chopped tomato, cheese, and chips over each salad and serve immediately.

NUTRITION INFO: 1 portion provides:

Protein: 1½ servings

Calcium: 1 serving

Vitamin C: 4 servings

Vitamin A: 3 servings

Whole grains and legumes: ½ serving

Iron: some

Fat: ½ serving

Steak Salad

SERVES 2

No need to trek over to your local steakhouse. Here are steak and a salad all on the same plate. You can substitute sliced grilled or roasted portobello mushrooms for the raw mushrooms.

1 strip steak or sirloin steak
  (about 1¼ inches thick, 12 ounces),
  trimmed of fat
Salt and cracked black pepper
1 teaspoon finely grated lemon zest
2 tablespoons fresh lemon juice
2 tablespoons mayonnaise
Black pepper
1 medium-size red onion, cut into
  ¼-inch-thick slices
4 cups (packed) arugula
1 cup thinly sliced white button
  mushrooms
1 roasted red bell pepper
  (leftover or from a jar), thinly sliced
½ cup Parmesan cheese shavings
  (about 2 ounces; see page 251)

1. Preheat the broiler or set up the grill and preheat it to high.

2. Season the steak all over with salt and cracked pepper. Broil or grill the steak until the internal temperature taken with an instant-read meat thermometer is 160°F, 3 to 5 minutes per side.

3. Meanwhile, place the lemon zest, lemon juice, and mayonnaise in a small bowl and whisk to mix. Season with salt and pepper to taste. Set the dressing aside.

4. Transfer the steak to a cutting board, leaving the broiler on or the grill lit. Let the steak rest for 5 minutes. Slice it into ¼-inch-thick strips. Reserve the meat juices.

5. Broil or grill the onion until cooked through and slightly charred, about 3 minutes per side. Place the cooked onions, arugula, mushrooms, and bell pepper in a large salad bowl and stir to mix. Add the dressing and toss to coat evenly.

6. Divide the arugula mixture between 2 plates. Arrange the steak slices on top and drizzle any meat juice over them. Sprinkle the Parmesan cheese over the salads and serve.

NUTRITION INFO: 1 portion provides:

Protein: 1½ servings

Calcium: 1 serving

Vitamin C: 2½ servings

Vitamin A: 3 servings

Other fruits and vegetables: 2 servings

Iron: some

Fat: 1 serving

Shrimp Caesar Salad

SERVES 2

Is chicken your go-to topper when you're making a a meal out of Caesar salad? It's time to go shrimp.

12 large shrimp, shelled and deveined
Salt, black pepper, and garlic powder
(optional)
2 teaspoons olive oil
4 cups shredded romaine lettuce
1 medium-size red bell pepper,
thinly sliced
1 cup small cherry or grape tomatoes
3 tablespoons Simple Caesar Dressing
or Tangy Caesar Dressing
(for both, see facing page)
½ cup grated Parmesan cheese,
plus more for serving
2 lemon wedges, for serving

1. Preheat the broiler. Line a large baking sheet with foil.

2. Place the shrimp in a bowl and toss with olive oil. Season with salt, pepper, and garlic powder, if using.

The Heart of the Matter

Love a good Caesar salad, but not so crazy about your post-Caesar breath? Removing the center core of the garlic before using it raw makes it easier on your breath—and your tummy. Or just substitute ⅛ teaspoon of garlic powder. Or skip the garlic altogether.

From the Test Kitchen

There's always room at the top of a Caesar for the old standard—grilled chicken breast. Grilled salmon's another tasty possibility—or sliced steak.

3. Transfer the shrimp to the baking sheet and arrange in a single layer, with no overlap.

4. Broil shrimp until cooked through and opaque, about 4 minutes. Set aside.

5. Place the lettuce, bell pepper, tomatoes, salad dressing, and Parmesan cheese in a salad bowl and toss to mix.

6. Divide the salad between 2 salad plates and top each with 6 shrimp. Serve with lemon wedges and more Parmesan, if desired.

NUTRITION INFO: 1 portion (without dressing) provides:

Protein: 1 serving

Calcium: 1 serving

Vitamin C: 4 servings

Vitamin A: 3 servings

Omegas: some

Simple Caesar Dressing

MAKES ABOUT ½ CUP

A traditional Caesar dressing made with raw or barely cooked egg is off the menu when you're expecting (unless the eggs are pasteurized). What's a pregnant Caesar-craver to do? Toss your salad with this creamy dressing, which swaps mayo for the eggs and oil. Not sold on anchovies? Add just a little at a time, or substitute a splash of Worcestershire sauce, which approximates the salty, briny flavor.

1 teaspoon chopped garlic (if raw garlic bothers you, see the box on page 262)
Salt
¼ cup fresh lemon juice
¼ cup mayonnaise
1 anchovy fillet, drained and coarsely chopped, plus more to taste (optional)
¼ cup grated Parmesan cheese, plus more to taste
Cracked black pepper

Place the garlic and ¼ teaspoon salt in a small bowl and mash with a fork to form a paste. Transfer to a blender or food processor, add the lemon juice, mayonnaise, anchovy, and Parmesan, and puree to form a smooth dressing. Season with more salt, Parmesan, and cracked pepper to taste.

NUTRITION INFO: 1 portion (¼ cup) provides:

Calcium: ½ serving

Vitamin C: ½ serving

Fat: 2 servings

Tangy Caesar Dressing

MAKES ABOUT 1 CUP

Here's a dressing that's full of flavor but not full of fat.

¼ cup buttermilk
¼ cup plain whole-milk yogurt
¼ cup grated Parmesan cheese, plus more to taste
2 tablespoons fresh lemon juice, plus more to taste
2 tablespoons mayonnaise or olive oil, plus more mayonnaise to taste
1 clove garlic, minced (if raw garlic bothers you, see the box on page 262)
1 teaspoon chopped shallot
2 anchovy fillets, drained (optional)
½ teaspoon Worcestershire sauce, plus more to taste
Salt and black pepper

Place the buttermilk, yogurt, Parmesan cheese, lemon juice, mayonnaise or oil, garlic, shallot, anchovies, if using, and Worcestershire in a blender or food processor and pulse until combined. Taste for seasoning, adding more Parmesan, lemon juice, mayonnaise, and/or Worcestershire as necessary, and salt and pepper to taste. If you prefer, you can toss more Parmesan with the salad rather than add it to the dressing.

NUTRITION INFO: 1 portion (¼ cup) provides:

Calcium: almost 1 serving

Fat: ½ serving

Salmon Salad Niçoise

SERVES 2

Have leftovers from last night's grilled salmon feast? Use them to top this delicious dinner (or lunchtime) salad.

12 asparagus stalks, cut into 3-inch pieces
4 cups shredded romaine lettuce
2 cooked skinless salmon fillets
    (each about 4 ounces)
4 small red potatoes, cooked and
    quartered
2 roma tomatoes, quartered
2 large hard-boiled eggs, quartered
¼ cup sliced pitted kalamata olives
2 teaspoons drained capers
3 tablespoons fresh lemon juice
3 tablespoons olive oil
2 teaspoons Dijon mustard
1½ teaspoons fresh tarragon leaves,
    chopped or ½ teaspoon dried
Salt and black pepper

1. Steam the asparagus (following the instructions on page 315) until crisp-tender, 4 to 6 minutes, depending on thickness. Pat dry with paper towels.

2. Divide the lettuce between 2 plates and place a salmon fillet on top of each. Surround the salmon with the asparagus, potatoes, tomatoes, eggs, and olives, dividing them equally between the plates. Top the salmon with the capers, dividing them equally.

3. Place the lemon juice, olive oil, mustard, and tarragon in a small bowl and whisk to mix. Season with salt and pepper to taste. Spoon the dressing over the salads, then serve.

NUTRITION INFO: 1 portion provides:

Protein: 1 serving plus

Vitamin C: 2 servings

Vitamin A: 2 servings

Fat: 1½ servings

Omegas: some

From the Test Kitchen

No leftover salmon in the fridge? Just open up a can. Can't find asparagus this time of year? Crisp-tender whole green beans make a classic substitute.

Shrimp and Mango Salad with Sesame Ginger Vinaigrette

SERVES 2

Do the dog days of summer have you panting for something refreshing? Chill out with this salad—super simple if you buy the shrimp already cooked. It's equally yummy with cubes of cooked chicken or turkey.

12 large shrimp, shelled and deveined

4 cups baby greens

1 Kirby (pickling) cucumber, peeled
and thinly sliced (you can substitute
¼ of a hothouse cucumber)

Sesame Ginger Vinaigrette
(recipe follows)

1 ripe mango, thinly sliced

1 medium-size red bell pepper,
thinly sliced

1. If the shrimp are not already cooked, steam them following the instructions on page 315 until they are cooked through and turn opaque, about 4 to 5 minutes. Transfer to a bowl and refrigerate until chilled. (You can also use grilled or broiled shrimp.)

2. Place the greens and cucumber in a salad bowl. Add ¼ cup of the Sesame Ginger Vinaigrette and toss to mix. Divide the greens between 2 salad plates.

3. Place the shrimp, mango, and bell pepper in the salad bowl. Toss with enough of the remaining vinaigrette to coat evenly. Top the greens with the shrimp mixture and serve.

NUTRITION INFO: 1 portion (without dressing) provides:

Protein: 1 serving

Vitamin C: 3 servings

Vitamin A: 3 servings

Other fruits and vegetables: ½ serving

Sesame Ginger Vinaigrette

MAKES ABOUT ½ CUP

The sweet and tangy punch of this Asian-inspired dressing comes from seasoned rice vinegar.

2 scallions (white and light green parts),
trimmed and thinly sliced

1 tablespoon grated peeled fresh ginger

1 tablespoon chopped fresh cilantro

¼ teaspoon chopped garlic (if raw garlic
bothers you, see the box on page 262),
optional

⅓ cup seasoned rice vinegar

1 tablespoon extra virgin olive oil

1 tablespoon low-sodium soy sauce

1 tablespoon sesame oil

Black pepper

Place the scallions, ginger, cilantro, garlic, if using, rice vinegar, olive oil, soy sauce, and sesame oil in a small bowl and whisk to mix. Add black pepper to taste.

NUTRITION INFO: 1 portion (¼ cup) provides:

Fat: 1 serving

From the Test Kitchen

Open, sesame: If you have sesame seeds handy (preferably toasted), toss a couple of tablespoons with the greens for a nutty crunch.

Pregnant Cobb Salad

SERVES 2

Craving a Cobb salad but concerned about how it fits into your pregnancy profile? It's easy. Just opt for fresh-cooked chicken or turkey instead of deli meat, and reach for pasteurized blue cheese (along with all the other fixings). Serve it with Southwest Russian Dressing (recipe follows) or Yogurt Ranch (or Yogurt Blue cheese); see page 291.

4 cups shredded romaine lettuce
8 ounces cooked chicken or turkey breast, cubed
2 small tomatoes, chopped, or 1 cup cherry tomatoes, halved
1 small ripe avocado, thinly sliced
2 ounces pasteurized blue cheese, crumbled
4 strips turkey bacon, cooked until crisp and crumbled (optional)
2 hard-boiled eggs, chopped

1. Divide the lettuce between 2 large bowls or plates.

2. Place half the chicken in each bowl, arranged in the center in a straight line.

3. Place half the tomatoes and avocado in a line on either side of the chicken, then distribute the blue cheese

crumbles, bacon, if using, and egg in lines across the top of the salad, in whatever order you'd like.

4. Serve with the dressing on the side.

NUTRITION INFO: 1 portion provides:

Protein: 1 serving plus

Calcium: 1 serving

Vitamin A: 2 servings

Omegas: some

Other fruits and vegetables: 1 serving

Southwest Russian Dressing

MAKES ABOUT 1 CUP

Pair your Pregnant Cobb Salad with this Russian dressing, which has a zippy taste of the Southwest and the tangy taste of buttermilk. It's also good with a simple chopped lettuce and tomato salad. Use any left over as a dip for veggies or a spread on sandwiches.

½ cup buttermilk
¼ cup store-bought mild salsa (preferably a chunky tomato one)
2 tablespoons mayonnaise
1 tablespoon chopped fresh flat-leaf (Italian) parsley
2 teaspoons fresh lemon juice
¼ teaspoon dry mustard
1 tablespoon sweet pickle relish
Salt and black pepper

From the Test Kitchen

Like your Russian dressing sweet? Add honey to taste. Like it spicy? Spike it with hot red pepper sauce.

Place the buttermilk, salsa, mayonnaise, parsley, lemon juice, and mustard in a blender and blend at low speed until smooth. Transfer the dressing to a bowl and stir in the pickle relish. Season with salt and pepper to taste. The dressing can be stored in the refrigerator, covered, for 2 days.

NUTRITION INFO: 1 portion (¼ cup) provides:

Fat: ½ serving

Building a Mason Jar Salad

Love a good salad for lunch—but not one that's good and soggy by the time you get around to eating it? Had one too many leaky dressing incidents in your car or on your clothes? Take your salad to work in a jar. That's right—a mason jar salad makes the perfect take-along lunch. No sog, no spills—just crunchy, fresh-tasting, perfectly dressed salad to go.

Think complicated pickling techniques (and your great-grandmother) when you think mason jars, aka "putting up"? Don't be put off. You're not sealing your salad for the winter—just for lunch. All you need to know is how hungry you'll be when lunch rolls around. A pint (16 ounces) will satisfy most salad cravings, but to fill a larger appetite, go for the quart size (32 ounces). Then get ready to layer.

Layer 1: Dressing. This ALWAYS goes on the bottom.

Layer 2: Proteins and grains. Grains like quinoa and farro, along with proteins such as chicken, steak, chickpeas, or edamame (basically anything large and chunky) go next. This allows your grains and proteins to marinate while protecting your more delicate top layers from getting soggy.

Layer 3: Everything else except leafy greens. Combinations such as cucumbers, halved cherry tomatoes, and shredded cheddar cheese can be packed atop cooked proteins.

Layer 4: Top your jar with leafy greens: mixed lettuces, chopped romaine hearts, baby spinach, arugula, baby kale, etc.

How to eat: Simply turn your mason jar salad upside down and gently shake to distribute your dressing. Twist off the top and eat right out of the jar. Or pour the ingredients into a bowl and stir to coat.

Winning Combinations:

1. Lemon-oregano vinaigrette, chopped grilled chicken breast, cucumber, cherry tomatoes, pecorino cheese, and chopped romaine hearts

2. Balsamic dressing, farro, edamame, cubed cooked beets or cooked sweet potato, and baby spinach

3. Creamy dressing, chickpeas, thinly sliced steak, quinoa, diced peppers, shaved parmesan, and baby kale

Pickled Vegetables

SERVES 10

Already polished off that jar of pickles and still craving more? How about pickles that satisfy more than your cravings? Just about any veggie can be pickled, but picking ones that pack in nutrients (say, carrots or cauliflower) gives you that pickled pleasure with a vitamin boost. Feeling fruity? Pickle some mango.

1 cup unseasoned rice vinegar

1 tablespoon salt

1 tablespoon sugar

2 bay leaves

2 teaspoons mustard seeds

2 teaspoons black peppercorns

2 teaspoons coriander seeds

4 thin slices fresh ginger, peeled

1 pound vegetables, such as trimmed
    green beans, cauliflower florets,
    quartered carrots, thinly sliced red
    onions, or cucumbers

1. Wash two wide-mouthed pint canning jars and their lids well with warm, soapy water; dry completely.

2. Place the vinegar, 1 cup water, the salt, and sugar in a medium-size nonreactive saucepan and bring to a boil over medium-high heat, stirring to dissolve the salt and sugar.

3. Divide the bay leaves, mustard seeds, peppercorns, coriander seeds, and ginger between the two jars. Tightly pack the vegetables into the jars. Carefully pour the vinegar mixture over the vegetables, filling to within ½ inch from the top. Seal tightly and let cool to room temperature. Refrigerate for 24 hours before serving. Pickled vegetables will keep refrigerated, tightly closed, for up to 2 months.

Meat

....

Has red meat always been your guilty pleasure? Well, lose the guilt—and bring on the pleasure. Red meat gets a green light when you're expecting, for a couple of reasons. First, cholesterol's not a concern for the pregnant set. Second, red meat is among the best sources of dietary iron, plus it packs plenty of protein and other pregnancy-friendly nutrients (like B vitamins) into every bite (omega-3s, too, if you use grass-fed beef or buffalo). Whether you're looking for a taste of nostalgia (in good old-fashioned dishes like Tomato-Layered Mini Meat Loaves and Slow-Cooker Roast Beef), or you're craving contemporary (like Pork Medallions with Arugula and Tomatoes or Beef Kebabs with Cumin Marinade), or you'd like to put an international spin on supper (with Ginger Beef Stir-Fry or Mexican Lasagna), there's a meat recipe for everyone in this section. So dig in like the carnivore you've always wanted to be.

Ginger Beef Stir-Fry

SERVES 2

Probably quicker than take-out, this stir-fry can be on your table in less than 20 minutes—without those leaky cardboard containers. A boldly sauced and delicious combination of beef sirloin, yellow or red bell pepper, carrots, and broccoli cooks up in no time flat, and packs in both protein and vitamins.

A bonus: The ginger is great for queasy days. Sniff some while you cook. The stir-fry is just as tasty prepared with chicken, turkey, lean pork, firm tofu, or shrimp. Have leftovers? Mix them in with soba or other whole-grain noodles and toss in another tablespoon or so of ginger sauce.

Cooking oil spray

3 teaspoons sesame oil

½ pound lean beef (such as boneless
    beef sirloin), thinly sliced

1 clove garlic, minced

1 medium-size or red bell pepper, sliced

1½ cups small broccoli florets

½ cup baby carrots

2 scallions (white and light green parts),
    trimmed and thinly sliced

¼ cup low-sodium beef broth

Ginger Sauce (recipe follows)

1 tablespoon chopped fresh cilantro

1 cup cooked brown rice, for serving
    (optional)

Cook It Once, Eat It All Week

If you cook a pound of brown rice or other whole grain once a week, you can simply reheat smaller portions in the microwave. It will take only a minute or two to reheat ½ cup rice.

Want to Beef Up?

Most of the recipes in this section call for 4 ounces of meat per serving, not only because that's all you need to net a protein serving, but also because smaller portions are easier for a pregnant tummy to handle. But if you've got the appetite for a bigger slab, knock yourself out with it—eat a 6-ounce portion and tally up 1½ protein servings . . . or on a really hungry day, tackle 8 ounces and count out 2 servings. Score omega-3's whenever you choose grass-fed beef.

1. Coat a large skillet with cooking oil spray. Add 1 teaspoon of the sesame oil and heat over medium-high heat. Add the beef and stir-fry until browned and cooked through, about 5 minutes. Remove the beef and set aside.

2. Add the remaining 2 teaspoons sesame oil to the skillet and heat over medium-high heat. Add the garlic and cook until the flavor releases, about 1 minute. Add the bell pepper, broccoli, carrots, and scallions and cook until slightly softened, about 2 minutes. Add the beef broth. Turn the heat down to medium, cover, and let cook, stirring occasionally, until the vegetables are tender but still slightly crunchy, about 3 minutes.

3. Return the beef to the skillet. Turn the heat to high, add the Ginger Sauce, and cook, stirring frequently, until heated through, about 2 minutes. Sprinkle the cilantro over the stir-fry. Serve over brown rice.

NUTRITION INFO: 1 portion (with sauce) provides:

Protein: 1 serving

Vitamin C: 3½ servings

Vitamin A: 3½ servings

Whole grains and legumes: 1 serving

Iron: some

Fat: ½ serving

Ginger Sauce

MAKES ABOUT ⅓ CUP

This assertive ginger-flavored sauce can be tossed with just about any stir-fry. If you like a little heat, include a dash or two of your favorite hot sauce.

**1 tablespoon grated peeled fresh ginger
  or ½ teaspoon ground ginger**
2 tablespoons rice vinegar
1 tablespoon low-sodium beef broth
2 teaspoons honey or brown sugar
2 tablespoons low-sodium soy sauce
2 teaspoons sesame oil

Place the ginger, rice vinegar, beef broth, honey, soy sauce, and sesame oil in a small bowl and whisk to mix.

Stir-Fry
Made Even Easier

Stir-frying is probably one of the quickest ways to get dinner on the table. The only time-consuming part is the chopping, grating, and slicing involved in prepping the ingredients for the wok or skillet. Fortunately for the perpetually time challenged, there's good news on that front: Almost everything you'd want to toss into a stir-fry can be bought pan-ready. Check your supermarket's meat case for pre-sliced beef, chicken, or turkey. Scan the produce section for chopped, sliced, shredded, or peeled fresh onions, garlic, broccoli, cauliflower, cabbage, carrots, and bell peppers. And if the produce section is running on empty, head to the frozen food aisle for some ready-to-use veggies.

Slow Cooker Beef Stew

SERVES 6

Entered the pregnancy hunger zone and trying to eat your way out? A big bowl of this hearty stew will get the job done, guaranteed. Let the slow cooker do the heavy lifting while you're at work or on the run, then get busy chowing down. Table for 2 (and a baby) tonight? You'll have plenty of leftovers to look forward to.

2 teaspoons olive oil, divided
1 boneless beef chuck roast
    (about 2 pounds), trimmed and
    cut into 1½-inch pieces
2 teaspoon kosher salt
½ teaspoon black pepper
2 teaspoon fresh thyme leaves
3 cups low sodium beef broth
1 cup sliced celery
2 cups chopped carrots
5 cloves garlic, peeled and crushed
1 cup uncooked farro
1 can (15 ounces) diced tomatoes,
    drained
2 tablespoons whole grain mustard
1 tablespoon red wine vinegar
1 cup frozen green peas, thawed

1. Heat 1 teaspoon oil in a large heavy skillet over high heat. Season beef with salt and pepper and place half of the beef in the skillet. Sear the beef on all sides until dark brown. Remove the beef from the skillet and set aside on a plate. Repeat with remaining oil and beef.

2. Pour 3 cups of the broth into the skillet, and bring to a boil, scraping up any brown bits from the bottom of the pan.

3. Pour broth into a 5-to-6 quart slow cooker. Stir in thyme, celery, carrots, garlic, farro, tomatoes and seared meat. Cook on LOW until beef and farro are tender, 7 hours. Stir in mustard, vinegar and peas. The stew can be refrigerated, covered, for up to 2 days.

NUTRITION INFO: 1 portion provides:

Protein: 1½ servings

Vitamin C: ½ serving

Vitamin A: 1 serving

Other fruits and vegetables: 1 serving

Whole grains and legumes: 1 serving

Iron: from the beef

Sheet-Pan Many Peppers Steak

SERVES 2

Many peppers, one pan makes for a super healthy version of a classic Asian dish that's almost as easy as ordering in. A variety of veggies add color and nutrients, while the cashews add crunch. Serve over brown rice.

½ pound boneless lean beef sirloin
    steak, thinly sliced
1 medium-size red bell pepper,
    cut into ¼-wide-wide strips
1 medium-size yellow bell pepper,
    cut into ¼-wide-wide strips
1 medium-size orange bell pepper,
    cut into ¼-wide-wide strips
1 medium-size green bell pepper,
    cut into ¼-wide-wide strips
½ cup shredded carrots
½ large red onion, thinly sliced
2 tablespoons olive oil
½ teaspoon kosher salt
¼ teaspoon black pepper
¼ teaspoon garlic powder
1 teaspoon ground ginger
¼ teaspoon crushed red pepper flakes
    (optional)
2 tablespoons low-sodium soy sauce
3 teaspoons light brown sugar
⅓ cup low-sodium beef broth
¼ cup toasted cashews (see page 217)
1 cup cooked brown rice

1. Place a rimmed baking sheet in the oven and preheat the broiler. (Do not remove the baking sheet while the broiler preheats.)

2. Place the steak, bell peppers, carrots, onion, olive oil, salt, pepper, garlic powder, ginger, and pepper flakes, if using, in a large bowl, stirring until well mixed. Transfer the meat to a separate bowl. Spread the vegetables in a single layer on the hot baking sheet. Broil until the vegetables are charred and mostly tender, about 10 minutes. Push the vegetables to the ends of the pan and spread the steak slices and any juices from the meat in a single layer in the center. Broil until the meat is charred and your desired degree of doneness, about 3 minutes for medium-rare.

3. Meanwhile, combine the soy sauce, brown sugar, and beef broth in a small saucepan and whisk to mix. Bring to a boil over high heat and cook for 2 minutes, until the sugar has dissolved and the sauce has slightly thickened. Stir in the cashews. Serve the steak and peppers over rice, if desired, pouring the sauce on top.

NUTRITION INFO: 1 portion provides:

Protein: 1 serving

Vitamin C: 4 servings

Vitamin A: 3 servings

Other fruits and vegetables: ½ serving

Whole grains and legumes: 1 serving

Iron: some

Fat: 1 serving

Beef Kebabs with Cumin Marinade

SERVES 2

Here's a meal on a stick—once you've placed the stick over some couscous, quinoa, brown rice, or other grain. You'll need to plan ahead a bit: The beef marinates for at least 3 hours (marinate in the morning, enjoy at night). Serving two is easy—just cut the recipe in half. If you are using wooden skewers, soak them in water first for a half-hour.

½ pound lean beef (such as top sirloin),
    well trimmed and cut into 1-inch
    pieces
2 tablespoons low-sodium soy sauce
2 tablespoons fresh lemon juice
1 tablespoon olive oil
1 teaspoon ground cumin
1 large red bell pepper, cut into 2-inch
    pieces
½ medium-size red onion, cut into 2-inch
    pieces
8 white button mushrooms, caps only,
    wiped clean
8 cherry or grape tomatoes

1. Place the beef, soy sauce, lemon juice, olive oil, and cumin in a bowl and stir to coat the beef evenly with the marinade. Cover the bowl with plastic wrap and refrigerate for at least 3 hours or as long as overnight.

2. Preheat the broiler or set up the grill and preheat it to high.

From the Test Kitchen

If you want sweet beef kebabs instead, substitute 2 tablespoons pineapple juice for the lemon juice, and use pineapple and mango chunks instead of the mushroom caps and tomatoes.

3. Remove the beef from the marinade and thread it onto 4 skewers, alternating bell peppers, pieces of onion, mushrooms, and tomatoes between the pieces of meat. Discard any remaining marinade.

4. Broil or grill the kebabs, turning occasionally, until the beef is tender, 8 to 10 minutes.

NUTRITION INFO: 1 portion provides:

Protein: 1 serving

Vitamin C: 2½ servings

Vitamin A: 1 serving

Other fruits and vegetables: 1½ servings

Iron: some

Tomato-Layered Mini Meat Loaves

SERVES 6

Classic comfort food, served up in mini form for maximum convenience. Leftovers can be easily rewarmed one mini loaf at a time, or sliced for a cold meat loaf sandwich.

2 pounds lean ground beef

1 cup shredded cheddar cheese

2 tablespoons ketchup

1 large egg, lightly beaten

3 tablespoons rolled oats

½ teaspoon dried oregano

¼ teaspoon garlic powder

¼ teaspoon salt

¼ teaspoon black pepper

2 medium-size ripe tomatoes, thinly sliced

1. Preheat the oven to 375°F.

2. Place the beef, cheddar, ketchup, egg, oats, oregano, garlic powder, salt, and pepper in a large bowl and mix them together with a fork. Press half of the beef mixture into six cups of a muffin tin, dividing it evenly among them. Top each meat loaf with a slice of tomato, then press the remaining beef mixture into the cups.

3. Bake the meat loaves until cooked through, about 20 minutes.

4. Remove the meat loaves from the tin immediately and serve. Wrap any leftover meat loaves in aluminum foil and refrigerate them. The baked meat loaves

From the Test Kitchen

Not in the mood for beef? Make the meat loaves with 2 pounds ground turkey breast or lean ground pork instead. Want to A-list your meat loaf? Mix in finely grated carrot.

can be refrigerated for 2 days, or frozen for up to 2 weeks. Defrost before reheating. To reheat the defrosted loaves, pop them, still wrapped in foil, in a preheated 350°F oven for 10 minutes, or remove the foil and heat in the microwave for 1 minute on high power. The meat loaves can also be frozen uncooked, wrapped in plastic wrap, for up to 1 month. To thaw before cooking, leave the meat loaves in the refrigerator overnight.

NUTRITION INFO: 1 portion provides:

Protein: 1½ servings

Calcium: almost 1 serving

Vitamin C: almost ½ serving

Iron: some

Mexican Lasagna

SERVES 6

Enchiladas, meet lasagna. This Mexican take on the traditional Italian favorite is like a fiesta for your eyes and your taste buds—plus, it layers on the nutrients.

2 teaspoons olive oil
1 medium-size onion, chopped
1 medium-size red bell pepper, chopped
2 cloves garlic, minced
1 pound extra-lean ground beef
¾ cup grated carrots
1 tablespoon chili powder
1½ teaspoons ground cumin
1 teaspoon dried oregano
1 cup fresh or frozen yellow corn kernels
1 cup prepared enchilada sauce
1 can (15 ounces) tomato sauce
    (preferably Mexican style)
1 container (16 ounces) low-fat cottage
    cheese
2 large eggs, lightly beaten
¼ cup grated Parmesan cheese
Black pepper
Cooking oil spray
12 small whole-grain corn or flour tortillas
1½ cups finely shredded cheddar cheese
Plain yogurt or sour cream, chopped
    fresh cilantro, chopped fresh tomato,
    and/or chopped black olives, for
    serving (optional)

1. Preheat the oven to 375°F.

2. Heat the olive oil in a large nonstick skillet over medium heat. Add the onion, bell pepper, and garlic and cook until softened, about 5 minutes. Add the beef, carrots, chili powder, cumin, and oregano and cook, chopping up the meat with a wooden spoon, until the meat cooks through, about 10 minutes. Stir in the corn, enchilada sauce, and tomato sauce and let simmer, stirring frequently, until the flavors blend, about 5 minutes.

3. Place the cottage cheese, eggs, and Parmesan in a bowl and stir to mix. Season lightly with black pepper. Set aside.

4. Coat a 9 x 13-inch baking dish with cooking oil spray. Place 6 of the tortillas on the bottom (they'll overlap slightly). Spread half of the meat mixture over the tortillas. Spread the cottage cheese mixture over the meat mixture. Arrange the remaining 6 tortillas on top of the cottage cheese mixture. Top the tortillas with the remaining meat mixture.

5. Bake the lasagna for 20 minutes. Remove it from the oven and sprinkle the cheddar evenly over the top. Return the lasagna to the oven and bake until the cheese is melted, about 10 minutes longer.

6. Let the lasagna stand for 10 minutes before serving. Top with yogurt, cilantro, tomato, and/or olives, if desired. The lasagna can be refrigerated, covered, for up to 3 days. Reheat leftovers in the microwave.

NUTRITION INFO: 1 portion provides:

Protein: 1½ servings

Calcium: 1 serving

Vitamin C: 1 serving

Vitamin A: 1 serving

Other fruits and vegetables: 1 serving

Whole grains and legumes: 2 servings

Iron: some

Pork Medallions
with Arugula and Tomatoes

SERVES 2

Here's a very quick dish that's impressive enough for company but easy enough for the busiest weekday. Sauté extra tenderloin while you're at it—leftovers make a yummy sandwich with fresh arugula and tomatoes.

Olive oil cooking spray
3 teaspoons olive oil
2 cloves garlic, minced (optional)
½ pound pork tenderloin,
    cut into 1-inch-thick slices
Salt and black pepper
2 tablespoons balsamic vinegar
4 ripe plum tomatoes, seeded and
    chopped
1 package (5 or 6 ounces) arugula or
    baby spinach
¼ cup coarsely grated Parmesan cheese

1. Coat a large nonstick skillet with cooking spray. Add 2 teaspoons of the olive oil and heat over medium heat. Add the garlic, if using, and cook, stirring, until golden, about 4 minutes.

2. Season the pork slices with salt and pepper and add them to the skillet. Increase the heat to medium-high and cook until the pork is well browned and cooked through, about 5 minutes per side. Transfer the pork to a plate and cover it with aluminum foil to keep warm.

3. Let the skillet cool for a minute, off the heat. Then heat the skillet over low heat and add the remaining 1 teaspoon oil and the balsamic vinegar, stirring to scrape up any brown bits. Add the tomatoes and stir for 1 minute, until the tomatoes are warmed through. Remove from the heat. Add the arugula and toss until wilted. Season with salt and pepper to taste.

4. Spoon the arugula and tomato mixture over the pork, sprinkle the Parmesan on top, and serve immediately.

NUTRITION INFO: 1 portion provides:

Protein: 1 serving

Calcium: ½ serving

Vitamin C: 2 servings

Vitamin A: 3 servings

Iron: some (if using spinach)

Fat: ½ serving

Omegas: some

Pacific Rim Pork Kebabs

SERVES 4

Looking for a super-easy dish with Hawaiian punch? These sweet and tangy pork kebabs are heady with grated ginger and zesty with lime. If you're using wooden skewers, soak them in water first for a half-hour. And try subbing chicken or shrimp for the pork.

1 pound lean pork tenderloin,
   cut into 1-inch cubes
2 medium-size red bell peppers,
   cut into 1-inch pieces
1 can (20 ounces) pineapple chunks
   in juice, drained, reserving ¼ cup
   of the juice
2 tablespoons fresh lime juice
2 teaspoons canola oil
2 teaspoons grated peeled fresh ginger
1 teaspoon curry powder
1 teaspoon minced garlic (optional)
2 cups cooked brown rice, quinoa, or
   another whole grain, for serving

1. Thread the pork, bell peppers, and pineapple onto 8 skewers, alternating pieces of each. Set the kebabs aside.

2. Place the pineapple juice, lime juice, oil, ginger, curry powder, and garlic, if using, in a large resealable plastic bag and squeeze the bag to blend the marinade. Add the kebabs, seal the bag, and gently shake and turn the bag to coat the kebabs evenly. Let the kebabs marinate for about 30 minutes.

3. Preheat the broiler or set up the grill and preheat it to high.

4. Remove the kebabs from the marinade and broil or grill until the pork is cooked through, turning occasionally, about 10 minutes. Discard any remaining marinade. Unskewer the kebabs and serve on top of the brown rice or quinoa.

NUTRITION INFO: 1 portion provides:

Protein: 1 serving

Vitamin C: 3 servings

Vitamin A: 1 serving

Whole grains and legumes: 1 serving

Sheet-Pan Pork Tenderloin with Sweet Potato and Apple

SERVES 2

This one-sheet meal is ready for the oven in minutes—the only hard part will be resisting the aroma of the sweet, savory, deliciously caramelized pork while you're waiting for it to rest after roasting.

Cooking oil spray
½ pound pork tenderloin
2 teaspoons olive oil
1 teaspoon kosher salt
½ teaspoon black pepper
1 medium-size sweet potato, peeled and
    cut into ¼-inch-thick slices
1 medium-size apple, cored and cut into
    ½-inch-thick slices
1½ tablespoons whole-grain mustard
2 teaspoons honey
Grated zest and juice of 1 lemon
1 teaspoon chopped fresh thyme leaves

1. Preheat the oven to 450°F. Coat a rimmed baking sheet with cooking oil spray.

2. Pat the pork dry with paper towels; rub evenly with 1 teaspoon of the oil. Sprinkle evenly with ½ teaspoon of the salt and ¼ teaspoon of the pepper. Place in the center of the baking sheet.

3. Toss together the sweet potato, apple, and the remaining 1 teaspoon oil, ½ teaspoon salt, and ¼ teaspoon pepper in a large bowl. Arrange the mixture evenly around the pork on the baking sheet.

4. Whisk together the mustard, honey, lemon zest and juice, and thyme in a small bowl. Brush the glaze evenly over the pork, sweet potato, and apple.

5. Bake for 15 minutes. Turn on the broiler to high and broil until the pork is browned on top and the internal temperature taken with an instant-read meat thermometer is 145°F, about 5 minutes. Remove from the oven and let rest for about 10 minutes.

6. Transfer the pork to a cutting board and slice. Serve with the sweet potato–apple mixture.

NUTRITION INFO: 1 portion provides:

Protein: 1 serving

Vitamin C: ½ serving

Vitamin A: 1 serving

Other fruits and vegetables: 1 serving

Poultry

....

Tired of the same old chicken that tastes, well, like chicken? Here's a flock of recipes that'll shake (and bake and sauté and grill) the way you feel about America's favorite bird. Want to fill your bucket with something healthy and crunchy? Try Oven-Fried Chicken Breasts. Take your bird on a round-the-world tour with Basque Chicken. Or play it safe—and soothing—with Apricot Ginger Glazed Chicken. Talking turkey? You will be once you try Turkey with Corn and Edamame Salsa and Turkey Cutlets in Mushroom Sauce. What's more, since most of these recipes serve 4, you can get 2 meals for half the cooking effort. Serve leftovers on salads or in sandwiches.

Rosemary Lemon Chicken

SERVES 4

A simple vinaigrette of fragrant fresh rosemary and tangy lemon brightens this super-simple chicken dish, making it perfect for a quick meal or leisurely dinner. Serve it hot the first night, and serve the leftovers (if there are any) cold the next night, perhaps sliced over a salad. Or, make a tasty sandwich or wrap for lunch.

1 tablespoon chopped fresh rosemary
1 tablespoon drained capers
1 teaspoon chopped garlic (optional)

1 teaspoon olive oil
Juice of 1 medium-size lemon, plus
   1 lemon, very thinly sliced
1 tablespoon pine nuts
4 skinless, boneless chicken breast
   halves (each 4 ounces)
Salt and black pepper

1. Preheat the oven to 350°F.

2. Place the rosemary, capers, garlic, if using, olive oil, lemon juice, and pine nuts in a small bowl and stir to mix. Set aside.

3. Place the lemon slices in a single layer in a baking dish large enough to hold the chicken breasts in a single layer. Season the chicken breasts with a pinch each of salt and pepper, then place them on top of the lemon slices. Spoon about a tablespoon of the rosemary mixture over each chicken breast. Bake the chicken until it registers 165°F at its thickest part, 20 to 25 minutes.

NUTRITION INFO: 1 portion provides:

Protein: 1 serving

Omegas: some

Oven-Fried Chicken Breasts

SERVES 2

Who needs to bring in a bucket? These chicken breasts are crunchy on the outside, moist on the inside, completely greaseless—and still finger-licking good.

½ cup whole-wheat bread crumbs
¼ cup grated Parmesan cheese
1 teaspoon paprika
½ teaspoon garlic powder
Salt and black pepper
⅓ cup buttermilk
1 tablespoon Dijon mustard (optional)
1 tablespoon mayonnaise
Olive oil cooking spray
2 skinless, boneless chicken breast
    halves (each 4 ounces)

1. Preheat the oven to 400°F.

2. Place the bread crumbs, Parmesan, paprika, and garlic powder in a large shallow bowl and stir to mix. Season with salt and pepper to taste.

3. Place the buttermilk, mustard, if using, and mayonnaise in another shallow bowl and stir to mix.

4. Coat a baking sheet with olive oil cooking spray. Dip the chicken breasts in the buttermilk mixture, then dredge them in the bread crumb mixture. Place the breasts on the baking sheet. Spray the breasts with a little olive oil, too. Bake the chicken until it registers 165°F at its thickest part, about 25 minutes.

NUTRITION INFO: 1 portion provides:

Protein: 1 serving

Calcium: ½ serving

Whole grains and legumes: 1 serving

Fat: ½ serving

Omegas: some

Bigger Breasts?

The recipes in this section call for 4 ounces of chicken or turkey per person—because that's all you need for 1 portion. Plus, petite portions are easier on pregnant digestion. But if you've got the appetite—and larger breasts in your refrigerator—go right ahead and enjoy. If you use 6-ouncers, count yourself in for 1½ protein servings. Or go for a full 8 ounces and score 2 full servings. Score extra omega-3s by choosing pasture-raised or free-range chicken.

Chunky Tomato Chicken Parmesan

SERVES 2

Mama mia! Baby's going to love this dish because it's nutritious—but you're going to love it because it's super easy and super yummy. Vitamin-packed roasted red peppers, rich tomato sauce, chopped fresh tomatoes, and a blanket of provolone top chicken breasts in a healthy remake of an old Italian favorite. Extra-hungry? Serve the chicken on pasta. Sandwich any leftovers into your favorite roll for a filling lunch.

¼ cup whole-wheat bread crumbs

2 tablespoons grated Parmesan cheese

2 skinless, boneless chicken breast
    halves (each 4 ounces)

Salt and cracked black pepper

½ teaspoon dried oregano

½ roasted red bell pepper
    (leftover or from a jar), cut into 4 strips

½ cup good-quality jarred tomato sauce

½ cup chopped seeded ripe tomatoes

2 slices provolone cheese
    (about 2 ounces total)

1. Preheat the oven to 350°F.

2. Place the bread crumbs and Parmesan cheese in a small bowl and stir to mix, then set aside.

3. Season the chicken breasts lightly with salt and pepper and the oregano. Place them in a baking dish. Sprinkle the bread crumb mixture evenly over the cheese. Top each chicken breast with 2 strips roasted pepper, half of the tomato sauce, and half of the tomatoes. Place a slice of provolone on top of each breast. Bake the chicken until it registers 165°F at its thickest part, about 25 minutes.

NUTRITION INFO: 1 portion provides:

Protein: 1 serving

Calcium: 1 serving

Vitamin C: 1½ servings

Vitamin A: ½ serving

Whole grains and legumes: ½ serving

Omegas: some

Apricot Ginger Glazed Chicken

SERVES 2

Craving something sweet but in the market for dinner, not dessert? Here's the ticket. An added bonus for queasy moms: The ginger is sure to soothe. Serve the chicken with a wild rice or quinoa pilaf tossed with dried apricots and toasted sliced almonds.

1 tablespoon all-fruit apricot preserves

½ tablespoon low-sodium soy sauce

½ teaspoon ground ginger

⅛ teaspoon cayenne pepper (optional)

2 skinless, boneless chicken breast
    halves (each 4 ounces)

Salt and black pepper (optional)

1. Place the apricot preserves, soy sauce, ginger, and cayenne, if using, in a small bowl and stir to mix. Divide the apricot and ginger glaze in half and set aside.

2. Preheat the broiler or set up the grill and preheat it to high.

3. Lightly season the chicken breast halves with salt and pepper, if desired, then brush one side of each with half of the glaze. Broil or grill the chicken glazed side up for 5 to 6 minutes. Turn the chicken over, brush the second side with the other portion of the glaze, and broil or grill until it registers 165°F at its thickest part, 5 to 6 minutes more.

NUTRITION INFO: 1 portion provides:

Protein: 1 serving

Omegas: some

Teriyaki Chicken

SERVES 2

Just about anything you're cooking—from turkey cutlets, to steak, to pork, to salmon, to firm tofu, to portobello mushrooms—tastes better prepared teriyaki style. Serve the chicken with brown rice and a veggie stir-fry. Turn leftovers into a sandwich: Layer chicken with salad greens, shredded carrot, and sliced cucumber on your favorite bread or wrap with a touch of mayo.

2 tablespoons low-sodium soy sauce
1 tablespoon honey
1½ teaspoons grated peeled fresh ginger
    or ½ teaspoon ground ginger
1 teaspoon sesame oil
1 tablespoon chopped fresh cilantro or
    ½ teaspoon ground coriander
2 skinless, boneless chicken breast
    halves (each 4 ounces)

1. Place the soy sauce, honey, ginger, sesame oil, and cilantro in a small bowl and whisk to mix.

2. Place the chicken in a baking dish and pour the teriyaki marinade over it, turning the breasts to coat them evenly. The chicken can marinate, covered, in the refrigerator for up to 8 hours.

3. Preheat the broiler or set up the grill and preheat it to high.

4. Broil or grill the chicken until it registers 165°F at its thickest part, 5 to 6 minutes per side.

NUTRITION INFO: 1 portion provides:

Protein: 1 serving

Omegas: some

Cooking in a Packet

Love a home-cooked meal but hate the cleanup that comes after? Skip the pots and pans, and cook your dinner in a packet! Most any combination of poultry, meat, or fish with vegetables and seasonings can be adapted to pouch cooking. All you need is a lot of aluminum foil and a little imagination. (You can also cook packets in parchment or parchment cooking bags. Don't overstuff, to allow the parchment to expand.) Here are some tips:

- Choose ingredients that cook quickly—boneless chicken breasts instead of legs; shredded carrots, not chunks; and summer squash rather than winter squash. Extra-firm tofu also works well in a packet.

- Tear off a square of heavy-duty aluminum foil large enough to completely enclose one portion of meat or fish and veggies and place it on a work surface.

- Layer the ingredients you want to cook on the foil, starting with the heaviest, such as sliced onions and strips of beef and ending with the lightest ones, like mushrooms. Top everything with herbs and other seasonings.

- Season aggressively, using generous amounts of spices and fresh herbs—more than you would ordinarily. They'll have to stand up to the steam created in the packet.

- If the ingredients aren't likely to form a sauce (tomatoes will, cabbage won't), pour a couple of tablespoons of broth, a little soy sauce, or a few squeezes of lemon, lime, or orange juice over everything. Citrus slices make an ideal addition to many fish and poultry packets.

- Fold the foil over the ingredients and crimp the edges all around to seal the packet very tightly. This will seal in the steam and those very intense flavors and aromas.

- Bake the packet on a rimmed baking sheet in a hot oven, 400°F. Cooking times will vary depending on the ingredients you use but will usually be between 15 and 25 minutes.

- For a dramatic and aromatic presentation, open the foil packet at the table, but do it carefully. The escaping steam is very hot, so keep your face and hands out of harm's way.

Chicken Enchiladas

SERVES 4

In this case, the whole enchilada offers a whole lot of nutrition—and flavor—but very little fat. Plus, leftovers reheat deliciously.

1 pound skinless, boneless chicken breasts, cut into ½-inch cubes
1 medium-size red bell pepper, cut into small dice
2 teaspoons chili powder
½ teaspoon dried oregano
Pinch of salt
1 tablespoon plus 2 teaspoons olive oil
1 can (14.5 ounces) diced tomatoes with mild green chiles, with their juices
1 can (about 15 ounces) black beans, drained and rinsed
1 can (10 ounces) enchilada sauce
4 large whole-grain corn tortillas (10-inch diameter)
1 cup shredded Colby-Jack cheese blend

1. Preheat the oven to 300°F.

2. Place the chicken, bell pepper, chili powder, oregano, salt, and 1 tablespoon of the olive oil in a large bowl and toss to mix.

3. Heat the remaining 2 teaspoons olive oil in a large nonstick skillet over medium heat. Add the chicken mixture and cook until the chicken registers 165°F at its thickest part, 5 to 7 minutes. Add the tomatoes with their juices and the black beans and cook until heated through, about 3 minutes.

4. Place the enchilada sauce in a small saucepan over medium heat and cook until heated through, 3 to 5 minutes.

5. Brush a tortilla with a little of the enchilada sauce. Spoon one-quarter of the chicken mixture into the center of a tortilla and roll it up. Place the filled tortilla in a 9 x 13-inch baking dish, seam side down. Repeat with the remaining tortillas and chicken mixture. Pour the remaining enchilada sauce over the filled tortillas and sprinkle the cheese on top.

6. Bake the enchiladas until the cheese melts, 15 to 20 minutes. If you are not ready to serve the enchiladas immediately, reduce the oven temperature to 200°F; the enchiladas will keep warm until you're ready to eat.

NUTRITION INFO: 1 portion provides:

Protein: 1½ servings

Calcium: 1 serving

Vitamin C: 2 servings

Vitamin A: 1 serving

Whole grains and legumes: 2 servings

Iron: some

Fat: ½ serving

Omegas: some

Basque Chicken

SERVES 2

In this rustic dish, the combination of tomatoes, kalamata olives, and bell peppers that have practically melted through slow cooking gives the chicken a distinctively Spanish flavor. Serve it over a bed of whole-grain rice or quinoa.

2 teaspoons olive oil

½ pound skinless, boneless chicken
   breasts, sliced into 1-inch-long strips

½ medium-size Spanish onion,
   thinly sliced

2 cloves garlic, thinly sliced

1 small red bell pepper, cut into
   julienne strips

1 small green bell pepper, cut into
   julienne strips

1 small yellow or orange bell pepper,
   cut into julienne strips

1 cup drained canned diced fire-roasted
   tomatoes

¼ cup pitted kalamata olives, halved

2 teaspoons fresh thyme leaves

1 teaspoon hot paprika or 1 teaspoon
   sweet paprika and a pinch of crushed
   red pepper flakes, plus more to taste

4 tablespoons chopped fresh flat-leaf
   (Italian) parsley

Salt and black pepper

1. Heat 1 teaspoon of the olive oil in a large nonstick skillet over medium heat. Add the chicken and sauté until it registers 165°F at its thickest part, 5 to 7 minutes. Remove the chicken from the skillet and set aside.

From the Test Kitchen

For a deeper flavor, substitute smoked paprika for the hot or sweet paprika. For a salty tang, top the chicken with crumbled pasteurized feta.

2. Add the remaining teaspoon of olive oil to the skillet along with the onion, garlic, and bell pepper, reduce the heat to medium-low, and cook until softened, about 8 minutes. Stir in the tomatoes, olives, thyme, paprika, and 2 tablespoons of the parsley. Cook, stirring frequently, until the flavors have blended, about 5 minutes. Season with salt, pepper, and additional paprika to taste. Add the cooked chicken, toss to coat with the sauce, and cook until heated through. Sprinkle the remaining 2 tablespoons parsley over the top.

NUTRITION INFO: 1 portion provides:

Protein: 1 serving

Vitamin C: 5 servings

Vitamin A: 1½ servings

Other fruits and vegetables: 1 serving

Fat: ½ serving

Omegas: some

Turkey Cutlets in Mushroom Sauce

SERVES 2

Love mushrooms? You're in for a treat in just minutes. This colorful and flavorful one-pot dish teams turkey with lots of mushrooms (use wild for even more flavor), peas, carrots, and fresh herbs. Complement this earthy entrée—or stretch any leftovers into a meal—by serving it on a bed of whole-grain noodles.

Whole-wheat flour
2 turkey cutlets (each 6 ounces,
    ½ inch thick; see Note)
Salt and black pepper
Olive oil cooking spray
1 teaspoon olive oil
2 teaspoons butter
2 shallots, finely minced
½ pound sliced wild or cultivated
    mushrooms (about 3 cups)
1 cup carrot matchsticks
½ cup frozen green peas
1 teaspoon minced fresh tarragon leaves
    or ¼ teaspoon dried
2 tablespoons chopped fresh flat-leaf
    (Italian) parsley, plus more for garnish
2 tablespoons minced fresh chives,
    plus more for garnish
¾ cup low-sodium chicken broth or
    mushroom broth

1. Place some flour in a shallow bowl. Season the turkey cutlets with salt and pepper, then lightly dredge both sides of each cutlet in the flour.

2. Coat a large, heavy nonstick skillet with olive oil spray. Place 1 teaspoon of the olive oil in the skillet and heat over medium heat. Cook the cutlets until browned but not cooked through, about 2 minutes per side. Remove the cutlets from the skillet and set aside.

3. Coat the skillet again with olive oil spray, add the butter, and melt it over medium-low heat. Add the shallots and cook until slightly softened, about 2 minutes. Increase the heat to medium-high, add the mushrooms, and cook for 2 minutes.

4. Add the carrots, peas, tarragon, parsley, chives, and broth and bring to a boil, then lower the heat and simmer for 2 minutes. Return the cutlets to the skillet. Let simmer, stirring frequently, until the sauce is slightly reduced and the turkey registers 165°F at its thickest part, about 2 minutes. Season with salt and pepper to taste, and garnish with more parsley and chives.

NOTE: If your turkey cutlets are more than ½ inch thick, pound them until they are an even ½ inch.

NUTRITION INFO: 1 portion provides:

Protein: 1½ servings

Vitamin C: ½ serving

Vitamin A: 2 servings

Other fruits and vegetables: 3 servings

Fat: ½ serving

Turkey with Corn and Edamame Salsa

SERVES 2

No need to wait until Thanksgiving for this turkey dish—and no need to wait hours for your bird to be ready. Make summer turkey season, too, with a tasty and quick-grilled turkey breast topped with a crisp, cool salsa. New to edamame? This will be a delicious introduction to chewy, nutritious soybeans.

4 roma tomatoes, seeded and chopped

1 cup cooked fresh corn kernels
    (or frozen corn, defrosted and drained)

1 cup cooked shelled edamame
    (soybeans)

1 teaspoon chili powder

2 tablespoons chopped fresh cilantro,
    plus more to taste

2 tablespoons olive oil

2 tablespoons fresh lime juice

Salt and black pepper

½ pound turkey cutlets

Garlic powder

Olive oil cooking spray

1 medium-size avocado (preferably
    Hass), sliced

4 lime wedges, for serving

1. Place the tomatoes, corn, edamame, chili powder, 1 tablespoon of the cilantro, 1 tablespoon of the olive oil, and the lime juice in a bowl and stir to mix. Season with salt and pepper to taste. Add additional cilantro, if desired. Set the salsa aside.

2. Brush the remaining tablespoon of olive oil on the turkey and season it with salt, pepper, and garlic powder.

From the Test Kitchen

Here's a time-saving tip: Grill a whole pound of turkey cutlets while you're at it, then have the leftovers in a sandwich (or in Fruity Turkey Salad, page 220).

3. Coat a large skillet with olive oil cooking spray and heat over medium-high heat. Add the turkey and cook until it registers 165°F at its thickest part, 2 to 4 minutes per side.

4. To serve, place the turkey on top of the salsa. Sprinkle the remaining tablespoon of cilantro over the turkey, then garnish with avocado slices and lime wedges.

NUTRITION INFO: 1 portion provides:

Protein: 1½ servings

Vitamin C: 1 serving

Other fruits and vegetables: 1½ servings

Whole grains and legumes: 1 serving

Fat: 1 serving

Slow-Cooker Chicken Mole

SERVES 4

Any day can be Taco Tuesday if you plan ahead. Don't be fooled by the long list of ingredients—the mole sauce blends together in moments. Then, once the slow cooker takes the wheel, the only fingers you'll have to lift are the ones that bring those tacos to your mouth. Double the recipe for double the dinners or lunch leftovers. You can also serve them cold on a salad.

1 dried ancho chile
4 boneless, skinless chicken thighs
    (each about 6 ounces)
1 teaspoon kosher salt
1 can (15 ounces) whole tomatoes,
    with their juices
1 medium-size onion, chopped
1 chipotle pepper with 1 tablespoon
    adobo sauce
½ cup toasted sliced almonds
    (see page 217)
½ cup dark chocolate chips
¼ cup raisins
¼ cup low-sodium chicken broth
3 cloves garlic, peeled and crushed
1 tablespoon ground cumin
1 teaspoon ground cinnamon
4 medium (8–10 inches) corn or
    whole-grain flour tortillas, toasted,
    for serving
Fresh cilantro leaves, for serving
½ cup shredded Monterey Jack cheese,
    for serving
1 lime, cut into wedges, for serving

1. Soak the ancho chile in hot water for 10 minutes. Drain, discarding the soaking water. Remove the stem and seeds; set aside the chile.

2. Place the chicken in a 5- to 6-quart slow cooker, and sprinkle with the salt.

3. Combine the tomatoes, onion, ancho chile, chipotle, adobo sauce, almonds, chocolate, raisins, chicken broth, garlic, cumin, and cinnamon in a food processor or blender; process until smooth.

4. Pour the sauce over the chicken. Cover and cook on LOW until the chicken is tender, about 8 hours.

5. Serve the chicken and sauce, sprinkled with cilantro, with the tortillas, cheese, and lime.

NUTRITION INFO: 1 portion provides:

Protein: 1½ servings

Vitamin C: 1 serving

Whole grains and legumes: 1½ servings

Omegas: some

Chicken Satay Lettuce Wraps

SERVES 2

Chicken breast can easily substitute for the dark meat chicken in this super fresh, multitextured wrap. The delicious peanut satay sauce makes enough to toss with your favorite noodles for a yummy chilled noodle salad lunch.

2 ounces uncooked whole-grain rice
    vermicelli noodles
2 skinless, boneless chicken thighs
    (6 ounces each)
¼ teaspoon kosher salt
¼ teaspoon black pepper
¼ cup creamy peanut butter
¼ cup well-shaken or stirred
    unsweetened canned coconut milk
1½ tablespoons fresh lime juice
1 tablespoon low-sodium soy sauce
½ tablespoon sriracha
6 medium Bibb lettuce leaves
½ cup thinly sliced red bell pepper
Thinly sliced scallions; chopped fresh
    basil leaves; chopped roasted,
    salted peanuts, for topping

1. Soak the rice noodles according to package directions.

2. Meanwhile, heat a grill pan or cast-iron skillet over high heat. Sprinkle the chicken with the salt and pepper. Cook until charred and no longer pink inside, 4 to 5 minutes per side. Transfer to a cutting board and let rest for 5 minutes. Thinly slice the chicken across the grain.

3. Whisk together the peanut butter, coconut milk, lime juice, soy sauce, and sriracha.

4. Drain the rice noodles. Divide the noodles and chicken slices among the lettuce leaves. Top each with red peppers and drizzle with 1 tablespoon of sauce (or more to taste). Top with scallions, basil, and peanuts; roll up and serve. Extra sauce can be refrigerated, tightly covered, for up to 3 days.

NUTRITION INFO: 1 portion provides:

Protein: 1½ servings

Vitamin C: 1 serving

Vitamin A: 1 serving

Whole grains and legumes: 1 serving

Fat: 2 servings

Omegas: some

Instant Pot Buffalo Chicken Lettuce Wraps

SERVES 4

Here's how to earn wings for your buffalo chicken—use breasts instead, and wrap them up in lettuce. Add crunch (and tradition) with celery and carrots, and a side of ranch.

½ cup low-sodium chicken broth
¼ cup Buffalo-style hot sauce
4 skinless, boneless chicken breasts
(each about 4 ounces)
¼ teaspoon kosher salt
6 medium-size butter lettuce leaves
1½ cups shredded carrots
1½ cups chopped celery
1 cup ranch dressing, recipe follows

1. Combine the chicken broth and hot sauce in a programmable pressure multicooker (such as an Instant Pot). Place the chicken in the liquid and sprinkle it with the salt. Cover the cooker with its lid and lock it in place. Turn the steam release handle to the SEALING position. Select the MANUAL/PRESSURE COOK setting. Select HIGH pressure for 4 minutes. (It will take about 5 minutes for the cooker to come up to pressure before cooking begins.)

2. Carefully turn the steam release handle to the VENTING position and let the steam fully escape. (This will take about 3 minutes.) Remove the lid from the cooker.

3. Remove the chicken from the sauce and use two forks to shred it. Stir the chicken back into the sauce. Serve the chicken and sauce on the lettuce leaves, topped with the carrots, celery, and ranch dressing.

NUTRITION INFO: 1 portion (1 wrap) provides:

Protein: 1 serving

Vitamin A: 1 serving

Other fruits and vegetables: 1 serving

Omegas: some

Yummy Yogurt Ranch Dressing

SERVES 4

Creamy, tangy, and super low-fat, this ranch salad dressing doubles as a dip.

½ cup whole buttermilk
6 tablespoons whole milk Greek yogurt
2 teaspoons cider vinegar
1 teaspoon Dijon mustard
1 tablespoon mayo (optional)
1½ teaspoons kosher salt
1 teaspoon onion powder
1 teaspoon garlic powder
½ teaspoon black pepper
4 teaspoons chopped fresh parsley
4 teaspoons chopped fresh chives

Whisk together all ingredients. Store in an airtight container in the refrigerator for up to 2 weeks.

NUTRITION INFO: 1 portion (1 cup) provides:

Calcium: 1 serving

From the Test Kitchen

Feeling blue? Add crumbled pasteurized blue cheese to the dressing.

Easy Tandoori Chicken

SERVES 4

This trimmed-down take on the Indian classic doesn't require a traditional clay oven or a long list of spices, so it translates well in any kitchen. Just marinate the chicken the night before, then bake before broiling so that it's juicy and tender on the inside, slightly crispy and charred on the outside.

1 cup plain full-fat yogurt

1 tablespoon minced garlic, optional

1 tablespoon ground cumin

2 teaspoons paprika

2 teaspoons ground ginger

Grated zest of 1 lime

2 teaspoons kosher salt

1½ teaspoons ground coriander

½ teaspoon ground turmeric

2 skinless, boneless chicken breasts
   (each about 8 ounces)

Cooking oil spray

¼ cup chopped fresh cilantro

Lime wedges, for serving

1. Combine the yogurt, garlic, if using, cumin, paprika, ginger, lime zest, salt, coriander, and turmeric in a small bowl. Place all but ¼ cup in a large resealable plastic freezer bag; cover the bowl containing the remainder and place in the refrigerator. Add the chicken to the marinade in the bag, seal the bag, and massage to coat the chicken. Marinate in the refrigerator for 8 to 24 hours, turning occasionally.

2. Preheat the oven to 400°F. Line a rimmed baking sheet with aluminum foil and place a wire rack on the foil. Coat the rack with cooking oil spray.

> ## From the Test Kitchen
>
> For an earthier flavor (and even simpler prep), swap out the cumin, paprika, ginger, coriander and tumeric for 3 tablespoons of curry powder.

3. Place the chicken on the rack. Discard any marinade in the bag. Bake the chicken until the internal temperature taken with an instant-read meat thermometer is 130°F, 12 to 15 minutes.

4. Turn on the broiler to high. Broil the chicken until the thermometer registers 165°F, 6 to 7 minutes, basting with the reserved marinade every 2 minutes. (There should be char after each basting.) Remove from the oven and let rest for 5 to 10 minutes. Cut the chicken into large chunks. Sprinkle with the cilantro and serve with lime wedges.

NUTRITION INFO: 1 portion provides:

Protein: 1 serving

Omegas: some

Coconut Chicken

SERVES 4

This simple poached chicken is the perfect make-ahead meal. Delicious cold or at room temperature with crunchy veggies and bright herbs, this is the opposite of Sad Desk Lunch. The "dressing" from the cooking liquid, along with the chicken, will keep in the refrigerator for up to 3 days.

2 cloves garlic, peeled and crushed
1 (2-inch) piece peeled fresh ginger, sliced
1 (2-inch) piece lemongrass stalk, thinly sliced
½ cup chopped fresh cilantro
1 can (13.5 ounces) unsweetened, full-fat coconut milk (sometimes labeled "classic")
½ teaspoon kosher salt
¼ teaspoon black pepper
2 skinless, boneless chicken breasts (each about 8 ounces)
¼ teaspoon red curry powder
Juice of 1 lime
4 cups (packed) chopped romaine hearts
1 cup thinly sliced hothouse (seedless English) cucumber
½ cup shredded peeled carrots
½ cup (packed) mixed fresh mint and basil leaves

1. Place the garlic, ginger, lemongrass, cilantro, coconut milk, salt, and pepper in a medium-size saucepan. Bring to a boil over medium-high heat. Add the chicken and reduce the heat to medium-low; keep the cooking liquid between 160°F and 180°F.

2. Cook the chicken until the internal temperature taken with an instant-read meat thermometer is 160°F, about 25 minutes. Remove the chicken from the cooking liquid and set aside to cool for 15 minutes. Shred the chicken.

3. Meanwhile, pour the cooking liquid through a fine-mesh strainer into a bowl; discard the solids. Return the cooking liquid to the saucepan. Stir in the curry powder and simmer for 5 minutes. Pour into a bowl, add the lime juice, cover with plastic wrap, and refrigerate for at least 30 minutes.

4. Combine the chicken, romaine, cucumbers, and carrots in a large bowl and toss with enough of the dressing to coat evenly. Gently stir in the mint and basil. Serve with any remaining dressing.

NUTRITION INFO: 1 portion provides:

Protein: 1 serving

Vitamin C: 2½ servings

Vitamin A: 2 servings

Other fruits and vegetables: 1 serving

Omegas: some

Fish and Seafood

....

Maybe you're a fish fan from way back. Or maybe you feel lukewarm about seafood—don't mind it, but you probably wouldn't make it your entree of choice. Or maybe you know you should embrace the seafood side of life (for its high-protein, low-fat benefits), but fish is a taste you're still waiting to acquire. No matter how you feel about fish and seafood, these recipes will win you over.

Looking for something exotic? Try Salmon Poached in Thai Carrot Broth. Going gourmet? How about Shrimp with Feta or Seared Scallops on White Beans and Kale. Fishing for a quick yet memorable meal? You'll find it here.

Ginger-Steamed Halibut

SERVES 2

Aluminum foil packets enclose an intensely flavored meal-in-one, steaming not only the halibut but also the couscous and a delicious mix of vegetables.

4 tablespoons uncooked whole-wheat
   couscous
½ large red bell pepper, thinly sliced
1 cup sugar snap peas, trimmed

½ cup sliced shiitake mushroom caps
1 cup (packed) baby spinach leaves
2 teaspoons grated peeled fresh ginger
Salt and black pepper
4 tablespoons low-sodium vegetable
   broth or fish broth
2 halibut or salmon fillets
   (each about 6 ounces)
4 fresh basil leaves (optional)

1. Preheat the oven to 450°F.

2. Tear off two pieces of heavy-duty aluminum foil, each 12 inches long. Place the pieces of foil on a work surface and put 2 tablespoons couscous in the center of each.

3. Place the bell pepper, sugar snap peas, mushrooms, spinach, and ginger in a bowl and stir to mix. Season the vegetable mix lightly with salt and black pepper, then place half in the center of each piece of foil.

4. Fold up the edges of each piece of foil slightly, then spoon 2 tablespoons broth into each.

5. Lightly season the fish fillets with salt and black pepper and place one on top of each mound of vegetables. Top each fish fillet with 2 basil leaves, if using.

6. Seal a packet by bringing together the two longest edges of the foil and double folding them, leaving room for air circulation inside. Crimp the edge to make a tight seal. Double fold and crimp the remaining 2 edges to finish sealing the packet. (There should be no gaps where juices can leak out.) Repeat with the remaining packet.

7. Transfer the foil packets to a rimmed baking sheet and bake until the fish is cooked through, 12 to 15 minutes, depending upon the thickness of the fillets. To test for doneness, carefully open a packet; when the fish is cooked through it will flake easily when pierced with a fork.

8. To serve, place the packets on serving plates and open them at the table, taking care to avoid the escaping hot steam.

Cucumber Sauce

This sauce is delish on any fish, whether it's roasted, poached, or grilled. Serve it as a dip for veggies, too, or in sandwiches or wraps.

½ cup plain whole-milk Greek
    yogurt
2 Kirby (pickling) cucumbers,
    peeled, cut in half lengthwise,
    and seeded
1 tablespoon chopped fresh dill or
    ½ teaspoon dried dill
1 ripe tomato, seeded and diced
Salt and black pepper

Place the yogurt, cucumbers, and dill in a food processor and process until just chunky. Fold in the tomato and season the sauce with salt and pepper to taste. Like a little bite? Add a teaspoon or two of well-drained prepared horseradish, and/or Dijon mustard. Minced fresh chives would also be a tasty addition.

NUTRITION INFO: 1 portion provides:

Protein: 1½ servings

Vitamin C: 2 servings

Vitamin A: 1 serving

Other fruits and vegetables: ½ serving

Whole grains and legumes: ½ serving

Iron: some

Omegas: some, if using salmon

Red Snapper with Mango Salsa

SERVES 2

Topping broiled red snapper with a snappy mango salsa gives the fish an authentic island kick. The mango salsa also goes well with turkey, beef, pork, or chicken and will keep nicely in the refrigerator for one or two days.

1 medium-size ripe mango,
   cut into small dice
½ medium-size red bell pepper,
   cut into small dice
2 scallions (white and light green parts),
   trimmed and thinly sliced
1 teaspoon minced fresh jalapeno pepper
   (optional)
2 tablespoons fresh lime juice
2 tablespoons chopped fresh cilantro
1 tablespoon olive oil
2 red snapper fillets
   (each about 6 ounces)
Salt and black pepper

1. Preheat the broiler.

2. Place the mango, bell pepper, scallions, jalapeño, if using, lime juice, cilantro, and 1 teaspoon of the oil in a bowl and stir to mix. Set the mango salsa aside.

From the Test Kitchen

Heartburn getting you down? Skip the heat: Substitute 1 teaspoon ground cumin for the jalapeno pepper.

3. Brush the fish fillets with the remaining oil and season with salt and black pepper. Broil them until they are cooked through and flake easily when pierced with a fork, 4 to 5 minutes per side.

4. Serve the fish with large spoonfuls of the mango salsa.

NUTRITION INFO: 1 portion provides:

Protein: 1½ servings

Vitamin C: 2 servings

Vitamin A: 1½ servings

Fat: ½ serving

Full of Fish?

Most recipes in this chapter call for 6-ounce fish fillets—because that's the size most commonly encountered at fish markets. That means you'll be racking up 1½ protein servings in each portion. But if that's too much fish for you, scale it back to 4-ounce portions, and you'll cut your protein serving down to 1. On the other hand, if you can never get your fill of fish, you can occasionally feast on 8 ounces—a portion that will yield 2 full protein servings.

Greek Salad Snapper

SERVES 2

Bake snapper in a snap with a delicious sauce that combines all of your favorite Greek salad ingredients—tomatoes, red pepper, capers, kalamata olives, oregano, and feta cheese.

1 tablespoon olive oil

2 scallions (white and light green parts), trimmed and thinly sliced

2 ripe roma tomatoes, cut into ½-inch pieces

½ large red bell pepper, cut into ½-inch pieces

1 teaspoon minced fresh oregano or ½ teaspoon dried oregano

1 teaspoon drained capers, or more to taste

6 pitted kalamata olives, chopped

¼ cup crumbled pasteurized feta cheese

2 tablespoons chopped fresh flat-leaf (Italian) parsley

Black pepper

Fresh lemon juice

Olive oil cooking spray

2 red snapper fillets (each about 6 ounces)

½ teaspoon chopped fresh dill

Salt

1. Preheat the oven to 400°F.

2. Heat the olive oil in a small skillet over medium-high heat. Add the scallions and cook until softened slightly, about 1 minute. Add the tomatoes, bell pepper, oregano, and capers and cook until the vegetables soften, about 4 minutes. Remove from the heat and add the olives and feta, then sprinkle parsley on top and season with black pepper and lemon juice to taste.

From the Test Kitchen

Not a red snapper fan? You can substitute haddock, tilapia, bass, cod, or flounder for any recipe that calls for red snapper.

3. Coat an 8-inch-square baking dish with olive oil spray. Place the fish fillets in the center of the baking dish, sprinkle the dill over them, and season with salt and black pepper. Spoon the vegetable and feta mixture on top. Cover the baking dish with aluminum foil and bake until the fish is cooked through and flakes easily when pierced with a fork, 8 to 10 minutes. Serve the fish with the vegetable and feta mixture.

NUTRITION INFO: 1 portion provides:

Protein: ½ serving

Calcium: ½ serving

Vitamin C: 1½ servings

Vitamin A: ½ serving

Fat: ½ serving

Roasted Mediterranean Sea Bass with Red Pepper and White Beans

SERVES 2

Here's a quick and easy way to bring the flavors of the Mediterranean to your table. White beans and red bell pepper pair up to provide a simple yet satisfying base for the bass.

4 scallions (white and light green parts), trimmed and chopped

½ cup loosely packed fresh flat-leaf (Italian) parsley leaves

¼ cup low-sodium vegetable broth

1 tablespoon olive oil

1 medium-size red bell pepper, thinly sliced

1 can (14 ounces) Great Northern beans, drained and rinsed

2 skinless sea bass or halibut fillets (each about 6 ounces)

1 lemon, halved and seeded (thinly slice 1 half)

1. Preheat the oven to 375°F.

2. Place the scallions, parsley, vegetable broth, and olive oil in a blender or food processor and puree them.

3. Place the bell pepper and beans in an 8-inch-square baking dish. Set aside 3 tablespoons of the scallion and parsley puree, then spoon the rest over the bell pepper and beans. Arrange the fish fillets on top and spoon the remaining scallion and parsley puree over the fish. Scatter the lemon slices on top.

4. Bake the fish until it is cooked through and flakes easily when pierced with a fork, about 15 minutes. Squeeze the remaining lemon half over the fish just before serving.

NUTRITION INFO: 1 portion provides:

Protein: 2 servings

Calcium: ½ serving

Vitamin C: 3 servings

Vitamin A: 2 servings

Whole grains and legumes: 2½ servings

Iron: some

Fat: ½ serving

Marinated Salmon Fillets with Ginger and Lime

SERVES 4

Simple broiled or grilled salmon is easy to prepare but much tastier—and just as easy—in this Pacific Rim–inspired dish. The lime and ginger marinade makes it fragrant and flavorful. (It's sassy on shrimp, too.) The recipe is easy to cut in half—or enjoy as leftovers the next day, perhaps over a bed of your favorite greens or grains.

Grated zest and juice of 2 limes
2 teaspoons olive oil
2 teaspoons low-sodium soy sauce
1 teaspoon sesame oil
1 teaspoon grated peeled fresh ginger
4 skinless salmon fillets
 (each about 6 ounces)
3 scallions (white and light green parts),
 trimmed and thinly sliced

1. Place the lime zest and juice, olive oil, soy sauce, sesame oil, and ginger in a small bowl and stir to mix.

2. Place the salmon in a 9 x 13-inch glass baking dish. Pour half of the lime and ginger mixture over the salmon; set the rest aside. Turn the salmon fillets to coat them evenly with the marinade.

3. Preheat the broiler or set up the grill and preheat it to high.

4. Broil or grill the salmon until it is cooked through and flakes easily when pierced with a fork, 3 to 5 minutes per side.

Minute Meals

For a fish dinner without any fuss (or unpleasant smells), turn to the microwave. Place a fish fillet (no more than ½ inch thick) in a microwave-safe baking dish. Season the fish with a combination of any of the following: grated lemon or orange zest, a sprinkling of chopped fresh herbs (such as tarragon and dill), and a coating of equal parts grainy mustard and mayonnaise. Cover the baking dish with plastic wrap, folding back one corner to allow the steam to escape. Microwave the fish on high power until it's cooked through, 2 to 3 minutes. Presto! With a squeeze of lemon or lime juice, dinner is ready.

5. Place the salmon fillets on serving plates and spoon the reserved lime and ginger marinade over them. Top the fillets with the scallions.

NUTRITION INFO: 1 portion provides:

Protein: 1½ servings

Fat: ½ serving

Omegas: some

Instant Pot Lemony Salmon with Sweet Potatoes and Kale

SERVES 2

Ready in an instant, but you'll want to sit down and savor this hearty, healthy, savory salmon dinner (it's a winner).

1 pound peeled sweet potatoes,
    cut in 2-inch pieces
1¼ teaspoons kosher salt
½ teaspoon black pepper
2 skinless center-cut salmon fillets
    (each about 6 ounces)
Grated zest of 1 lemon
1 tablespoon fresh lemon juice
5 cups (packed) chopped kale,
    thick stems removed
1 tablespoon olive oil
2 teaspoons minced garlic
2 teaspoons unsalted butter

1. Place the sweet potatoes, 1 cup water, ¾ teaspoon of the salt, and ¼ teaspoon of the pepper in a programmable pressure multicooker (such as an Instant Pot).

2. Sprinkle the salmon on both sides with the lemon zest and the remaining ½ teaspoon salt and ¼ teaspoon pepper. Place the salmon on top of the potatoes. Cover the cooker with its lid and lock it in place. Turn the steam release handle to the SEALING position. Select the MANUAL/PRESSURE COOK setting. Select HIGH pressure for 4 minutes. (It will take about 5 minutes for the cooker to come up to pressure before cooking begins.)

3. Carefully turn the steam release handle to the VENTING position and let the steam fully escape. (This will take about 3 minutes.) Remove the lid from the cooker.

4. While the cooker is venting, massage the kale with the lemon juice and oil in a large bowl until the kale is softened.

5. Remove the salmon from the cooker and set aside. Select the SAUTÉ setting. Select the HIGH temperature setting and allow the cooker to preheat. Add the kale and garlic to the potatoes. Cook, stirring occasionally, until most of the liquid has evaporated, 4 to 5 minutes. Add the butter and cook, stirring and smashing the potatoes with a wooden spoon, for about 1 minute. Serve immediately with the fish.

NUTRITION INFO: 1 portion provides:

Protein: 1½ serving

Vitamin C: 3 servings

Vitamin A: 5 servings

Fat: ½ serving

Iron: some

Omegas: some

Roast Salmon on a Bed of Lentils

SERVES 2

Earthy lentils provide a nutritious bed for roast salmon. The result is a hearty dish that's sure to satisfy.

2 skinless salmon fillets
   (each about 6 ounces)
2 teaspoons olive oil
2 teaspoons fresh thyme leaves
Pinch each of salt and black pepper
Warm Lentil Ragout (recipe follows)
1 tablespoon minced fresh flat-leaf
   (Italian) parsley

1. Preheat the oven to 450°F.

2. Place the salmon fillets in an 8-inch-square baking dish and rub the olive oil all over them. Sprinkle the thyme, salt, and pepper on top of the salmon.

3. Bake the salmon until it is cooked through and flakes easily when pierced with a fork, 10 to 15 minutes.

4. Spoon a serving of lentils onto each of two serving plates and place a salmon fillet on top. Sprinkle parsley over each fillet and serve.

NUTRITION INFO: 1 portion salmon (without lentils) provides:

Protein: 1½ servings

Warm Lentil Ragout

SERVES 4

This recipe makes twice as much as you'll need for the salmon. So tomorrow you can serve a broiled chicken breast over the leftovers.

2 teaspoons olive oil
1 medium-size onion, chopped
2 cloves garlic, minced
2 medium-size carrots, diced
1 cup green lentils
1 sprig fresh thyme
1 bay leaf
3 cups low-sodium chicken broth or
   vegetable broth
Salt and black pepper

1. Heat the olive oil in a medium-size saucepan over medium-low heat. Add the onion and garlic and cook until they just begin to soften, 3 minutes.

2. Add the carrots and cook, stirring frequently, until they soften slightly, about 3 minutes. Add the lentils, thyme, and bay leaf and cook, stirring to mix well, for about 1 minute.

3. Stir in the chicken broth, raise the heat to medium-high, and bring to a boil. Reduce the heat, and let simmer until the lentils are tender, about 20 minutes. Season with salt and pepper to taste. Remove and discard the thyme sprig and bay leaf before serving. The lentils can be refrigerated, covered, for up to 5 days.

NUTRITION INFO: 1 portion provides:

Protein: ½ serving

Vitamin A: 1 serving

Other fruits and vegetables: ½ serving

Whole grains and legumes: 1½ servings

Iron: some

Omegas: some

Mustard Glazed Salmon

SERVES 2

Fishing for an easy dinner? Serve this salmon: It's sweet, salty, a little spicy, and ready to savor in a matter of minutes. Pair it with quickly sautéed greens and brown rice (always keep a stash in your freezer). Leftovers make a scrumptious salad topper.

2 tablespoons maple syrup

1½ teaspoons low-sodium soy sauce

1½ teaspoons spicy brown mustard

½ teaspoon rice vinegar

Pinch of crushed red pepper flakes

2 skin-on salmon fillets
    (each about 6 ounces)

2 (¼-inch-thick) unpeeled orange slices,
    cut into half-moons

2 teaspoons olive oil

¼ teaspoon kosher salt

1 teaspoon toasted sesame seeds
    (see page 217)

1. Preheat the broiler to high. Line a rimmed baking sheet with heavy-duty aluminum foil.

2. Whisk together the maple syrup, soy sauce, mustard, vinegar, and pepper flakes in a small bowl. Arrange the salmon skin side down in the center of the baking sheet; brush evenly with 2 tablespoons of the glaze. Place 2 orange pieces on each salmon fillet; brush evenly with the remaining glaze.

3. Broil the salmon until it is cooked through and flakes easily when pierced with a fork, about 8 minutes. Sprinkle evenly with sesame seeds and serve immediately.

NUTRITION INFO: 1 portion provides:

Protein: 1½ servings

Omegas: some

Roasted Salmon with a Mild Mustard Crust

SERVES 2

Salmon's rich taste stands up beautifully to this flavorful mustard coating. But don't shy away from trying this crust on a milder fish, like halibut. For that matter, try it on chicken breasts.

Olive oil cooking spray

2 skinless salmon fillets
    (each about 6 ounces)

Salt and black pepper

1½ tablespoons grainy mustard

2 teaspoons mayonnaise

2 teaspoons chopped fresh dill

1. Preheat the oven to 375°F.

2. Coat the bottom of an 8-inch-square baking dish with olive oil cooking spray. Place the salmon fillets in the baking dish and lightly season them with salt and pepper.

3. Place the mustard, mayonnaise, and dill in a small bowl and stir to mix.

4. Spread the mustard mixture on the salmon fillets.

5. Bake the salmon until it is cooked through and flakes easily when pierced with a fork, about 10 minutes.

NUTRITION INFO: 1 portion provides:

Protein: 1½ servings

Omegas: some

From the Test Kitchen

For a sweet-and-pungent taste, skip the dill and add 2 teaspoons all-fruit apricot preserves to the mustard mixture.

Roast This

When fish is so fresh you can taste it, don't cover it up with fancy sauces or coatings. Instead, try the simplest and most satisfying way to prepare fish—roast it. Arrange fish fillets on a bed of fresh herbs, such as sprigs of rosemary, thyme, or sage, in a baking dish and sprinkle more herbs on top. Fennel seeds are a nice addition, too. Brush the fish with some olive oil, season with sea salt and cracked pepper, and scatter thin lemon slices over and around the fish. Bake the fish at 450°F until it is cooked through and flakes easily when pierced with a fork.

Another delicious way to roast fish is on a bed of vegetables. Toss slices or chunks of carrots, beets, butternut squash, potatoes (white or sweet), and/ or fennel with a little olive oil, fresh thyme leaves, and a little salt and pepper. Spread the vegetables out in a baking dish and roast them in a 450°F oven until tender, about 20 minutes. Spoon the roasted vegetables into the center of the baking dish so they can act as a bed for the fish. Place fillets on top, sprinkle them with herbs and lemon as above, and bake until the fish is done for a rustic fish dinner.

Salmon with Basil and Tomatoes

SERVES 2

Tomatoes and basil, a classic combo, make these salmon fillets moist, fragrant, and flavorful. How can so little effort result in something so tasty? Take a few minutes to get these packets ready for the oven, and you'll find out.

Olive oil cooking spray
2 skinless salmon fillets
　(each about 6 ounces)
12 ripe cherry tomatoes, halved
12 fresh basil leaves
1 tablespoon olive oil
Salt and black pepper

1. Preheat the oven to 450°F.

2. Tear off two pieces of heavy-duty aluminum foil, each 12 inches long. Place the pieces of foil on a work surface and coat them with olive oil spray.

3. Place a salmon fillet in the center of each piece of foil. Top each fillet with 12 cherry tomato halves and 6 basil leaves. Drizzle 1½ teaspoons olive oil over each fillet, then season with salt and pepper.

4. Seal a packet by bringing together the two longest edges of the foil and double folding them, leaving room for air circulation inside. Crimp the edge to make a tight seal. Double fold and crimp the remaining 2 edges to finish sealing the packet. (There should be no gaps where juices can leak out.) Repeat with the remaining packet.

From the Test Kitchen

Make a double batch and you'll have tomorrow's dinner, too. Flake the salmon into penne pasta, then fold in the cooked cherry tomatoes along with your favorite jarred tomato sauce, and top with a sprinkling of Parmesan cheese.

5. Transfer the foil packets to a rimmed baking sheet and bake until the salmon is cooked through, 15 to 20 minutes, depending upon the thickness of the fillets. To test for doneness, carefully open a packet; when the salmon is cooked through it will flake easily when pierced with a fork and will have turned light pink inside.

6. To serve, place the packets on serving plates and open them at the table, taking care to avoid the escaping hot steam.

NUTRITION INFO: 1 portion provides:

Protein: 1½ servings

Vitamin C: 1 serving

Fat: ½ serving

Omegas: some

Salmon Poached in Thai Carrot Broth

SERVES 2

Intensely and intriguingly flavored with sweet carrots, pungent ginger, cilantro, and tangy lime, this light-as-air salmon dish gives spa food a good name.

2 cups bottled carrot juice

1 cup diced carrots

1 tablespoon minced peeled fresh ginger

2 teaspoons grated lemon zest

1 teaspoon grated lime zest

2 tablespoons fresh lime juice,
     plus more to taste

3 scallions (white and light green parts),
     trimmed and sliced

2 skinless salmon fillets
     (each about 6 ounces)

2 tablespoons chopped fresh cilantro,
     plus more for garnish

Salt and black pepper

1. Place the carrot juice, carrots, and ginger in a medium-size saucepan that is large enough to hold the salmon fillets without crowding and bring to a boil over medium-high heat. Reduce the heat and let simmer until the carrots are tender, about 5 minutes. Add the lemon and lime zests, lime juice, and scallions and let simmer until heated through, about 1 minute.

2. Add the salmon fillets, return to a simmer, cover, and cook until the salmon is just cooked through and flakes easily when pierced with a fork, about 10 minutes. Spoon the carrot broth over the fillets periodically.

> ## From the Test Kitchen
>
> The carrot broth is too good to save for just salmon. Try poaching halibut, sea bass, shrimp, scallops, or skinless, boneless chicken breast halves in it, too. Not sold on the taste of cilantro? Substitute basil or flat-leaf parsley.

3. Place the salmon fillets in shallow bowls. Add the cilantro to the carrot broth, then season it with salt and pepper to taste and add more lime juice, if desired. Pour the carrot broth and carrots over the salmon, garnish with cilantro, and serve.

NUTRITION INFO: 1 portion provides:

Protein: 1½ servings

Vitamin A: 2 servings; plus 4 more if you sip half the carrot broth

Omegas: some

Salmon Cakes with Tropical Salsa

MAKES 6 CAKES; SERVES 3

Don't have the time (or the stomach) to stop by the fish market for fresh fillets? No harm in fishing some salmon out of a can. In fact, the soft bones in canned salmon provide a calcium bonus—and you'll never notice them once they're mashed up. If there are any salmon cakes left over, you can have them cold for lunch.

1 can (14.75 ounces) pink salmon, drained, mashed with a fork
1 medium-size red bell pepper, cut into small dice
½ cup grated carrot
1 tablespoon drained capers
1 large egg
Grated zest of ½ lemon
¼ cup whole-wheat bread crumbs
2 tablespoons ground flaxseed
¼ teaspoon black pepper
2 teaspoons olive oil
1 cup pineapple chunks, fresh or drained canned
1 cup ripe mango chunks (1 large mango)
2 tablespoons balsamic vinegar
Pinch of crushed red pepper flakes

1. Place the salmon, half of the bell pepper, the carrot, capers, egg, and lemon zest in a bowl and stir to mix.

2. Place the bread crumbs and flaxseed in a small bowl and whisk to mix. Add half of the bread crumb mixture to the salmon mixture and mix well. Season with black pepper, then stir well to combine.

3. Divide the salmon mixture into 6 equal portions and pat into cakes, each about ½ inch thick. Dredge both sides of the salmon cakes in the remaining bread crumb mixture.

4. Heat the oil in a large skillet over medium-high heat. Add the salmon cakes and cook until golden brown and heated through, about 4 minutes per side. To check for doneness, insert a knife into the center of a salmon cake; if the knife feels hot when removed, the cake is done.

5. Meanwhile, place the remaining bell pepper and the pineapple, mango, balsamic vinegar, and red pepper flakes in a bowl and stir to mix.

6. Spoon the salsa onto serving plates and top with the salmon cakes.

NUTRITION INFO: 1 portion (2 cakes) provides:

Protein: 1 serving

Vitamin C: 2 servings plus

Calcium: 1 serving if made with bones

Vitamin A: 1 serving

Whole grains and legumes: ½ serving

Omegas: some

Speedy Salsas

Looking for a way to dress up protein? Try any of these salsas on grilled or broiled fish, meat, or poultry:

- Chopped seeded ripe tomato, olives, basil, red onion, garlic, and lemon juice

- Chopped seeded ripe tomato, fresh yellow peaches or nectarines, fresh mint, balsamic vinegar, and olive oil

- Chopped fresh or canned, drained pineapple, red bell pepper, jalapeno pepper, and fresh cilantro

- Chopped seeded ripe tomato, roasted corn kernels, chopped roasted red bell pepper, red onion, fresh cilantro, and lime juice

- Diced mango, yellow bell pepper, jalapeño pepper, ground cumin, lime juice, and olive oil

- Black beans (drained and rinsed), chopped ripe tomato, yellow bell pepper, cilantro, scallions, lime juice, and olive oil

Seared Sea Scallops on Succotash

SERVES 2

Silken sea scallops love nothing more than a good bed, and crunchy succotash makes a beautiful one.

½ pound sea scallops
2 teaspoons fresh lemon juice
2 teaspoons olive oil
¾ teaspoon minced fresh tarragon, or
    ¼ teaspoon dried tarragon
Edamame Succotash (page 331)
Grated zest of ½ lemon
½ teaspoon minced fresh dill
½ teaspoon minced fresh flat-leaf
    (Italian) parsley
Salt and cracked black pepper

1. Place the scallops in a mixing bowl. Add the lemon juice, olive oil, and tarragon and stir to coat the scallops evenly. Let the scallops marinate in the refrigerator, covered, for up to 30 minutes.

2. Preheat the broiler or set up the grill and preheat it to high.

3. Broil or grill the scallops until they are just cooked through, springy to the touch, and have a golden brown edge, 2 to 3 minutes per side.

4. Toss the succotash with the lemon zest, dill, and parsley and divide it evenly between 2 serving plates. Season the cooked scallops lightly with salt and pepper. Divide them between the plates and serve at once.

NUTRITION INFO: 1 portion (without the succotash) provides:

Protein: 1 serving

Seared Scallops on White Beans and Kale

SERVES 2

This Spanish-influenced dish marries delicate scallops with a robust ragout of beans, tomatoes, and greens. The result is hearty, satisfying, and speedy to prepare, thanks to the canned beans and tomatoes.

2 teaspoons olive oil
1 small onion, chopped
2 cloves garlic, minced (optional)
1 bay leaf
1 can (14.5 ounces) diced tomatoes,
    drained
2 cups chopped kale, thick stems
    removed first
1 cup drained canned navy or cannellini
    beans, rinsed
1 tablespoon chopped fresh flat-leaf
    (Italian) parsley, plus more for garnish
    (optional)
Salt and black pepper
2 teaspoons fresh lemon juice, plus more
    for seasoning the beans
1 teaspoon butter
½ pound sea scallops

1. Heat the olive oil in a large nonstick skillet over medium-low heat. Add the onion, garlic, if using, and bay leaf and cook, stirring frequently, until the onion is softened and golden brown, about 10 minutes. Add the tomatoes and kale and cook, stirring frequently, until they soften, about 10 minutes. Add the beans and parsley, stir to mix, and season to taste with salt, pepper, and if desired, fresh lemon juice. Set the bean mixture aside, covered, to keep warm.

2. Preheat the broiler.

3. Melt the butter in a small saucepan over low heat. Stir in the lemon juice. Place the scallops in a broiling pan and

From the Test Kitchen

Make the white beans again, or cook extra—just about any roasted or grilled fish (halibut, salmon, sea bass), seafood (shrimp, calamari), poultry (chicken, turkey), or meat (pork, beef, lamb) will be tasty served on top.

brush the tops with half of the lemon butter. Broil the scallops close to the heat until browned, 2 to 3 minutes. Turn the scallops and brush them with the remaining lemon butter. Broil the second side until the scallops are just cooked through and springy to the touch, 2 to 3 minutes.

4. Divide the bean mixture between two serving plates. Lightly season the scallops with salt and pepper, then arrange them on top of the beans. Sprinkle additional chopped parsley on top, if desired.

NUTRITION INFO: 1 portion provides:

Protein: 1½ servings

Vitamin C: 1½ servings

Vitamin A: 2 servings

Other fruits and vegetables: ½ serving

Whole grains and legumes: 1 serving

Iron: some

Fat: ½ serving

Shrimp and Watermelon Kebabs

SERVES 4

When watermelon meets heat, its texture softens, and its sweetness deepens, making this expectant-mom favorite fruit an unexpectedly complementary companion for savory shrimp—especially when sriracha adds spice to the mix. Serve the kebabs over brown rice, farro, or whole-grain couscous, or toss with arugula and pasteurized feta for a satisfying dinner salad.

1 pound shelled and deveined large
    shrimp
2 tablespoons sriracha
1 tablespoon olive oil
1 tablespoon orange juice
1 tablespoon low-sodium soy sauce
1 tablespoon honey
1 teaspoon minced garlic
4 cups cubed seedless watermelon
    (1-inch pieces)
½ medium-size red onion, cut into
    1-inch pieces
1 teaspoon kosher salt
1 tablespoon chopped fresh basil

1. If you are using wooden or bamboo skewers, soak in water for 10 minutes so they won't burn.

2. Place the shrimp, sriracha, olive oil, orange juice, soy sauce, honey, and garlic in a large bowl. Stir to coat the shrimp evenly with the marinade. Cover the bowl with plastic wrap and refrigerate for up to 30 minutes.

3. Preheat the broiler or heat a grill to high. Remove the shrimp from the marinade and thread them onto 8 skewers, alternating pieces of watermelon and red onion between the shrimp. Discard any leftover marinade. Sprinkle the kebabs with the salt.

4. Broil or grill until the shrimp turn pink and are cooked through, turning occasionally, 3 to 4 minutes total. Sprinkle evenly with the basil before serving.

NUTRITION INFO: 1 portion provides:

Protein: 1 serving

Vitamin C: 1 serving

Iron: some

Omegas: some

Shrimp with Feta

SERVES 2

Here's a traditional Greek dish that's bound to become a tradition in your home, too—especially when you see how easy it is to make. Serve the shrimp over whole-wheat orzo, farro, quinoa, brown rice, or the whole grain of your choice.

1 tablespoon olive oil

1 medium-size red bell pepper, chopped

1 small fennel bulb, trimmed, halved, and
  thinly sliced crosswise

3 cloves garlic, minced (optional)

4 ripe roma tomatoes, seeded and
  chopped

1 tablespoon minced fresh oregano or
  1 teaspoon dried oregano

¾ pound shelled and deveined large
  shrimp

Fresh lemon juice

Black pepper

½ cup crumbled pasteurized feta cheese

¼ cup toasted pine nuts (see page 217;
  optional)

Salt

2 tablespoons chopped fresh flat-leaf
  (Italian) parsley

1. Heat the olive oil in a large skillet over medium-high heat. Add the bell pepper, fennel, and garlic, if using, and cook, stirring frequently, until the vegetables are softened, about 5 minutes. Add the tomatoes and oregano and cook, stirring frequently, until the tomatoes are slightly softened, about 2 minutes. Stir in the shrimp and cook until they are cooked through and turn opaque, about 4 minutes.

From the Test Kitchen

Don't feel like splurging on shrimp? Try substituting an equal amount of cubed skinless, boneless chicken breast or turkey tenders—or cubed firm tofu for a good vegetarian alternative. Just cook the chicken or turkey until it's cooked through before adding it to the sauce. Add the tofu after the tomatoes and oregano.

---

2. Season the shrimp and vegetables to taste with lemon juice and black pepper. Add the feta, stir well, and let simmer until the cheese begins to melt, about 30 seconds. Stir in the pine nuts, if using, and season with salt to taste (you may not need any since the feta is salty). Sprinkle the parsley on top and serve.

NUTRITION INFO: 1 portion provides:

Protein: 1½ servings

Calcium: 1 serving

Vitamin C: 3 servings

Vitamin A: 1 serving

Fat: ½ serving

Iron: some

Omegas: some

Shrimp Remoulade Toast

SERVES 2

The Big Easy classic made, well, easy. And this shrimp remoulade isn't just a lighter lift, it's lighter, too. And has long been a New Orleans staple. Top your toast first with a little shredded Romaine for some extra nutrition.

½ pound shelled and deveined medium-size shrimp

2 teaspoons olive oil

2 tablespoons mayonnaise

2 cups shredded romaine lettuce (optional)

¼ cup plain low-fat Greek yogurt

¼ cup buttermilk

1½ tablespoons chopped fresh flat-leaf (Italian) parsley

1½ teaspoons prepared horseradish, drained

1½ teaspoons fresh lemon juice

1½ teaspoons chopped drained capers

½ teaspoon paprika

¼ teaspoon black pepper

4 slices whole-grain bread, toasted

2 cups shredded romaine lettuce (optional)

1. Preheat the broiler to high.

2. Toss the shrimp with the olive oil in a bowl. Arrange the shrimp in a single layer on a baking sheet. Broil until the shrimp are cooked through and turn opaque, about 3 minutes, turning after 2 minutes. Remove from the oven and cool completely.

3. Whisk together the mayonnaise, yogurt, buttermilk, parsley, horseradish, lemon juice, capers, paprika, and pepper in a medium-size bowl. Set aside.

4. Stir the shrimp into the remoulade. To serve, top the toast with romaine, if desired, about ½ cup each. Spoon the shrimp and sauce on top of the toast and serve.

NUTRITION INFO: 1 portion provides:

Protein: 1 serving

Vitamin C: 1 serving if using romaine

Vitamin A: 1 serving if using romaine

Whole grains and legumes: 2 servings

Fat: 1 serving

Iron: some

Omegas: some

Pan-Fried Trout with Tomatoes and Spinach

SERVES 2

A delicious cornmeal crust adds crunch to trout. Then it's topped with a warm salad of tomato and spinach. This is what happens when fish leaves the campfire and goes uptown on the stove.

½ cup whole-grain (non-degerminated) cornmeal
2 tablespoons grated Parmesan cheese (optional)
1 teaspoon grated lemon zest
Salt and black pepper
Garlic powder
1 large egg
¼ cup buttermilk
2 large boneless trout fillets (each about 6 ounces)
Olive oil cooking spray
1½ tablespoons olive oil
1 tablespoon fresh lemon juice
4 ripe roma tomatoes, seeded and chopped
2 teaspoons chopped fresh tarragon, or ½ teaspoon dried
1 package (5 to 6 ounces) baby spinach
2 teaspoons minced fresh chives
Lemon wedges, for serving

1. Place the cornmeal, Parmesan cheese, if using, lemon zest, and a pinch each of salt, pepper, and garlic powder in a shallow dish and stir to mix. Place the egg and the buttermilk in another shallow dish and gently whisk to combine.

2. Dip each trout fillet in the egg mixture, then in the cornmeal mixture, turning it to coat evenly and thoroughly.

3. Coat a large skillet with olive oil cooking spray, then heat 1½ teaspoons of the olive oil in it over medium heat. Add the trout and cook until the coating is browned and the fish is cooked through, about 4 minutes per side. Transfer the trout to a platter and cover with aluminum foil to keep warm.

4. Add the remaining 1 tablespoon olive oil and the lemon juice to the skillet and scrape up the browned bits. Add the tomatoes and tarragon, reduce the heat to low, and cook until the tomatoes soften slightly, about 2 minutes. Add the spinach and cook, stirring, until barely wilted, about 2 minutes. Season with salt and pepper to taste. Top the trout with the tomato and spinach mixture, sprinkle with chives, and serve with lemon wedges.

NUTRITION INFO: 1 portion provides:

Protein: 1½ servings

Vitamin C: 2 servings

Vitamin A: 3 servings

Whole grains and legumes: 1 serving

Iron: some

Fat: ½ serving plus

From the Test Kitchen

The combination of trout and nuts goes way back. For a change of pace, replace the cornmeal breading for the pan-fried trout with a combination of ¼ cup ground toasted pecans or hazelnuts (see page 217), ⅓ cup dry whole-wheat bread crumbs, ¼ cup minced fresh flat-leaf (Italian) parsley, 1 teaspoon grated lemon zest, and a pinch each of salt and black pepper. Skip the egg and buttermilk bath; just moisten the trout fillets with milk before dredging them in the nut mixture. Pan-fry the fish in a combination of 1½ teaspoons butter and 1½ teaspoons olive oil. Sprinkle the trout with minced chives and lemon juice, and serve with lemon wedges and a pilaf instead of the tomato and spinach mixture.

Veggies, Beans, and Grains

S eeking sweet potato fries with that snapper? Broccoli with that beef? A pilaf bed for your chicken? Or a meatless main that highlights grains—or legumes, or veggies? Whether you're searching for the perfect side for your meat, poultry, fish, or seafood or planning plant-focused meals, you'll find just what you're looking for in this batch of veggie, bean, and grain recipes. Side dishes that aren't besides the point, instead standing out in nutrition and taste—like Smoky Roasted Carrots with Lime Cream, Cheesy Roasted Cauliflower, and Kale and Shiitake Mushroom Salad, Farro Risotto with Mushrooms. And easy, tasty meatless meals that could satisfy even confirmed carnivores, like Sheet-Pan Tofu with Broccolini and Sweet Potatoes. Add an egg, some cheese, and any of these veggie sides can become a light meal, too.

Broccoli Vinaigrette

SERVES 4

As much a salad as a veggie side, this delicious hybrid tops steamed broccoli with a zesty vinaigrette. Coarsely chopped nuts add a crunchy crowning touch. Want to crown your broccoli twice? Add a sprinkle of grated Parmesan. The broccoli is delicious the next day, too.

3 cups broccoli florets

1 teaspoon minced shallot

2 tablespoons fresh lemon juice, plus
    more to taste

2 tablespoons extra virgin olive oil

2 teaspoons Dijon mustard, optional

2 teaspoons minced fresh chives

Salt and black pepper

¼ cup coarsely chopped toasted
    pistachios or walnuts (see page 217)

1. Steam the broccoli following the instructions in the box below until crisp-tender, 4 to 5 minutes. Place the broccoli in a large bowl.

2. Place the shallots, lemon juice, olive oil, mustard, if using, and chives in a small bowl and whisk to mix, then season with salt and pepper to taste. Pour the vinaigrette over the broccoli and toss well to coat. Sprinkle the pistachios over the broccoli just before serving.

NUTRITION INFO: 1 portion provides:

Vitamin C: 1 serving

Vitamin A: 1½ servings

Fat: ½ serving

Omegas: some

Steaming Savvy

When it comes to vegetables, steaming beats boiling hands down. First, it retains far more nutrients. When you boil vegetables, the nutrients end up in the cooking water; that's fine if you're going to drink the cooking water—as in a soup—but not so fine if you'll be pouring the water down the drain. Second, steaming eliminates 2 steps: there's no waiting for a big pot of water to boil; and there's no draining afterwards. Third, and possibly most important, steaming preserves flavor and texture.

If those aren't enough reasons to switch to steaming, here's one more: It couldn't be easier. Just pour water to a depth of 1 inch into a large pot with a tight-fitting cover and bring it to a boil. Season the veggies now if you won't later. Place the veggies in the steamer basket, lower the basket into the pot, cover the pot, and steam the vegetables until they are just tender. Serve them as is with just a squeeze of lemon, or toss them into any recipe that calls for cooked veggies. (Steaming is also an easy way to cook shrimp.) For microwave steaming tips, see page 322.

Asparagus and Parmesan Curls

SERVES 2

Serve this asparagus alongside a fish, chicken, or meat dish or as an elegant start to any meal.

½ pound asparagus stalks
2 teaspoons olive oil
Juice and grated zest of ½ lemon
Salt and black pepper
¼ cup Parmesan or provolone cheese
    shavings (about 1 ounce; see page 251)

1. Trim off and discard the tough stem ends of the asparagus stalks.

2. Steam the asparagus following the instructions in the box on page 315 until just tender, 4 to 6 minutes, depending on the thickness of the asparagus.

3. Pat the asparagus dry and divide them evenly between two serving plates. Drizzle the olive oil and lemon juice over the asparagus, and top it with the lemon zest. Season with salt and pepper to taste, then top with the cheese shavings.

From the Test Kitchen

Steam twice as much asparagus as you want to serve, then chill the leftovers for the next day's salad. It's delicious tossed with a little lemon vinaigrette, as in Broccoli Vinaigrette (page 315). Or skip the steaming, and roast the asparagus in a hot oven (see the box on the next page). Like a green leafy option? Substitute broccoli or baby broccoli (broccolini) for the asparagus.

NUTRITION INFO: 1 portion provides:

Calcium: ½ serving

Vitamin C: 1 serving

For Veggies with the Most, Just Roast

So long, steaming! To get the most from your veggies, roast them. From Brussels sprouts to cauliflower, carrots to butternut squash, broccoli to mushrooms, pretty much every vegetable takes on a deeper, sweeter, more complex taste and earthy, almost meaty texture when roasted. Plus, the prep and cleanup couldn't be easier. Just preheat the oven to 425°F and line a large baking sheet with parchment paper. Then place your veggies, cut into bite-size pieces (small florets for cauliflower and broccoli, halved Brussels sprouts, small chunks of winter squash; asparagus can be roasted whole) in one layer on the sheet. Spray or drizzle with olive oil and sprinkle with salt, coarse black pepper, and if desired, fresh herbs (say, thyme leaves or rosemary springs, chopped Italian parsley or sage), and toss to coat. Roast the veggies until tender and golden, even a little charred around the edges, stirring once during baking. Roasting times will vary, but average 20 to 30 minutes. Serve your veggies hot or at room temperature, straight up or with a vinaigrette, a squeeze of lemon, or some grated cheese. Leftovers (if you don't end up eating them all) can be served cold in a salad the next day, or right from the fridge as a snack.

Roast Butternut Squash

SERVES 4

Getting a vitamin A plus was never this easy or yummy. Leftovers warm up easily the next day.

Olive oil cooking spray

1 package (16 ounces) cubed peeled butternut squash

2 tablespoons olive oil

1 tablespoon fresh thyme leaves or 1 teaspoon dried thyme

½ cup grated Parmesan cheese

1. Preheat the oven to 400°F.

2. Coat a 9 x 13-inch baking dish with olive oil cooking spray, then add the squash. Drizzle the olive oil over the squash, sprinkle the thyme on top, and toss gently to coat evenly.

3. Bake the squash until tender and golden brown, about 25 minutes. Sprinkle the Parmesan over the squash before serving.

NUTRITION INFO: 1 portion provides:

Calcium: ½ serving

Vitamin C: 2 servings

Vitamin A: 4 servings

Fat: ½ serving

Smoky Roasted Carrots with Lime Cream

SERVES 2

If smoky and sweet had a baby (carrot), this would be the delicious result. Warm, roasted spice is cooled by a tangy, creamy topping, with a sprinkle of almonds adding crunch and a toasty note.

¾ pound small carrots
    (about 12 carrots) peeled, stems
    removed
1 teaspoon olive oil
½ teaspoon ground cumin
½ teaspoon smoked paprika
¼ teaspoon chili powder
¼ teaspoon kosher salt
3 tablespoons light sour cream
1 tablespoon fresh lime juice
¼ cup chopped roasted unsalted
    almonds or shelled pistachios
1 tablespoon chopped fresh cilantro
    leaves

1. Preheat the oven to 425°F. Line a rimmed baking sheet with parchment paper.

2. Toss together the carrots, oil, cumin, paprika, chili powder, and salt in a medium bowl, rubbing the spices into the carrots. Spread out the carrots on the prepared baking sheet in a single layer. Roast until tender, about 15 minutes.

3. Meanwhile, stir together the sour cream and lime juice in a small bowl.

4. Transfer the carrots to a serving platter and top with the sour cream mixture, almonds, and cilantro. Serve immediately.

NUTRITION INFO: 1 portion provides:

Vitamin A: 3 servings

Fat: ½ serving

Omegas: some

Lemon Carrots with Rosemary

SERVES 2

Baby carrots with a twist of lemon and a sprinkling of aromatic rosemary make a classic companion to roast chicken or store-bought rotisserie chicken. They're also delish with fish.

2 teaspoons olive oil or butter
1½ cups baby carrots
¼ cup low-sodium chicken broth or
  vegetable broth
1 clove garlic, minced
2 teaspoons fresh chopped rosemary or
  ½ teaspoon dried rosemary
1 teaspoon grated lemon zest
Salt and black pepper
Fresh lemon juice

1. Heat 1 teaspoon of the olive oil or melt the butter in a large nonstick skillet over medium heat. Add the carrots and cook until they begin to soften, about 2 minutes. Stir in the broth and bring to a boil. Reduce the heat, cover the skillet, and let the carrots simmer until they are tender, about 10 minutes. Transfer the carrots to a bowl and set aside, covered, to keep warm.

2. Heat the remaining 1 teaspoon olive oil in the same skillet over medium heat. Add the garlic and cook until it begins to soften, about 1 minute. Add the rosemary and lemon zest. Return the cooked carrots to the pan and stir to coat them.

From the Test Kitchen

Using thyme leaves in the Lemon Carrots in place of the rosemary makes them a perfect partner for poultry. Feeling fishy? Substitute 2 teaspoons chopped fresh dill or ½ teaspoon dried dill.

3. Remove the carrots from the heat. Season with salt, pepper, and lemon juice to taste and serve.

NUTRITION INFO: 1 portion provides:

Vitamin A: 3 servings

Fat: ½ serving

Balsamic Braised Red Cabbage

SERVES 4

Braising red cabbage with balsamic vinegar helps preserve its color and infuses it with a delectably sweet and complex flavor. Fresh and dried cranberries contribute to the color scheme as well as to the nutritional content and tangy taste. Team this traditional holiday favorite with the Christmas goose, the Thanksgiving turkey—or Tuesday night's pork chop.

4 cups thinly sliced red cabbage
  (about 1 small head)
2 cups low-sodium vegetable broth or
  chicken broth
¼ cup balsamic vinegar
1 tablespoon honey
1 cup fresh or frozen cranberries
⅓ cup dried cranberries

1. Preheat the oven to 400°F.

2. Place the cabbage, vegetable broth, balsamic vinegar, honey, and fresh and dried cranberries in a large mixing bowl and stir to mix. Transfer the cabbage mixture to a flameproof baking dish. Bring the mixture to a boil over medium heat.

From the Test Kitchen

Don't have an hour to spare? Simply place all of the ingredients for Balsamic Braised Red Cabbage in a large saucepan over medium heat and bring them to a simmer. Cover the pan and let the cabbage cook until tender, about 10 minutes. Another tip: Make this dish up to 2 days in advance—the flavors will deepen. Warm the braised cabbage before serving, or just let it return to room temperature.

3. Carefully cover the baking dish with aluminum foil and transfer it to the oven. Bake until the cabbage is tender, about 45 minutes. Serve warm or at room temperature. The cabbage can be stored in the refrigerator, covered, for up to 2 days.

NUTRITION INFO: 1 portion provides:

Vitamin C: 1 serving

Other fruits and vegetables: 1 serving

Cheesy Roasted Cauliflower

SERVES 4

Even the most resolute vegetable resister will relent to this homey dish of cauliflower topped with a creamy cheese sauce that's packed with calcium and flavor.

1 small head cauliflower, rinsed, patted
    dry, and cut into florets (about 2 cups)
2 tablespoons olive oil
1 cup milk
2 tablespoons all-purpose flour
1 cup grated cheddar or Gruyère cheese
Salt and white pepper

1. Preheat the oven to 400°F.

2. Toss the cauliflower with the oil in a medium-size bowl until coated. Spread in a single layer on a baking sheet and roast for 25 to 30 minutes, until tender and the edges are golden brown.

3. Meanwhile, place the milk and flour in a small saucepan and stir until the flour dissolves. Bring to a boil over medium-high heat, then reduce the heat and let simmer, stirring occasionally, until the sauce thickens, about 4 minutes.

From the Test Kitchen

Say "cheese" two ways: You can also use a combination of Parmesan and cheddar in the sauce for the cauliflower. And because broccoli loves cheese, too, try this cheese sauce on roasted broccoli. Or make a combo of broccoli and cauliflower. Time extra short? Use the cheese sauce over steamed-in-the-bag cauliflower or broccoli.

4. Remove the saucepan from the heat. Add the cheese and stir until it melts. Season with salt and pepper to taste, then pour the sauce over the roasted cauliflower.

NUTRITION INFO: 1 portion provides:

Calcium: 1 serving

Vitamin C: 1 serving

Fat: ½ serving

That's Italian Green Beans

SERVES 2

Any green vegetables take a turn for the Tuscan when prepared with tomatoes, Italian herbs, and Parmesan cheese. Steamed broccoli is also tasty prepared this way. Add extra cheese on top for a calcium fix.

½ pound green beans, trimmed
½ cup canned Italian seasoned diced
   tomatoes, drained
1½ teaspoons minced fresh oregano or
   ½ teaspoon dried
1½ teaspoons minced fresh basil or
   ½ teaspoon dried
2 tablespoons grated Parmesan cheese
Pinch of crushed red pepper flakes
   (optional)

1. Steam the green beans following the instructions on page 315 until just tender but still crisp, 4 to 5 minutes.

2. Transfer the green beans to a saucepan, add the tomatoes, oregano, basil, Parmesan, and red pepper flakes, if using, and stir to mix. Cook over medium heat until heated through, about 1 minute.

NUTRITION INFO: 1 portion provides:

Vitamin C: ½ serving

Other fruits and vegetables: 1 serving

Vegetables in a Flash

You can't beat steaming when it comes to retaining the nutrients found in vegetables, but you can beat the clock by using a microwave to bring freshly cooked vegetables to the table in 4 minutes or less. When you need to save even more time and effort, choose ready-to-cook vegetables in a bag (you can shave off even more time by buying steam-in-the-bag veggies and zapping them according to the package directions).

Ready to make microwave magic? Arrange the vegetables (the pieces should be uniform in size) in a single layer in a microwave-safe dish. Add 2 tablespoons vegetable or chicken broth (you can also use water). Season the vegetables if you like with herbs, garlic powder, a sprinkle of lemon juice, a dash of salt and pepper, even a spoonful or two of chopped fresh or canned tomatoes—or nothing at all, if you like your veggies naked, or you'll be adding the steamed veggies to another recipe or topping them with a sauce later. Tent the dish with microwave-safe plastic wrap, punctured to allow steam to escape (don't let the plastic touch the veggies). Or skip the plastic wrap and cover with a microwave-safe plate. Or, best option: Invest in a microwave steamer dish that comes with a cover.

Microwave veggies on high until just tender, 1½ to 4 minutes, depending on the thickness and how crisp you like them; larger amounts of vegetables may need longer cooking times. Let the vegetables stand for 3 to 5 minutes before serving.

Minty Peas, Carrots, and Mushrooms

SERVES 2

The unexpected addition of mint and shiitake mushrooms to peas and carrots gives you a deliciously sophisticated take on the standard school cafeteria version. You'll eat every carrot and pea on your plate when they're cooked this way. (And make it faster still by using frozen or steam-in-the-bag peas and carrots.)

¾ cup shelled fresh green peas, or
     ¾ cup frozen green peas
½ cup thinly sliced carrots
1 tablespoon olive oil or butter
1 cup sliced shiitake mushroom caps
1 teaspoon minced shallot, optional
1 tablespoon chopped fresh mint
Salt and black pepper

1. Cook the peas and carrots separately until crisp-tender, following the steaming instructions on page 315 or the microwave oven instructions on the facing page, about 2 minutes for steamed peas or 1½ minutes in the microwave, and 3 minutes for steamed carrots or 2½ minutes in the microwave.

2. Heat the olive oil in a saucepan over medium heat. Add the mushrooms and shallot and cook until they begin to soften, about 2 minutes. Add the peas, carrots, and mint and stir gently until heated through. Season with salt and pepper to taste and serve.

NUTRITION INFO: 1 portion provides:

Vitamin C: ½ serving

Vitamin A: 1 serving

Other fruits and vegetables: 1 serving

Fat: ½ serving

Kale and Shiitake Mushroom Salad

SERVES 2

Is it a salad, or is it a stir-fry? Don't try to label it—just enjoy it, along with a day's worth of green and yellow vegetables and a bonus of soy protein.

1 small bunch kale (8 ounces), thick stems and tough center veins removed, rinsed well
2 tablespoons low-sodium vegetable broth
1 tablespoon low-sodium soy sauce
1 tablespoon sesame oil
1 cup frozen shelled edamame (soybeans)
1¾ cups sliced shiitake mushroom caps
¼ cup carrot matchsticks
2 tablespoons seasoned rice vinegar
2 teaspoons olive oil or canola oil
1 tablespoon toasted sesame seeds (see page 217)

1. Cut the kale into ½-inch strips.

2. Place the vegetable broth, soy sauce, and sesame oil in a large skillet over medium-low heat and bring to a simmer. Add the kale and edamame and toss to coat. Cover the skillet and cook just until the kale begins to wilt, 2 to 3 minutes. Transfer the vegetables to a salad bowl.

3. Add the shiitake mushrooms and carrots to the skillet and cook until just tender, 2 to 3 minutes. Add the mushroom mixture to the kale mixture and let cool to room temperature.

4. Just before serving, place the rice vinegar and oil in a small bowl and whisk to mix. Drizzle it over the vegetable mixture and toss to coat. Sprinkle the sesame seeds on top and serve.

NUTRITION INFO: 1 portion provides:

Protein: ½ serving

Calcium: 1 serving

Vitamin C: 1½ servings

Vitamin A: 4 servings

Other fruits and vegetables: 1½ servings

Whole grains and legumes: 1 serving

Iron: some

Fat: 1 serving

Italian Swiss Chard

SERVES 2

This tasty sauté brings out the best in sturdy green leafy vegetables; try it with kale, too.

1 bunch Swiss chard (about 1 pound),
    rinsed and patted dry
¾ cup low-sodium chicken broth or
    vegetable broth
2 teaspoons olive oil
1 clove garlic, minced
2 teaspoons minced shallot
¼ cup grated Parmesan cheese
2 tablespoons toasted pine nuts
    (see page 217)
Salt and black pepper

1. Slice the leaves off the stems of the Swiss chard. Coarsely chop the leaves and cut the stems crosswise into pieces about ½ inch wide and 2 inches long.

2. Place the chicken broth in a small saucepan and bring to a simmer over medium heat. Add the Swiss chard stems, reduce the heat to low, and cook until just tender, 8 to 10 minutes. Drain and set aside.

3. Heat the olive oil in a large nonstick skillet over medium-low heat. Add the garlic and shallot and cook, stirring occasionally, until softened, about 2 minutes. Add the Swiss chard leaves and cooked stems and cook, stirring, until the leaves are just wilted, 1 to 2 minutes.

4. Add the Parmesan and pine nuts to the Swiss chard and stir to mix. Season with salt and pepper to taste and serve.

NUTRITION INFO: 1 portion provides:

Calcium: ½ serving

Vitamin C: ½ serving

Vitamin A: 2 servings

Iron: some

Great Greens

Many greens that you're used to eating raw in salads wilt well—and tastily. And since the greens cook down, you can pack far more vitamin power into an average portion. Try arugula or baby spinach, following the recipe for Italian Swiss Chard, starting with Step 3, since these do not have tough stems. Tender greens like these wilt in no time. Serve wilted greens as a side dish or as a delicious bed for fish or chicken.

Oven-Roasted Potatoes

SERVES 2

You don't need a trip through the golden arches when these golden but nearly greaseless potatoes are just twenty-five minutes from your plate.

Olive oil cooking spray
2 medium-size Yukon Gold or red
   potatoes (about ¾ pound total)
1 tablespoon olive oil
Salt and cracked black pepper

1. Preheat the oven to 425°F. Coat a large rimmed baking sheet with olive oil cooking spray.

2. Cut the potatoes into ¼-inch-thick slices, then pat them dry with paper towels. Place the potatoes in a bowl, drizzle the olive oil over them, then toss to coat evenly.

3. Arrange the potato slices on the baking sheet in a single layer and lightly season them with salt and cracked pepper.

4. Bake the potato slices until golden brown on top, about 15 minutes. Turn the potatoes over and continue baking until the second side is golden brown and the potato slices are tender, 10 to 15 minutes longer. If you like crisper potatoes, let them bake a little longer but watch them carefully so they don't burn.

From the Test Kitchen

Fries with that? Cut potatoes into thick french fry–shaped sticks. Toss them with olive oil, then place them in a single layer on a rimmed baking sheet that has been coated with cooking oil spray. Bake the potatoes in an oven preheated to 400°F for 15 minutes. Stir the potatoes to turn and continue baking for another 10 minutes. For extra-crisp potatoes, stir them every 5 minutes. You can shake things up a bit by sprinkling some grated Parmesan cheese, garlic powder, or chili powder over them—or whatever flavor you fancy.

NUTRITION INFO: 1 portion provides:
Vitamin C: 1 serving
Fat: ½ serving

Green Mashers

SERVES 2

Festive on St. Patrick's Day, but so delicious you'll want to serve them all year round. The green—and a healthy dose of protein—comes from the edamame the potatoes are mashed with.

1 cup frozen shelled edamame (soybeans)
2 small Yukon Gold potatoes, cut into 1-inch chunks
1 can (14.5 ounces) low-sodium chicken broth or vegetable broth
⅓ cup milk or buttermilk, plus more as needed
2 teaspoons olive oil (optional)
¼ cup grated Parmesan cheese, or more to taste (optional)
Salt and black pepper

1. Bring a saucepan of water to a boil over high heat, add the edamame, and return to a boil. Reduce the heat to medium and cook the edamame until very soft, about 12 minutes. Drain and set aside.

2. Place the potatoes and enough broth to cover them in a small saucepan. Bring to a boil over high heat, then reduce the heat and let simmer until the potatoes are tender, 10 to 15 minutes. Drain, reserving the cooking liquid.

3. Place the milk in a small microwave-safe bowl and microwave at medium-high-power until heated through, about 45 seconds (or warm the milk in a small saucepan).

4. Place the cooked edamame and a few tablespoons of the reserved potato cooking liquid in a food processor and process until smooth, then transfer to a bowl. Add the cooked potatoes, warm milk, olive oil, and Parmesan, if using. Using a potato masher, mash to the desired consistency, adding more cooking liquid or warm milk as needed. Season with salt and pepper to taste and serve immediately.

NUTRITION INFO: 1 portion provides:

Protein: ½ serving

Calcium: ½ serving if made with Parmesan cheese

Vitamin C: 1½ servings

Whole grains and legumes: 1 serving

Iron: some

Roasted Herbed Sweet Potatoes

SERVES 2

Pop sweet potatoes in the oven when you're roasting poultry or meat, then pop the fragrant, golden brown wedges in your mouth anytime. If you can find them, try using purple sweet potatoes.

Olive oil cooking spray
1 medium-size sweet potato
   (about ½ pound), unpeeled
1 tablespoon olive oil
1 teaspoon chopped fresh rosemary
1 tablespoon chopped fresh oregano or
   1 teaspoon dried oregano
Dash of ground nutmeg
Dash of ground cumin
Salt and black pepper

1. Preheat the oven to 425°F. Coat a small baking dish with olive oil cooking spray.

2. Cut the sweet potato in half lengthwise. Cut each half into 6 wedges.

3. Place the sweet potato wedges, olive oil, rosemary, oregano, nutmeg, cumin, and a sprinkle each of salt and pepper in a large bowl and toss gently to coat evenly.

4. Place the sweet potato wedges in the baking dish in a single layer and bake, uncovered, until tender and golden brown, about 45 minutes, gently stirring them halfway through.

Microbaked Potatoes

Craving the creaming comfort of a baked potato without the wait? Skip the baking and head for the microwave instead. To microbake a large potato, scrub well, pat dry, and poke 4 or 5 times with a paring knife (to allow steam to escape and avoid a potato explosion). Place on a microwave-safe dish. Microwave on high power for about 7 minutes (12 minutes for 2 potatoes), flipping halfway through cooking (use a mitt—the potato will be hot). Feeling sweet? You can microbake a scrubbed, poked sweet potato on high in 5 to 6 minutes, flipping carefully halfway through. Check any potato for doneness by sticking a fork in—it should be soft through. If it's too firm, continue microwaving a minute at a time.

NUTRITION INFO: 1 portion provides:

Vitamin C: ½ serving

Vitamin A: 1 serving

Fat: ½ serving

Sweet Potato Chips

SERVES 2

Bet you can't stop at just one Sweet Potato Chip—and there's no good reason why you should. You can get a chip fix and a hefty dose of vitamin A in the bargain.

Olive oil cooking spray
1 medium-size sweet potato
   (about ½ pound)
1 tablespoon olive oil
2 tablespoons grated Parmesan cheese
1 teaspoon chopped fresh thyme
Salt and black pepper (optional)

1. Preheat the oven to 425°F. Coat a large rimmed baking sheet with olive oil cooking spray.

2. Peel the sweet potato, then cut into ¼-inch-thick slices. Pat the slices dry with paper towels. Arrange the sweet potato slices on the baking sheet in a single layer and brush the tops with the olive oil.

3. Bake the sweet potato slices until the tops brown slightly, about 15 minutes. Turn the slices over and continue baking until the second side is lightly browned and the sweet potatoes are tender, 10 to 15 minutes longer. If you like crisper sweet potatoes, let them bake a little longer but watch them carefully so they don't burn.

4. Sprinkle the Parmesan, thyme, and salt and pepper, if desired, over the sweet potatoes before serving.

NUTRITION INFO: 1 portion provides:

Vitamin C: ½ serving

Vitamin A: 1 serving

Fat: ½ serving

Roasted Roots

SERVES 4

You'll want to return to these roots over and over again, and to make extra so that you'll have leftovers (served cold, they'd make a delicious addition to a salad or sandwich, too). For easy cleanup, line your pan with parchment paper before coating with oil.

Olive oil cooking spray
1 medium-size sweet potato, halved, each half quartered
4 medium-size parsnips, peeled
4 medium-size carrots, peeled
½ pound beets, trimmed, peeled, and cut into 1-inch chunks
1 large fennel bulb, trimmed and quartered
2 tablespoons olive oil
1 tablespoon fresh thyme leaves
Salt and freshly ground black pepper
Grated zest of 1 lemon (optional)

1. Preheat the oven to 425°F. Coat a roasting pan with olive oil cooking spray (or line the pan with parchment paper for easier cleanup).

2. Arrange sweet potatoes, parsnips, carrots, beets, and fennel in a single layer in the roasting pan. Brush the vegetables with the olive oil and sprinkle the thyme over them. Season with salt and pepper. Cover the roasting pan with aluminum foil.

3. Roast the vegetables until they begin to soften, about 25 minutes. Uncover the pan and stir the vegetables. Roast them uncovered until tender and golden brown, about 20 minutes longer.

From the Test Kitchen

Roasting brings out the best flavor in just about every vegetable. You can use any of the following in place of, or in addition to, those in Pan-Roasted Vegetables: chunks of red onion, turnips, celery root, rutabaga, acorn squash and/or butternut squash, and whole peeled pearl onions. Just be sure that they are roughly the same size, or cut into comparable-size pieces.

And don't stop there. Roast cauliflower with cumin seeds, green beans with oregano, tomatoes with basil, and just about any vegetable with rosemary or sage. See page 317 for more.

4. Place the vegetables on a platter and sprinkle the lemon zest, if using, over them. The vegetables can be refrigerated, covered, for up to 2 days. Reheat in the oven at 350°F until hot, about 10 minutes. They can also be enjoyed at room temperature or straight out of the fridge for a snack.

NUTRITION INFO: 1 portion provides:

Vitamin C: ½ serving

Vitamin A: 3 servings

Other fruits and vegetables: 2 servings

Fat: ½ serving

Edamame Succotash

SERVES 4

A far cry from the mushy cafeteria variety, this succotash—made with crisp asparagus, bright red bell pepper, sweet corn, and chewy edamame—is fresh tasting and packed with protein. Terrific, too, as a bed for fish fillets or chicken breasts.

1 tablespoon olive oil

½ cup chopped red bell pepper

1 cup low-sodium vegetable broth

12 asparagus stalks, trimmed and
** cut into ½-inch chunks**

1 cup shelled frozen edamame
** (soybeans)**

1 cup yellow corn kernels
** (fresh or thawed frozen)**

2 tablespoons chopped fresh flat-leaf
** (Italian) parsley**

Salt and cracked black pepper

Heat the olive oil in a medium-size nonstick skillet over low heat. Add the bell pepper and cook until it begins to soften, about 3 minutes. Add the vegetable broth, raise the heat to medium, and bring to a simmer. Add the asparagus, edamame, corn, and parsley. Cover the skillet, reduce the heat to low, and let simmer until just tender, about 4 minutes. Season the succotash with salt and cracked pepper to taste before serving.

NUTRITION INFO: 1 portion provides:

Protein: ½ serving

Vitamin C: 1 serving

Vitamin A: 1 serving

Whole grains and legumes: ½ serving

Other vegetables and fruits: ½ serving

Iron: some

Fat: ½ serving

Grilled Tofu

SERVES 2

Extra-firm tofu takes on an almost meaty texture when it's grilled, making this dish a great vegetarian alternative when you feel like passing on the sirloin. It's more like a meal than a side dish, especially when served over Spicy Greens with Ginger Dressing (page 256). Don't have a grill? Cook this dish on a grill pan heated to medium-high on the stovetop.

1 package (14 ounces) extra-firm tofu,
　　drained well on paper towels
¼ cup low-sodium soy sauce or tamari
2 teaspoons sesame oil
1 teaspoon canola oil
1 tablespoon honey
2 teaspoons minced garlic (optional)
1 teaspoon chile-garlic sauce, or sriracha
　　plus more to taste (optional)

1. Cut the tofu crosswise into 8 even slices. Place the tofu slices in a baking dish large enough to hold all of them in a single layer.

2. Place the soy sauce, sesame oil, canola oil, honey, and the garlic, and chile-garlic sauce or sriracha, if using, in a small bowl and stir to mix. Taste and add more chile-garlic sauce if desired. Pour the marinade over the tofu slices. Cover and let marinate in the refrigerator for 10 minutes, turning the tofu several times.

3. Meanwhile, set up the grill and preheat it to medium-high.

From the Test Kitchen

For a delicious nutty taste and crunch, try sprinkling the marinated tofu with untoasted sesame seeds before grilling it.

4. When you're ready to cook, oil the grill grate. Remove the tofu from the marinade and set the marinade aside. Grill the tofu until it's heated through and starts to brown, 3 to 4 minutes per side, brushing with reserved marinade as it grills.

NUTRITION INFO: 1 portion provides:

Protein: 1 serving

Calcium: ½ serving

Vitamin C: 1 serving

Iron: some

Fat: ½ serving

Broccoli and Tofu Stir-Fry

SERVES 2

You don't have to be a vegan to veg out on this nutritious Chinese favorite. It makes a meaty meatless meal, particularly when it's teamed with brown rice or soba noodles.

¾ cup plus 2 tablespoons low-sodium vegetable broth
2 tablespoons low-sodium soy sauce
2½ teaspoons all-purpose flour
2 teaspoons unseasoned rice vinegar
2 teaspoons sesame oil
1 tablespoon canola oil
8 ounces extra-firm tofu, drained well on paper towels and cut into ½-inch cubes
Pinch of salt
2 cups broccoli florets
2 teaspoons minced garlic
1 tablespoon grated peeled fresh ginger (optional)
1 cup sliced shiitake mushrooms
Crushed red pepper flakes (optional)

1. Place 2 tablespoons of the vegetable broth and the soy sauce, flour, rice vinegar, and sesame oil in a small bowl and whisk to mix. Set the sauce mixture aside.

2. Heat the canola oil in a large nonstick skillet over medium heat. Add the tofu and salt. Cook, stirring frequently, until the tofu is golden brown all over, about 8 minutes. Remove the tofu from the skillet.

3. Add the broccoli, the remaining ¾ cup broth, the garlic, and the ginger, if using, to the skillet. Cover and cook, stirring occasionally, until the broccoli is crisp-tender, about 4 minutes. Uncover the skillet, add the mushrooms and cook until softened, about 2 minutes. Add the sauce mixture and browned tofu to the broccoli and stir gently to coat. Season with red pepper flakes to taste, if desired. Cook, stirring occasionally, until the sauce thickens, about 2 minutes.

NUTRITION INFO: 1 portion provides:

Protein: ½ serving

Vitamin C: 2 servings

Vitamin A: 2 servings

Other fruits and vegetables: 1 serving

Iron: some

Fat: 1 serving

Sheet-Pan Tofu 3-Ways

SERVES 2

This simple technique will take your extra-firm tofu to places you never thought possible: crispy, meaty, flavorful. Baked tofu is incredibly versatile—use it with your favorite sauce or in your favorite recipe—from curry to teriyaki. Toss it into your favorite pasta dish, or in place of your usual protein in your sandwich or wrap. Or try it one of three delicious ways suggested here.

1 package (14 ounces) extra-firm tofu
1 tablespoon oil of your choice
1 tablespoon low-sodium soy sauce
1 tablespoon cornstarch or arrowroot
   starch

1. Preheat the oven to 400 degrees. Line a large baking sheet with parchment paper.

2. Place the tofu block on a clean kitchen towel or paper towels. Cover with another towel and place a skillet on top to weigh it down. Let the tofu drain for at least 10 minutes or up to 30 minutes. Transfer to a cutting board. Cut the block crosswise into 1-inch-thick slices and transfer to a medium bowl.

3. Drizzle tofu with oil of your choice and 1 tablespoon low-sodium soy sauce.

From the Test Kitchen

Leftover baked tofu keeps in the fridge for up to 3 days and reheats well in the microwave. Even better, toss it in the oven or toaster oven to resurrect its crispy edges.

Sprinkle with 1 tablespoon cornstarch or arrowroot starch and toss gently until the tofu is covered evenly. You can also sprinkle with seasoning, if you like—curry powder if you'll be making a curry, a little dried oregano and garlic powder if you're going Italian, chili powder if you'll be making Mexican.

4. Place the tofu on prepared baking sheet in a single layer. Bake for 25 to 30 minutes, carefully turning tofu over halfway, until tofu is golden brown and crispy around the edges.

Broccolini and Sweet Potatoes

SERVES 2

1 medium sweet potato (peeled or
   unpeeled) sliced lengthwise into
   ¾ wedges
2 tablespoons oil
1 teaspoon salt
½ teaspoon pepper
1 large bunch broccolini

1. Toss the sweet potato wedges in a bowl with 1 tablespoon oil, ½ teaspoon salt, ¼ teaspoon pepper, and place on a rimmed baking sheet. Transfer to preheated oven with tofu and bake 30 to 35 minutes, flipping wedges halfway through.

2. While potato wedges cook, toss the broccolini with 1 tablespoon oil, ½ teaspoon salt, ¼ teaspoon pepper, and add to the baking sheet with sweet potato wedges about halfway through and cook for the remaining 15 to 20 minutes until the sweet potatoes are browned and the broccolini is crisp-tender. If you are using regular broccoli, you'll need to add it a few minutes earlier.

3. Serve with Sheet-Pan Tofu and chopped, salted, roasted peanuts (if desired).

NUTRITION INFO: 1 portion provides:

Vitamin C: 1 serving

Vitamin A: 3 servings

Fat: 1½ servings

Iron: some

Peanut Sauce with Red Bell Peppers and Green Beans

SERVES 2

1 sliced large red bell pepper
6 ounces green beans (about ½ bag
    pre-packaged fresh green beans)
1 tablespoon oil
½ teaspoon salt
¼ teaspoon pepper
¼ cup creamy peanut butter
¼ cup well-shaken unsweetened canned
    coconut milk
1½ tablespoons lime juice
1 tablespoon low-sodium soy sauce
½ tablespoon sriracha

1. Toss bell pepper with green beans, oil, salt, and pepper. Transfer to a rimmed baking sheet and put in preheated oven with tofu. Cook for 15 minutes, or until vegetables are crisp-tender.

2. Meanwhile, in a small bowl whisk together the peanut butter, coconut milk, lime juice, soy sauce, and sriracha.

3. Serve roasted vegetables with Sheet-Pan Tofu and drizzle with desired amount of peanut sauce.

NUTRITION INFO: 1 portion provides:

Vitamin A: 3 servings

Other: 2 servings

Fat: 2½ servings

Protein: 1 serving

Curried Cauliflower

SERVES 2

1 tablespoon yellow curry paste
    (such as Thai Kitchen)
1 tablespoon water
1 tablespoon low-sodium soy sauce
2 teaspoons brown sugar
1 teaspoon chile-garlic sauce
1½ cups fresh cauliflower florets
3 tablespoons fresh cilantro
2 tablespoons toasted cashews
    (see page 217)

1. In a large bowl, whisk together the yellow curry paste, water, soy sauce, brown sugar, and chile-garlic sauce.

2. Add the cauliflower florets to bowl and toss until coated with curry mixture. Transfer to a rimmed baking sheet and add to preheated oven with tofu. Cook until browned and crisp-tender, about 20 minutes.

3. Serve with Sheet-Pan Tofu, garnished with the cilantro, and cashews (see page 217).

NUTRITION INFO: 1 portion provides:

Protein: 1 serving

Vitamin C: 2 servings

Cauliflower Fried "Rice" with Pickled Peppers

SERVES 2

Never thought of fried rice as health food? Think outside the greasy take-out box, and take in this tasty dish, packed with flavor and nutrients, but not with fat. The peppers spice things up (and they're pickled, always a pregnancy plus), while the peanuts add crunch. It partners well with chicken, pork, fish, or shrimp.

3 tablespoons vegetable oil

2 cups small broccoli florets

¼ cup thinly sliced shallots

2 large eggs, lightly beaten

1 (10-ounce) package riced cauliflower
   (2½ cups), thawed if frozen

2 tablespoons low-sodium soy sauce

1 tablespoon sesame oil

¼ teaspoon sugar

¼ teaspoon black pepper

½ cup Peppadew/Piquante pickled
   peppers or pickled banana peppers

2 tablespoons chopped fresh cilantro

2 tablespoons chopped roasted salted
   peanuts

1. Heat 1 tablespoon of the oil in a large nonstick skillet over medium-high heat. Add the broccoli and cook for 4 to 5 minutes, stirring occasionally, until it is bright green and slightly tender. Add the shallots and cook for 30 seconds more. Remove the skillet from the heat and transfer the vegetables to a plate.

From the Test Kitchen

Want some real rice with your veggie rice? Add ½ cup cooked brown or other whole-grain rice, or legume "rice," after the cauliflower rice is cooked.

2. Wipe the skillet clean (careful, it will be hot). Return it to the stove over medium heat and add 1 tablespoon of the remaining oil. Add the eggs and cook 2 to 3 minutes, until set, stirring once or twice. Transfer the eggs to a cutting board and cut into ½-inch pieces.

3. Raise the heat under the skillet to medium-high. Add the remaining 1 tablespoon oil. Add cauliflower and cook, undisturbed, until softened and lightly toasted, about 4 minutes. Remove from the heat. Stir in the soy sauce, sesame oil, sugar, pepper, broccoli mixture, and eggs. Divide between two serving plates and top with the pickled peppers, cilantro, and peanuts.

NUTRITION INFO: 1 portion provides:

Vitamin C: 4 servings

Vitamin A: 2 servings

Fat: 2 servings

Farro Risotto with Mushrooms

SERVES 2

Creamy and cheesy, this dish has all the best elements of a traditional risotto, making it a hearty sidekick for chicken or fish. Or serve the full recipe as a vegetarian main dish for one. The nutritious twist? Farro stands in for Arborio rice, lending more fiber and protein.

1 tablespoon olive oil or butter

1 tablespoon minced shallot

2 cups coarsely chopped mushrooms, such as portobello, brown, oyster, shiitake, or white button

1½ tablespoons chopped fresh flat-leaf (Italian) parsley

2 teaspoons fresh thyme leaves, or ½ teaspoon dried thyme

2 cloves garlic, minced

½ cup farro

2½ cups low-sodium vegetable broth or chicken broth, plus more as needed

1 tablespoon tomato paste

¾ cup grated Parmesan cheese

Salt and black pepper

1. Heat the olive oil in a medium-size nonstick saucepan over medium heat. Add the shallot and cook until softened, about 4 minutes.

2. Add the mushrooms and cook until browned, stirring occasionally, about 10 minutes.

3. Add the parsley, thyme, garlic, and farro, and cook, stirring, until heated slightly, about 1 minute.

4. Add 2 cups of the broth and bring to a boil. Reduce the heat, cover the pan, and let simmer until the liquid is almost absorbed and the farro is almost tender, 20 to 25 minutes.

5. Add the remaining ½ cup broth and the tomato paste. Cook uncovered, stirring occasionally, until the farro is tender and creamy, about 5 minutes. If the farro becomes too dry, add a little more vegetable broth.

6. Stir in the Parmesan and season with salt and pepper to taste. Serve.

NUTRITION INFO: 1 portion provides:

Protein: ½ serving

Calcium: 1½ servings

Other fruits and vegetables: 2 servings

Whole grains and legumes: 1 serving

Iron: some

Fat: ½ serving

Quinoa with Wild Mushrooms

SERVES 2

This protein-rich grain is easier to cook than to figure out how to pronounce (it's KEEN-wah). And you'll pronounce it delicious alongside poultry or beef.

1 cup low-sodium vegetable broth or
    chicken broth
½ cup quinoa, rinsed and drained
1 teaspoon fresh thyme leaves
⅛ teaspoon salt
1 tablespoon olive oil
2 cups sliced shiitake mushroom caps
1 shallot, minced
1 tablespoon chopped fresh flat-leaf
    (Italian) parsley
2 teaspoons sherry vinegar

1. Place the vegetable broth in a medium-size saucepan and bring to a boil over high heat. Add the quinoa, thyme, and salt, then let the broth return to a boil.

Reduce the heat to low, cover the pan, and cook until the quinoa is tender, about 15 minutes.

2. Meanwhile, heat the olive oil in a nonstick skillet over medium heat. Add the mushrooms, shallot, and parsley and cook until the mushrooms are softened, about 5 minutes. Add the sherry vinegar and cook just until heated through, about 30 seconds. Toss the cooked quinoa with the mushrooms and serve.

NUTRITION INFO: 1 portion provides:

Protein: ½ serving

Other fruits and vegetables: 2 servings

Whole grains and legumes: 1 serving

Iron: some

Fat: ½ serving

The Grain Game

There's a whole world of whole grains. Sure, right now you may not know how to pronounce some of them, never mind cook them, but there's no need to be intimidated. Actually, preparing whole grains isn't any trickier than preparing pasta, though in some cases the cooking time is a lot longer—from 30 minutes to as much as an hour. To save yourself time, consider cooking large batches, then refrigerating leftovers to be reheated in the microwave for hot cereal, pilaf, or stuffing or served cold in salads. They'll keep for up to one week. So experiment! Have fun! And remember, no matter how you serve whole grains, you'll be serving yourself a healthy dose of fiber, protein, B vitamins, and trace minerals. Prefer to stay grain-free? Substitute legume "rice" for any grain—just cook according to package directions before saucing.

Leek and Tomato Quinoa

SERVES 2

An easy and cheesy way to explore this intriguing high-protein grain.

½ cup quinoa, rinsed and drained
1 cup plus 2 tablespoons low-sodium
    vegetable broth
1 tablespoon olive oil
1 large leek (white and pale green parts),
    trimmed, rinsed well, and finely
    chopped
1 medium-size ripe tomato, seeded and
    chopped
2 tablespoons chopped fresh basil or
    flat-leaf (Italian) parsley
½ tablespoon fresh lemon juice, plus
    more to taste
Salt and black pepper
¼ cup grated Parmesan cheese

1. Place the quinoa and 1 cup of the vegetable broth in a medium-size saucepan and bring to a boil over high heat. Reduce the heat to low, cover the pan, and let simmer until the quinoa is tender, about 15 minutes (or follow instructions on the package.) Drain if necessary and set aside.

2. Meanwhile, heat the olive oil in a large nonstick skillet over medium heat. Add the leek and cook until it begins to soften, about 5 minutes.

3. Add the remaining 2 tablespoons vegetable broth, cover the skillet, and let simmer until the leek is tender, about 5 minutes.

4. Add the cooked quinoa to the leek and cook, stirring, until heated through, about 3 minutes.

5. Add the tomato, basil or parsley, and lemon juice and gently stir to mix. Taste for seasoning, adding more lemon juice as necessary and salt and pepper to taste. Sprinkle the Parmesan on top and serve.

NUTRITION INFO: 1 portion provides:

Protein: ½ serving

Calcium: ½ serving

Vitamin C: ½ serving

Whole grains and legumes: 1 serving

Iron: some

Fat: ½ serving

Red Peppers Stuffed with Quinoa

SERVES 4

These tasty and colorful bundles, packed with the goodness of grains and veggies, make a super side or a super supper (especially if you top with shredded cheese before baking, for a calcium and protein boost).

¼ cup quinoa
1 cup low-sodium vegetable broth
Pinch of salt
1 cup fresh or thawed frozen corn kernels (about 2 ears)
2 tablespoons chopped fresh cilantro
1 tablespoon fresh lime juice, plus more to taste
1 teaspoon chopped peeled fresh ginger
2 scallions (white and light green parts), chopped
½ cup chopped ripe fresh tomato
½ cup chopped yellow bell pepper
1 tablespoon olive oil
Salt and black pepper
2 large red bell peppers, cut in half lengthwise, stems, seeds, and ribs removed

1. Preheat the oven to 375°F.

2. Place the quinoa in a large saucepan over medium heat and cook, stirring frequently, until the seeds are golden brown and fragrant, 5 to 7 minutes.

3. Add the vegetable broth and salt and bring to a boil. Cover the pan, reduce the heat to medium-low, and let simmer until the liquid is almost absorbed, about 20 minutes.

4. Add the corn to the quinoa and cook until heated through, about 5 minutes. Remove the saucepan from the heat. Add the cilantro, lime juice, ginger, scallions, tomato, yellow bell pepper, and olive oil to the quinoa and corn mixture and stir gently to mix. Season to taste with salt, pepper, and more lime juice if desired. Mound the pilaf in the bell pepper halves, dividing it evenly between them.

5. Place the stuffed pepper halves on a baking sheet and bake until golden brown, 20 to 25 minutes.

NUTRITION INFO: 1 portion provides:

Vitamin C: 3 servings

Vitamin A: 1 serving

Other vegetables and fruits: ½ serving

Whole grains and legumes: ½ serving

Iron: some

Three-in-One Pilaf

SERVES 4

Bulgur, quinoa, and roasted buckwheat groats team up here for a deliciously different—and nutritious—pilaf. Peas or edamame add even more nutrients and a touch of color.

1 tablespoon canola oil
1 small shallot, chopped
½ cup coarse bulgur
¼ cup quinoa, rinsed and drained
¼ cup roasted whole buckwheat groats
2¾ cups low-sodium vegetable broth
Salt and black pepper
½ cup thawed frozen green peas or
    shelled edamame (soybeans)

1. Heat the oil in a medium-size non-stick skillet over medium heat. Add the shallot and cook until it begins to soften, about 2 minutes.

2. Add the bulgur, quinoa, and buckwheat groats to the skillet and cook, stirring, until coated, about 2 minutes.

3. Add the vegetable broth and a pinch each of salt and pepper and bring to a boil. Cover the skillet, reduce the heat, and let simmer until almost all of the liquid is absorbed and the grains are tender, about 20 minutes.

4. Add the peas and let simmer until the peas are heated through, about 2 minutes. Season with more salt and pepper to taste before serving. Leftovers can be stored, covered, in the refrigerator for up to 3 days.

NUTRITION INFO: 1 portion provides:

Whole grains and legumes: 1 serving

Iron: some

"Mocktails" and Smoothies

....

T hink the party's over just because you're pregnant? Not so. Whether you're stocking your bar for a weekend brunch, a July Fourth barbecue, or a New Year's open house, don't forget to fill a pitcher or blender with your favorite "mocktail" or smoothie so you can toast the occasion, too. But don't wait for a toast to enjoy these drinks. Sip them anytime you're thirsty (or in the case of smoothies, hungry) for a tasty treat. Some make satisfying before-dinner drinks, while others can stand in for—or supplement—breakfast when you're in a hurry or too queasy to face solids.

Iced Watermelon Water

MAKES ABOUT 3 QUARTS

R efreshingly different—and just plain refreshing. It will be especially soothing to sip when you're queasy.

1 cup loosely packed fresh mint leaves

3 tablespoons calcium-fortified orange juice (optional)

4 cups diced seeded watermelon

2 cups ice cubes

Place the mint and a couple of tablespoons water in a 4-quart pitcher and muddle them with a wooden spoon. Add the orange juice, if using, the watermelon, ice cubes, and 6 cups of water. Stir to mix. To serve, pour into glasses. Nibble on the fruit while you sip for a dose of vitamin C.

First Blush

SERVES 2

So sweet and satisfying, your First Blush may lead to a second. Substitute thawed frozen or fresh strawberries and add a little sparkling water if you'd like a more sippable drink.

1 cup diced seedless watermelon
½ cup frozen strawberries
1 cup calcium-fortified orange juice
8 fresh mint leaves (optional)
½ cup sparkling water (optional)

Place the watermelon, strawberries, orange juice, and mint leaves, if using, in a blender or food processor and process until the fruit is pureed and the mixture is well blended. Divide the drinks evenly between two tall glasses, stir ¼ cup cold sparkling water into each, if desired, and serve.

From the Test Kitchen

Turn your First Blush into a first-class smoothie by adding 1 cup vanilla yogurt. You'll also turn a half serving of calcium into a whole one, and add protein if your yogurt is Greek.

NUTRITION INFO: 1 portion provides:

Calcium: ½ serving

Vitamin C: 2 servings plus

Get Juiced Without the Acid

The high acid levels in regular orange juice can definitely trigger tummy troubles in some expectant moms, particularly during the queasy early months. If that's true for you, shake up your shake without shaking up your stomach by using low-acid OJ or substituting another kinder, gentler juice, such as white grape. Many low-acid juices also come fortified with calcium.

Citrus Blueberry Blast

SERVES 2

Very berry, very nutritious, very delicious—blissful blueberries, packed with antioxidants, combine with white grape and orange juice to make this "mocktail" a blast to drink.

1 cup frozen blueberries
½ cup unsweetened vitamin C–fortified white grape juice
1 cup calcium-fortified orange juice
1 cup sparkling water

Place the blueberries, grape juice, and orange juice in a blender or food processor and process until the fruit is pureed and the mixture is well blended. Divide the drinks evenly between two tall glasses, stir ½ cup sparkling water into each, and serve.

NUTRITION INFO: 1 portion provides:

Calcium: ½ serving

Vitamin C: 1½ servings

Other vegetables and fruits: 1 serving

Tropical Temptation

SERVES 1

Drink your vitamins. With a unique combo of flavors—orange, carrot, and peach or mango—this "mocktail" provides a taste of the tropics and a whole lot of nutrition.

½ cup calcium-fortified orange juice
½ cup carrot juice
1 cup sliced fresh ripe or frozen yellow peaches or mango
1 tablespoon pineapple juice (optional)

Place the orange juice, carrot juice, peaches, and pineapple juice, if using, in a blender or food processor and process until the fruit is pureed and the mixture is well blended. Pour into a tall glass and serve.

NUTRITION INFO: 1 portion provides:

Calcium: ½ serving

Vitamin C: 1 serving if made with peaches; 3 servings if made with mango

Vitamin A: 3 servings if made with peaches; 4 servings if made with mango

Other fruits and vegetables: 1 serving if made with peaches

Ocean Breeze Smoothie

SERVES 2

Here's another taste of the tropics, with more vitamins than you can shake one of those little paper umbrellas at. Almond milk can help relieve heartburn, but feel free to use cow's milk instead. For a thicker smoothie, use vanilla Greek yogurt.

1 cup frozen mango chunks
1 cup frozen pineapple chunks or drained canned pineapple
½ cup almond milk or cow's milk
1 cup vanilla yogurt
2 fresh mint sprigs

Place the mango, pineapple, milk, and yogurt in a blender or food processor and process until the fruit is pureed and the mixture is well blended. Divide the drinks evenly between two tall glasses, garnish each glass with a mint sprig, and serve.

NUTRITION INFO: 1 portion provides:

Calcium: 1 serving

Vitamin C: 2 servings

Vitamin A: 1 serving

Apple and Spice Smoothie

SERVES 1 VERY GENEROUSLY

Spice up your morning while calming your morning sickness with this big mama smoothie. Add yogurt—and maybe some flaxseed or wheat germ—if you'd like to make it a meal. Using frozen banana slices will make the smoothie even thicker.

1 cup pineapple juice
1 cup frozen pineapple chunks
1 small apple, peeled, cored, and chopped
1 ripe banana, sliced
1 piece (1-inch) fresh ginger, peeled and thinly sliced

Place the pineapple juice, pineapple, apple, banana, and ginger in a blender or food processor and process until the fruit is pureed and the mixture is well blended. Pour into a tall glass and serve.

NUTRITION INFO: 1 portion provides:

Vitamin C: 3 servings

Other fruits and vegetables: 2 servings

Soothing Smoothies

The name says it all—smoothies go down easily even when you're feeling a little rough. They can stand in for a meal when you don't feel like cooking or eating. Here are some general tips for making successful smoothies:

- Start with a liquid: fruit juice, cow's milk, almond milk, or plant-based milk. For a smoothie that's more sippable, use at least 1 cup liquid. For a thick smoothie worthy of a spoon— and an extra jolt of calcium—substitute regular or Greek yogurt for part of the liquid or use some in addition. Whenever possible, opt for juice that's been calcium fortified.

- To make the smoothie creamy and custardy, use frozen fruits instead of fresh, or freeze cut-up fresh fruit first.

- Boost the smoothie's nutritional profile by adding a tablespoon or two of wheat germ, oat bran, ground flaxseed, or soft tofu.

- Turn any yogurt smoothie vegan by substituting soft tofu for the yogurt. Just sweeten to taste with your natural sweetener of choice. Or use your favorite vanilla plant-based milk.

- Ginger snaps the queasies for many women; try tossing a tablespoon of sliced peeled fresh ginger into any smoothie before blending.

- Like your smoothies really sweet? Add some honey, maple syrup, or other sweetener of choice, from Splenda to Swerve (see page 74). Extra ripe frozen banana also adds sweetness, plus a thick creaminess.

Razzleberry

SERVES 2

Serve this drink thick and creamy—or thin it and make it fizz by adding sparkling water. Either way, it's yummy.

1⅓ cups frozen raspberries
1 cup calcium-fortified orange juice
12 fresh mint leaves (optional)
2 tablespoons soft tofu
1 tablespoon honey or maple syrup, or to taste
1 cup sparkling water (optional)

Place the raspberries, orange juice, mint leaves, if using, tofu, and honey in a blender or food processor and process until the fruit is pureed and the drink is thick and creamy. Divide the drinks evenly between two tall glasses. If you want a thinner consistency, add ½ cup sparkling water to each before serving.

NUTRITION INFO: 1 portion provides:

Protein: ½ serving

Vitamin C: 2 servings

It's Easy Being Green Smoothie

SERVES 1

Feeling too green to eat your greens in a salad? Here's your sweet revenge: a green smoothie that doesn't taste like a green smoothie. Switch up the fruit to fit today's preferred flavor profile (that's why you've stashed away so many different varieties in your freezer, right?).

1 cup frozen pineapple chunks
1 cup 1-inch pieces spinach, stems removed
1 cup unsweetened almond milk or cow's milk, plus more as needed
1 small ripe banana
½-inch slice fresh ginger, peeled and grated (optional)

Combine the pineapple, spinach, milk, banana, and ginger, if using, in a blender. Blend until combined and smooth, adding additional milk as needed. Serve immediately.

NUTRITION INFO: 1 portion provides:

Calcium: 1 serving

Vitamin C: 2½ servings

Vitamin A: 1 serving

Other fruits and vegetables: 1 serving

Iron: some

Breakfast Booster Shake

SERVES 1 GENEROUSLY

No time to eat breakfast? Drink it instead. This breakfast in a blender may be just the ticket, too, when solids don't appeal—or just aren't staying down.

1 cup vanilla yogurt
½ cup almond milk or cow's milk
½ cup cubed fresh or frozen mango
    (about ½ medium-size mango)
½ cup frozen or fresh blueberries
½ ripe banana, sliced (see Note)
3 ice cubes (optional; see Note)

Place the yogurt, milk, mango, blueberries, banana, and ice, if using, in a blender or food processor and process until the fruit is pureed and the drink is thick and creamy. Pour the drink into a tall glass and serve.

NOTE: If you like a really thick shake, freeze the banana slices first (you can keep a stash in the freezer). If you are using fresh mango and blueberries and an unfrozen banana, add the ice cubes to chill the shake.

NUTRITION INFO: 1 portion provides:

Calcium: 1½ servings

Vitamin C: 2 servings

Vitamin A: 1 serving

Other fruits and vegetables: 1½ servings

From the Test Kitchen

BOOST YOUR BREAKFAST

Give your shake a bigger boost by trying these tips:

- Add 1 or 2 tablespoons wheat germ or ground flaxseed.

- Add 1 tablespoon almond butter or peanut butter.

- Add ¼ cup soft tofu—you'll get an extra protein boost without any change in flavor.

- Substitute ¼ cup peach or apricot slices for the mango.

- Sweeten your smoothie, if you like, with honey, maple syrup, or the sweetener of your choice to taste.

Mango Tango

MAKES 1 TALL DRINK

This super-nutritious drink will have your taste buds dancing all the way to the tropics. It's like paradise in a glass.

1 cup frozen mango chunks
1 cup chilled pineapple juice
½ cup vanilla yogurt
½ teaspoon vanilla extract
2 or 3 ice cubes (optional)

Place the mango, pineapple juice, yogurt, vanilla extract, and ice cubes, if using, in a blender or food processor and process until the fruit is pureed and the ice is crushed. Pour into a tall glass and serve.

From the Test Kitchen

For a dairy-free smoothie, substitute ½ cup soft tofu for the yogurt. Sweeten to taste with honey or another sweetener, or use vanilla almond milk.

NUTRITION INFO: 1 portion provides:

Calcium: ½ serving

Vitamin C: 4 servings

Vitamin A: 2 servings

Mango and Strawberry Smoothie Bowl

SERVES 1

Cold cereal leaving you cold? Swap out that bowl of ho-hum with this bowl of yum—you'll also be knocking off a couple fruit servings (plus you'll score an A from the mango).

1 cup frozen mango chunks
½ cup frozen strawberries, plus
    2 to 3 tablespoons for serving
½ cup unsweetened almond milk or
    cow's milk
1 tablespoon maple syrup or honey
1 frozen banana
2 tablespoons chopped walnuts,
    for serving
1 tablespoon unsweetened flaked
    coconut, for serving

Combine the mango, ½ cup strawberries, milk, banana, and maple syrup in a blender. Process on high speed until smooth, about 1 minute. Pour into a serving bowl. Garnish with the remaining strawberries, the walnuts, and the coconut.

NUTRITION INFO: 1 portion provides:

Calcium: ½ serving

Vitamin C: 3 servings

Vitamin A: 2 servings

Other fruits and vegetables: 1 serving

Omegas: some

Peanut Butter, Banana, and Chocolate Smoothie

SERVES 1

What's peanut butter without banana? And what's either without chocolate? Stop questioning and start blending this match made in smoothie heaven. Add ice to make it thick enough to eat with a spoon—the perfect excuse for sprinkling salted peanuts and dark chocolate chips on top.

½ cup frozen ripe banana slices
    (about 1 large banana)
½ cup Greek vanilla yogurt
2 tablespoons creamy peanut butter
1 tablespoon unsweetened cocoa powder

Combine the banana slices, peanut butter, and cocoa in a blender. Blend until combined and smooth. Serve immediately.

NUTRITION INFO: 1 portion provides:

Protein: ½ serving

Calcium: ½ serving

Other fruits and vegetables: 1 serving

Fat: 2 servings

Go Bananas

If there's one smoothie ingredient you should always have on hand, it's frozen ripe bananas. They'll make your smoothie sweet, thick, and extra satisfying. Peel ripe bananas (the peels should be well-speckled, without a hint of green) and cut into thirds before storing them in a container or freezer bag. Another use for your frozen banana stash: Coat them in melted dark chocolate for a decadent treat.

Carrot Cake Smoothie Bowl

SERVES 1

Craving carrot cake—and a healthy, speedy way to start your day (or to get you through a long afternoon)? Have your cake and drink it, too, in this yummy smoothie.

1 cup unsweetened vanilla almond milk or
   cow's milk
2 tablespoons almond butter
½ cup grated carrot
¼ cup frozen pineapple
¼ teaspoon ground nutmeg
¼ cup ice
1 tablespoon raisins
1 tablespoon unsweetened coconut
   flakes
1 tablespoon toasted chopped walnuts
   (see page 217)

Combine the almond milk, almond butter, carrot, pineapple, nutmeg, and ice into a food processor or blender and process until smooth. Pour into a serving bowl. Garnish with raisins, coconut, and walnuts.

Nutrition Info 1 portion provides:

Protein: 1 serving

Calcium: 1 serving

Vitamin C: ½ serving

Vitamin A: 2 servings

Fat: 2 servings

Omegas: some

Desserts

....

Healthy isn't the first thing that usually comes to mind when you think dessert. Sweet, yes. Tempting, yes. But healthy? Not often . . . unless your idea of dessert is a ripe peach. Fortunately, with the recipes in this chapter, healthy desserts aren't just a pipe dream. On the pages that follow you'll find delicious popsicles, cookies, cakes, pies, and cobblers designed to fill your nutritional requirements with whole grains and fruit while filling your sweet tooth with joy. Does having such nutritious treats just a short recipe away (or stashed in the freezer) mean that you'll never want to reach for a truly decadent dessert like that molten chocolate cake or glazed tart? Maybe not. But it's nice to know you can have the option of reaching for a second slice of cake or a third cookie without a second thought. So dig in!

Fruity Oatmeal Cookies

MAKES ABOUT 30 COOKIES

These are way chewier than your average oatmeal cookie and a lot more nutritious, too. Handle them with care, or you'll find out just how this cookie crumbles (of course, the crumbs taste just as good as the cookie).

2 cups old-fashioned rolled oats

¼ cup ground flaxseed

¼ cup wheat germ

2 teaspoons ground cinnamon

6 tablespoons (¾ stick) butter, melted

1 large egg

¾ cup honey

½ cup raisins, chopped

⅓ cup chopped toasted pecans or walnuts (see page 217)

1. Preheat the oven to 325°F.

2. Place the oats, flaxseed, wheat germ, and cinnamon in a large bowl and stir to mix well. Add the butter and stir to combine.

3. Whisk together the egg and honey in another bowl until blended. Pour the egg mixture over the oat mixture and stir well. Add the raisins and nuts and stir to mix.

4. Drop the dough by tablespoonfuls about 1 inch apart onto two nonstick cookie sheets, then flatten slightly with the back of a fork (wet the fork slightly if the dough sticks to it) to make irregular circles.

5. Bake the cookies until they are lightly browned and the edges are firm, about 15 minutes. Let the cookies cool completely on the cookie sheets before serving. The cookies can be stored in an airtight container for up to 5 days or frozen for up to 1 month.

NURITION INFO: 1 portion (2 cookies) provides:

Whole grains and legumes: ½ serving

Iron: some

Fat: ½ serving

Omegas: some

Cooking with Alternative Sweeteners

Looking to sweeten the pot (or the cake or muffin or pancake batter) without sugar? Whether you're looking to alternative sweeteners to cut calories or to control blood sugar, it's not just a matter of taste. Some sweeteners are better suited to cooking and baking than others, but happily most (including Sucralose, stevia, monk fruit, and xylitol) are heat stable. Saccharin (Sweet'n Low) and aspartame (NutraSweet, Equal) aren't, but they're not well suited for pregnancy use, anyway.

Something else to seek in a sweetener: a 1 to 1 ratio when swapping for sugar. If the taste is sweeter, spoon for spoon, than sugar, you'll need to use less. Less sweet than sugar? You'll need to use more. Also look for a taste that approximates sugar well, keeping in mind that taste (and sweetness) can vary from brand to brand.

Finally, if curbing carbs is your goal—especially if it's on doctor's orders—be mindful of the carb count. Scan the Nutrition Facts to get the scoop on the sweetener you're scrutinizing. Some sweeteners, particularly baking blends, may contain some sugar.

For more about alternative sweeteners, see page 74.

Gingerbread Mom

MAKES ONE 9-INCH CAKE (8 TO 12 SERVINGS)

Ginger makes this cake especially soothing for a queasy tummy—and especially hard to resist.

Cooking oil spray
1 cup whole-wheat flour
¼ cup ground flaxseed
¼ cup old-fashioned rolled oats or wheat germ
2 teaspoons ground ginger
1 teaspoon ground cinnamon
2 teaspoons baking soda
½ cup molasses
½ cup (packed) brown sugar
2 large eggs
¼ cup canola oil
2 teaspoons minced peeled fresh ginger

1. Preheat the oven to 350°F. Lightly coat a nonstick 9-inch-square cake pan with cooking oil spray.

2. Combine the flour, flaxseed, oats, ground ginger, cinnamon, and baking soda in a medium-size bowl.

3. Place the molasses, brown sugar, eggs, oil, and fresh ginger in another bowl and beat with an electric mixer on low speed or with a whisk until well mixed.

4. Add the flour mixture to the molasses mixture, beating at low speed just until thoroughly blended. Pour the batter into the prepared cake pan.

5. Bake until the top of the cake springs back when lightly pressed, about 30 minutes.

6. Let the cake cool slightly in the pan before turning it out onto a wire rack to cool completely, or let it cool and serve straight from the pan. For instructions on storing the cake, see the box below.

NUTRITION INFO: provides:

Whole grains and legumes: 1 serving

Iron: some

Fat: ½ serving

Pop Them into Your Freezer

No one expects you to eat an entire cake at one sitting (though you might be tempted to do so every now and then). Instead, bake the cake, cut it into individual servings, wrap the pieces in aluminum foil, and store them in the freezer for an easy dessert or anytime snack. (Don't forget to eat one slice first!) The cake slices will keep for up to a month in the freezer. To serve, simply let cake slices thaw at room temperature or in the fridge.

Almond Flour Brownies

MAKES 9 TO 12 BROWNIES

These chewy, gooey brownies are gluten-free, but no one will notice. Plus, almond flour adds protein power, scoring you extra brownie points, even if you're not adding gluten.

Cooking oil spray
1⅓ cups semisweet chocolate chips
⅔ cup (packed) light brown sugar
2 large eggs
5 tablespoons avocado oil (or canola oil)
1 teaspoon vanilla extract
⅔ cup blanched almond flour
2 tablespoons unsweetened cocoa powder
½ teaspoon baking powder
¼ teaspoon salt

1. Preheat the oven to 350°F. Lightly coat a nonstick 8-inch-square cake pan with cooking oil spray.

2. In a small saucepan, melt ⅔ cup of the chocolate chips over low heat until smooth and glossy. Remove from the heat and set aside to cool slightly.

3. Whisk together the brown sugar, eggs, oil, and vanilla in a medium-size bowl. Stir the almond flour, cocoa, baking powder, and salt together in a small bowl. Slowly whisk the flour mixture into the egg and sugar mixture. Whisk in the melted chocolate.

4. Fold in the remaining ⅔ cup chocolate chips. Pour the batter into the prepared pan and smooth the surface with a rubber spatula. Bake for 20 to 24 minutes, until the edges are set and the center is still ever so slightly underdone and a toothpick inserted in the center comes out with a few moist crumbs stuck to it. Allow the brownies to cool in the pan before cutting into squares. Store in an airtight container for up to 3 days.

NUTRITION INFO: 1 portion (1 2-inch brownie) provides:

Fat: ½ serving

Omegas: some

Not Nuts for Nuts?

Nuts provide a healthy host of vitamins, minerals, and vital fatty acids. But if you'd like to leave them out of these recipes because you're not nuts for the taste, you have a nut allergy, or your doctor has advised you to avoid nuts during pregnancy, go right ahead. Omitting chopped nuts from a recipe won't affect the outcome significantly (toss in unsweetened coconut flakes if you like). If a recipe calls for ground nuts, substitute an equal amount of ground flaxseed, wheat germ, oats, or flour.

Poached Pears with Ginger

SERVES 4

Yes, these elegant pears are perfect for company. But why should company have all the fun? They're easy enough to make midweek, too. Have the leftovers for breakfast or as a snack.

4 Bosc pears
3 cups unsweetened vitamin C–fortified
    apple juice
¼ cup brown sugar
1 teaspoon vanilla extract
1 piece (1 inch) fresh ginger, peeled and
    thinly sliced
4 small wedges aged cheddar cheese
    (1 to 1½ ounces each)

1. Peel the pears, then arrange them, stem end up, in a deep saucepan just big enough to hold them tightly in place. Add the apple juice, sugar, vanilla, ginger, and just enough water to cover the pears.

2. Place the saucepan over medium-high heat and bring the poaching liquid to a boil. Reduce the heat, partially cover the pan, and let the pears simmer until soft but not mushy, about 20 minutes.

3. Let the pears cool to room temperature in the poaching liquid. Remove them and set aside.

4. Place the saucepan over high heat, bring the poaching liquid to a boil, and continue boiling until reduced by half, about 10 minutes.

5. To serve, place the pears on serving plates and drizzle some of the poaching liquid over them. Serve a wedge of cheddar alongside each pear.

NUTRITION INFO: 1 portion provides:

Calcium: 1 serving

Vitamin C: 2 servings

Other fruits and vegetables: 2 servings

Strawberry Mint Slushie

SERVES 1

Not your average syrupy slushie, this one delivers icy refreshment that's just sweet enough, especially if the strawberries you use are extra ripe. Frozen strawberries will work, too, as will frozen or fresh blueberries. But why stop with berries? Just about any fruit is nice with ice.

1½ cups chopped ripe fresh or frozen strawberries
2 teaspoons fresh mint
1 cup ice
¼ cup sparkling water (more, as needed)

Combine strawberries, mint, and ice in a food processor or blender and process until the ice is completely crushed (some larger, crushed pieces may remain), stopping as needed to scrape down the sides. Pour sparkling water in and process for a few more seconds until the consistency resembles a slushie. Add more sparkling water as needed to reach desired consistency.

From the Test Kitchen

Not sweet enough after all? Add a sprinkle of your favorite sweetener.

NUTRITION INFO: 1 portion provides:

Vitamin C: 4 servings

Yogurt Banana Popsicles

MAKES 8 POPSICLES

Searching for a sweet frozen treat that's actually healthy to eat? You'll go bananas for these easy-to-prep popsicles—keep a stash for dessert, snacks . . . hey, even breakfast.

4 cups sliced ripe bananas
(about 2 large bananas)
4 tablespoons sugar
(or Splenda or Swerve)
½ cup plain whole-milk Greek yogurt
3 tablespoons heavy cream

1. Place the bananas and 2 tablespoons of the sugar in a blender and blend until smooth, about 1 minute, stopping to scrape down the sides as needed.

2. Place the yogurt, heavy cream, and the remaining 2 tablespoons sugar in a bowl and stir to mix well. Add the banana puree and whisk to mix well. Spoon the mixture into 8 (4-ounce) ice pop molds. Insert popsicle sticks into the molds and freeze until solid, 4 hours to overnight.

From the Test Kitchen

Swap out 1 cup of bananas for 1 cup of your favorite fruit. Strawberries, blueberries for a berry blast or mangos or pineapple if you're feeling tropical.

3. Just before serving, run the molds briefly under hot water to release the popsicles.

NUTRITION INFO: 1 portion (1 popsicle) provides:

Other fruits and vegetables: ½ serving

Spicy and Sweet Popsicles

MAKES 8 POPSICLES

Cool, creamy, and sassy with a balance of sweet and heat, in case you're craving both. Sub chopped raspberries or blueberries.

2 cups fresh or frozen strawberries
(about 8 ounces)
1 tablespoon light brown sugar
5 tablespoons honey
½ teaspoon cayenne pepper
2 (2-inch-long) strips lemon peel
2¼ cups plain whole-milk Greek yogurt

1. Place the berries and brown sugar in a small saucepan over medium heat. Cook, stirring occasionally to mix well and pressing to break up the berries, until they fully release their juices, 10 to 12 minutes. Cool completely.

2. Meanwhile, place ⅓ cup water, the honey, cayenne, and lemon peel in a small saucepan. Cover and bring to a boil over medium-high heat. Remove from the heat; let stand for 15 minutes. Pour the syrup through a fine-mesh strainer into a bowl; discard the solids. Cool completely, about 10 minutes.

3. Stir the yogurt into the syrup. Alternately spoon the yogurt and the berry mixtures into 8 (4-ounce) ice pop molds, beginning and ending with the yogurt mixture. Insert popsicle sticks into the molds and freeze until solid, 4 hours to overnight.

4. Just before serving, run the molds briefly under hot water to release the popsicles.

NUTRITION INFO: 1 portion (1 popsicle) provides:

Calcium: ½ serving

Vitamin C: ½ serving

Conversion Table

Approximate Equivalents

1 stick butter = 8 tbs = 4 oz = ½ cup

1 cup all-purpose presifted flour or
dried bread crumbs = 5 oz

1 cup granulated sugar = 8 oz

1 cup (packed) brown sugar = 6 oz

1 cup confectioners' sugar = 4½ oz

1 cup honey or syrup = 12 oz

1 cup grated cheese = 4 oz

1 cup dried beans = 6 oz

1 large egg = about 2 oz = about 3 tbs

1 egg yolk = about 1 tbs

1 egg white = about 2 tbs

Weight Conversions

U.S.	METRIC	U.S.	METRIC
½ oz	15 g	7 oz	200 g
1 oz	30 g	8 oz	250 g
1½ oz	45 g	9 oz	275 g
2 oz	60 g	10 oz	300 g
2½ oz	75 g	11 oz	325 g
3 oz	90 g	12 oz	350 g
3½ oz	100 g	13 oz	375 g
4 oz	125 g	14 oz	400 g
5 oz	150 g	15 oz	450 g
6 oz	175 g	1 lb	500 g

NOTE: All conversions are approximate but close enough to be useful when converting from one system to another.

Liquid Conversions

U.S.	IMPERIAL	METRIC
2 tbs	1 fl oz	30 ml
3 tbs	1½ fl oz	45 ml
¼ cup	2 fl oz	60 ml
⅓ cup	2½ fl oz	75 ml
⅓ cup + 1 tbs	3 fl oz	90 ml
⅓ cup + 2 tbs	3½ fl oz	100 ml
½ cup	4 fl oz	125 ml
⅔ cup	5 fl oz	150 ml
¾ cup	6 fl oz	175 ml
¾ cup + 2 tbs	7 fl oz	200 ml
1 cup	8 fl oz	250 ml
1 cup + 2 tbs	9 fl oz	275 ml
1¼ cups	10 fl oz	300 ml
1⅓ cups	11 fl oz	325 ml
1½ cups	12 fl oz	350 ml
1⅔ cups	13 fl oz	375 ml
1¾ cups	14 fl oz	400 ml
1¾ cups + 2 tbs	15 fl oz	450 ml
2 cups (1 pint)	16 fl oz	500 ml
2½ cups	20 fl oz (1 pint)	600 ml
3¾ cups	1½ pints	900 ml
4 cups	1¾ pints	1 liter

Oven Temperatures

°F	GAS	°C	°F	GAS	°C
250	½	120	400	6	200
275	1	140	425	7	220
300	2	150	450	8	230
325	3	160	475	9	240
350	4	180	500	10	260
375	5	190			

NOTE: Reduce the temperature by 25°F (14°C) for fan-assisted (convection) ovens.

Index

N

W

Recipe Index

Additional front cover photographs by (clockwise from top left): Mark Gillow/E+/ Getty Images, Kevin Summers/Photographer's Choice/Getty Images, Anna Kucherova/ Shutterstock.com, Ermak Oksana/Shutterstock.com, Tim UR/Shutterstock.com, Maks Narodenko/Shutterstock.com, Thai Breeze/Shutterstock.com, GSDesign/Shutterstock. com, Nik Merkulov/Shutterstock.com, xpixel/Shutterstock.com, Artem Kutsenko/ Shutterstock.com, Smit/Shutterstock.com, Tim UR/Shutterstock.com, Poh Kim Yeoh/ EyeEm/Getty Images, Lev Kropotov/Shutterstock.com, Drozhzhina Elena/Shutterstock. com, Spalnic/Shutterstock.com, Eivaisla/iStock/Getty Images, Tim UR/Shutterstock.com, © Chernetskaya/Dreamstime, Nattika/Shutterstock.com, koosen/Shutterstock.com, Roman Samokhin/Shutterstock.com, MarcoFood/Shutterstock.com, Asya Nurullina/Shutterstock .com, Nyura/Shutterstock.com

Additional back cover photographs by (clockwise from top left): Eivaisla/iStock/Getty Images, Ermak Oksana/Shutterstock.com, Asya Nurullina/Shutterstock.com, Thai Breeze/ Shutterstock.com, Drozhzhina Elena/Shutterstock.com, Spalnic/Shutterstock.com, Roman Samokhin/Shutterstock.com, Scisetti Alfio/Shutterstock.com, MarcoFood/Shutterstock .com, Nyura/Shutterstock.com, Spalnic/Shutterstock.com, Artem Kutsenko/Shutterstock .com, Jakob Fridholm/Getty Images, Mark Gillow/E+/Getty Images, Lev Kropotov/ Shutterstock.com, Kevin Summers/Photographer's Choice/Getty Images, Poh Kim Yeoh/ EyeEm/Getty Images, Tim UR/Shutterstock.com, Anna Kucherova/Shutterstock.com, Smit/Shutterstock.com, Nattika/Shutterstock.com, koosen/Shutterstock.com, GSDesign/ Shutterstock.com, xpixel/Shutterstock.com, Nik Merkulov/Shutterstock.com, Maks Narodenko/Shutterstock.com, Tim UR/Shutterstock.com, © Chernetskaya/Dreamstime

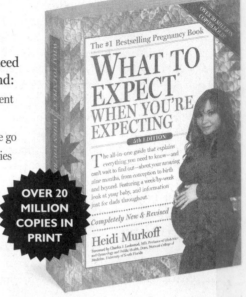
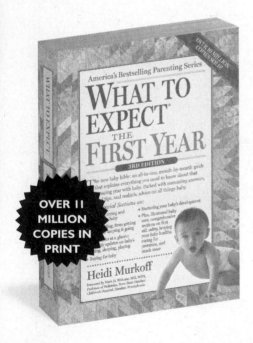